Y0-BIV-299

REFERENCE

DO NOT REMOVE FROM LIBRARY

SOUTH UNIVERSITY
709 MALL BLVD.
SAVANNAH, GA 31406

Obesity
SOURCEBOOK

Health Reference Series

First Edition

Obesity
SOURCEBOOK

Basic Consumer Health Information about Diseases and Other Problems Associated with Obesity, and Including Facts about Risk Factors, Prevention Issues, and Management Approaches

Along with Statistical and Demographic Data, Information about Special Populations, Research Updates, a Glossary, and Source Listings for Further Help and Information

Edited by
Wilma Caldwell and Chad T. Kimball

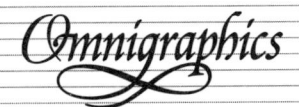

Omnigraphics

615 Griswold Street • Detroit, MI 48226

Bibliographic Note

Because this page cannot legibly accommodate all the copyright notices, the Bibliographic Note portion of the Preface constitutes an extension of the copyright notice.

Each new volume of the *Health Reference Series* is individually titled and called a "First Edition." Subsequent updates will carry sequential edition numbers. To help avoid confusion and to provide maximum flexibility in our ability to respond to informational needs, the practice of consecutively numbering each volume will be discontinued.

Edited by Wilma Caldwell and Chad T. Kimball

Health Reference Series

Karen Bellenir, *Series Editor*
Peter D. Dresser, *Managing Editor*
Maria Franklin, *Permissions Assistant*
Joan Margeson, *Research Associate*
Dawn Matthews, *Verification Assistant*
Jenifer Swanson, *Research Associate*

EdIndex, Services for Publishers, *Indexers*

Omnigraphics, Inc.

Matthew P. Barbour, *Vice President, Operations*
Laurie Lanzen Harris, *Vice President, Editorial Director*
Kevin Hayes, *Production Coordinator*
Thomas J. Murphy, *Vice President, Finance and Comptroller*
Peter E. Ruffner, *Senior Vice President*
Jane Steele, *Marketing Coordinator*

Frederick G. Ruffner, Jr., Publisher

© 2001, Omnigraphics, Inc.

All rights reserved. No part of this publication may be reproduced or transmitted in any form or by any means, electronic or mechanical, including photocopy, recording, or any information retrieval system, without permission in writing from the publisher.

Library of Congress Cataloging-in-Publication Data

Obesity sourcebook : basic consumer health information about diseases and other problems associated with obesity, and including facts about risk factors, prevention issues, and management approaches; along with statistical and demographic data, information about special populations, research updates, a glossary, and source listings for further help and information / edited by Wilma Caldwell and Chad T. Kimball.--1st ed.
    p. cm. -- (Health reference series)
  Includes bibliographical references and index.
  ISBN 0-7808-0333-7
  1. Obesity--Popular works. I. Caldwell, Wilma. II. Kimball, Chad T. III. Series.
RC628 .O297 2000
616.3'98--dc21

                                                                  00-050122

∞

This book is printed on acid-free paper meeting the ANSI Z39.48 Standard. The infinity symbol that appears above indicates that the paper in this book meets that standard.

Printed in the United States

Table of Contents

Preface ix

Part I: General Information about Obesity

Chapter 1—What Is Obesity? 3
Chapter 2—Obesity Epidemic Increases Dramatically
    in the United States 5
Chapter 3—Do You Know the Health Risks of Being
    Overweight? 9
Chapter 4—Understanding Adult Obesity 15
Chapter 5—Bariatric Medicine and Obesity 23
Chapter 6—Why Aren't Obesity Treatments Tax
    Deductible? 29
Chapter 7—Obesity as a Disability 33
Chapter 8—Obesity and Health Insurance 39
Chapter 9—Courts Weigh in on Obesity 41

Part II: Diseases Linked to Obesity

Chapter 10—Health Effects of Obesity 45
Chapter 11—Lifetime Risks and Costs of Heart Disease
    Are Much Higher for Obese People 55
Chapter 12—How to Prevent High Blood Pressure 57
Chapter 13—Obesity and Sleep Apnea 67

Chapter 14—Obesity and Diabetes 71
Chapter 15—Dieting and Gallstones 75
Chapter 16—Cushing's Syndrome 81
Chapter 17—Obesity before Pregnancy Is a Risk Factor
 for Cesarean Delivery 91
Chapter 18—Extra Weight Could Complicate Surgery
 Recovery 93
Chapter 19—Excess Pounds May Lead to Asthma 97
Chapter 20—Getting to Know Gout 99

Part III: Managing Obesity

Chapter 21—Setting Goals for Weight Loss 107
Chapter 22—Weight Loss for Life 113
Chapter 23—Choosing a Safe and Successful
 Weight-Loss Program 123
Chapter 24—The Facts about Weight Loss Products
 and Programs 127
Chapter 25—Weight-Loss Aids and Dietary Changes 133
Chapter 26—Food Labels Make Good Eating Easier 139
Chapter 27—Very Low-Calorie Diets 145
Chapter 28—Weight Control through Exercise:
 Tips and Guidelines 149
Chapter 29—Guide to Behavior Change 159
Chapter 30—You Can Control Your Weight As You
 Quit Smoking 163
Chapter 31—Smoking Cessation and Overweight 169
Chapter 32—Prescription Medications for the
 Treatment of Obesity 171
Chapter 33—Orlistat for Obesity 181
Chapter 34—"Fen-Phen" Update 183
Chapter 35—Questions and Answers about Withdrawal
 of Fenfluramine and Dexfenfluramine 185
Chapter 36—Warnings about the Drug Promotion of
 "Herbal Fen-Phen" for Weight Loss 191
Chapter 37—Dieter's Brews Make Tea Time a
 Dangerous Affair 193
Chapter 38—A Fat Regulator in the Body 199
Chapter 39—New Drugs, Safer Surgery May Help
 Overcome Overweight and Obesity 203

Chapter 40—Gastric Surgery for Severe Obesity 209

Part IV: Obesity Issues for Special Populations and the Prevention of Obesity

Chapter 41—Obesity in Minority Populations 219
Chapter 42—Women and Obesity 223
Chapter 43—Native Americans: Helping Researchers
             Understand Obesity 229
Chapter 44—Helping Your Overweight Child 235
Chapter 45—Promoting Healthier Lifestyles and
             Active Living for Childhood Obesity 245
Chapter 46—Diet and Exercise Guidelines for
             Overweight Children 251
Chapter 47—Television-Watching Is Associated with
             Obesity 253
Chapter 48—Growing Older, Eating Better 255
Chapter 49—Obesity in Older Persons 263

Part V: Additional Help and Information

Chapter 50—Glossary of Terms Related to Obesity
             and Its Management 277
Chapter 51—Practical Dietary Therapy Information 297
Chapter 52—References 329
Chapter 53—Resources 333

Index 345

Preface

About This Book

Obesity and overweight have afflicted Americans in the past three decades more than at any other time in American history. During the 1990s, an obesity epidemic every bit as serious as an infectious disease epidemic rapidly spread across all states, regions, and demographic groups in the United States. This epidemic is still spreading today. Defined as being over 30 percent above ideal body weight, obesity is linked to heart disease, diabetes, high blood pressure, stroke, gall bladder disease and several cancers.

This Sourcebook provides laypeople with the basic information needed to assess health risks, set reasonable goals for weight loss, develop exercise and dietary plans, and communicate with physicians regarding new prescription drugs for weight loss, including updates on the status of "Fen-Phen." It details the health and economic costs of obesity; obesity-related medical conditions; legal issues for the obese; and obesity in women, children, minority populations, and the elderly. A glossary and resource listing are included for additional help and information.

How to Use This Book

This book is divided into parts and chapters. Parts focus on broad areas of interest. Chapters are devoted to single topics within a part.

Part I: General Information about Obesity introduces and defines obesity, describes bariatric medicine, and outlines basic health risks for obesity and overweight. It also provides information about the legal and medical issues involved with obesity.

Part II: Diseases Linked to Obesity presents information about various diseases which are associated with obesity including heart disease, high blood pressure, sleep apnea, diabetes, gallstones, Cushing's syndrome, asthma, and gout. It also describes the risks obesity poses for cesarean delivery and surgery recovery.

Part III: Managing Obesity focuses on weight loss and weight management. It surveys various weight loss programs as well as giving guidelines for evaluating diets and weight loss products and programs. Chapters on exercise, smoking and overweight, gastric surgery, and prescription medications for obesity are also included.

Part IV: Obesity Issues for Special Populations and the Prevention of Obesity discusses obesity as it relates to women, children, elderly, Native Americans, and other minorities.

Part V: Additional Help and Information includes a glossary of obesity-related terms, a bibliography of reliable publications and articles, and a list of resources for people seeking further information about obesity. It also contains a chapter with practical dietary information including low-fat menus and shopping lists, tips for eating out, and the Body Mass Index (BMI) table.

Bibliographic Note

This volume contains documents and excerpts from publications issued by the following U.S. government agencies: Centers for Disease Control and Prevention (CDC), National Institute of Diabetes and Digestive and Kidney Diseases (NIDDK), Weight-Control Information Network (WIN), National Heart, Lung, and Blood Institute (NHLBI), National Institutes of Health (NIH), Food and Drug Administration (FDA), Federal Trade Commission (FTC), National Association of Attorneys General (NAAG), Center for Drug Evaluation and Research (CDER), and the United States Department of Agriculture (USDA).

In addition, this volume contains copyrighted documents from the following organizations: American Dietitic Association, American Obesity Association, American Society of Bariatric Physicians, Manissess

Communications Group, Inc., and the Mayo Foundation. Copyrighted articles from *American Family Physician*, *The American Surgeon*, *Better Nutrition*, *Business and Health*, *Consumers Research Magazine*, *Environmental Nutrition*, *Nutrition Research Newsletter*, and *Tufts University Health and Nutrition Letter* are also included.

Full citation information is provided on the first page of each chapter. Every effort has been made to secure all necessary rights to reprint the copyrighted material. If any omissions have been made, please contact Omnigraphics to make corrections for future editions.

Acknowledgements

In addition to the organizations listed above, special thanks are due to document engineer Bruce Bellenir, researchers Jenifer Swanson and Joan Margeson, verification assistant Dawn Matthews, and permissions specialist Maria Franklin.

Note from the Editor

This book is part of Omnigraphics' *Health Reference Series*. The series provides basic information about a broad range of medical concerns. It is not intended to serve as a tool for diagnosing illness, in prescribing treatments, or as a substitute for the physician/patient relationship. All persons concerned about medical symptoms or the possibility of disease are encouraged to seek professional care from an appropriate health-care provider.

Our Advisory Board

The *Health Reference Series* is reviewed by an Advisory Board comprised of librarians from public, academic, and medical libraries. We would like to thank the following board members for providing guidance to the development of this series:

Dr. Lynda Baker, Associate Professor of Library and Information Science, Wayne State University, Detroit, MI

Nancy Bulgarelli, William Beaumont Hospital Library, Royal Oak, MI

Karen Imarasio, Bloomfield Township Public Library, Bloomfield Township, MI

Karen Morgan, Mardigian Library, University of Michigan-Dearborn, Dearborn, MI

Rosemary Orlando, St. Clair Shores Public Library, St. Clair Shores, MI

Health Reference Series *Update Policy*

The inaugural book in the *Health Reference Series* was the first edition of *Cancer Sourcebook* published in 1992. Since then, the *Series* has been enthusiastically received by librarians and in the medical community. In order to maintain the standard of providing high-quality health information for the lay person, the editorial staff at Omnigraphics felt it was necessary to implement a policy of updating volumes when warranted.

Medical researchers have been making tremendous strides, and it is the purpose of the *Health Reference Series* to stay current with the most recent advances. Each decision to update a volume will be made on an individual basis. Some of the considerations will include how much new information is available and the feedback we receive from people who use the books. If there is a topic you would like to see added to the update list, or an area of medical concern you feel has not been adequately addressed, please write to:

Editor
Health Reference Series
Omnigraphics, Inc.
615 Griswold Street
Detroit, MI 48226

The commitment to providing on-going coverage of important medical developments has also led to some format changes in the *Health Reference Series*. Each new volume on a topic is individually titled and called a "First Edition." Subsequent updates will carry sequential edition numbers. To help avoid confusion and to provide maximum flexibility in our ability to respond to informational needs, the practice of consecutively numbering each volume has been discontinued.

Part One

General Information about Obesity

Chapter 1

What Is Obesity?

Obesity is a disease that affects 39 million Americans: nearly one-quarter of all adults and one in five children. The number of overweight and obese Americans has continued to increase since 1960, a trend that is not slowing down. Today, 55% of adult Americans (97 million) are categorized as being overweight or obese. Each year, obesity causes at least 300,000 excess deaths in the U.S. and healthcare costs of American adults with obesity amount to more than $200 billion. Obesity is the second leading cause of unnecessary deaths.

Despite its toll taken in death and disability, obesity does not receive the attention it deserves from the government, the health care profession, or the insurance industry. Research is severely limited by a shortage of funds, inadequate insurance coverage for treatment, and discrimination and mistreatment of people with obesity.

- Obesity is a chronic disease with a familial component.

- Obesity increases one's risk of developing conditions such as high blood pressure, diabetes, heart disease, stroke, gall bladder disease, and cancer of the breast, prostate, and colon.

- Health insurance providers rarely pay for treatment of obesity, despite its serious effects on health.

From the American Obesity Association website, http://www.obesity.org/what.htm, revised April 24, 2000, copyright 1999 American Obesity Association. Reprinted with permission of the American Obesity Association.

- The tendency toward obesity is fostered by our American lifestyle: lack of physical activity combined with high-calorie, convenience foods and large portion sizes.

- If maintained, even small weight losses (as little as 10% of body weight) improve your health.

- The National Institutes of Health annually spends less than 1.0% of its budget on obesity research.

- Persons with obesity are victims of employment and other discrimination and are penalized for their condition despite many federal and state laws and policies.

What Is Body Mass Index (BMI)?

Body Mass Index, or BMI, is a mathematical calculation used to determine whether a patient is overweight. BMI is calculated by dividing a person's body weight in kilograms by their height in meters squared (weight [kg] + height [m]^2), or by using the conversion with pounds and inches squared (weight [lbs] + height [in]^2 x 704.5). This number, however, can be misleading for very muscular people, or for pregnant or lactating women.

Being obese and being overweight are not the same condition. A BMI of 30 or greater is considered obese and a BMI between 25–29.9 is considered overweight. There are several variables that have an impact on a person's health risk relative to their BMI such as a person's waist size, whether a person smokes, the types of foods someone eats regularly, whether someone exercises regularly, and the medical conditions associated with obesity, including diabetes, high blood pressure, high cholesterol, and coronary heart disease.

The Role of the American Obesity Association

In the past, no one has spoken out for people with obesity. The American Obesity Association has been formed to address obesity as a public health concern, and to remove the barriers to effective treatment through vigorous advocacy and education.

Chapter 2

Obesity Epidemic Increases Dramatically in the United States

A growing obesity epidemic is threatening the health of millions of Americans in the United States, according to CDC (Centers for Disease Control and Prevention) research published in the October 27, 1999, issue of *The Journal of the American Medical Association* (*JAMA*).

According to the findings, the obesity epidemic spread rapidly during the 1990s across all states, regions, and demographic groups in the United States. Obesity (defined as being over 30% above ideal body weight) in the population increased from 12% in 1991 to 17.9% in 1998. The highest increase occurred among the youngest ages (18- to 29-year-olds), people with some college education, and people of Hispanic ethnicity. By region, the largest increases were seen in the South with a 67% increase in the number of obese people. Georgia had the largest increase—101%. The findings also show that a major contributor to obesity—physical inactivity—has not changed substantially between 1991 and 1998.

"Overweight and physical inactivity account for more than 300,000 premature deaths each year in the U.S., second only to tobacco-related deaths. Obesity is an epidemic and should be taken as seriously as any infectious disease epidemic, " says Jeffrey P. Koplan, director of the CDC, and one of the authors of the *JAMA* article. "Obesity and overweight are linked to the nation's number one killer—heart disease—as well as diabetes and other chronic conditions."

Centers for Disease Control and Prevention (CDC), http://www.cdc.gov/od/oc/media/pressrel/r991026.htm, October 1999.

A national effort is needed to control the epidemic, according to Koplan.

"While obese individuals need to reduce their caloric intake and increase their physical activity, many others must play a role to help these individuals and to prevent a further increase in obesity," Koplan says. "Health-Care providers must counsel their obese patients; workplaces must offer healthy food choices in their cafeterias and provide opportunities for employees to be physically active on site; schools must offer more physical education that encourages lifelong physical activity; urban policymakers must provide more sidewalks, bike paths, and other alternatives to cars; and parents need to reduce their children's TV and computer time and encourage outdoor play. In general, restoring physical activity to our daily routines is critical."

According to surveys conducted in 1977-78 and 1994-96, reported daily caloric intakes increased from 2239 Kcal (calories) to 2455 Kcal in men, and from 1534 Kcal to 1646 Kcal in women. Eating more frequently is encouraged by innumerable environmental changes: more food and foods with higher caloric content, the growth of the fast food industry, the increased numbers and marketing of snack foods, increased time for socializing, and a custom of socializing with food and drink.

At the same time, there are fewer opportunities in daily life to burn calories: children watch more television daily; many schools have done away with or cut back on physical education; many neighborhoods lack sidewalks for safe walking; the workplace has become increasingly automated; household chores are assisted by labor-saving machinery; and walking and cycling have been replaced by automobile travel for all but the shortest distances.

According to Koplan, the American lifestyle of convenience and inactivity has had a devastating toll on every segment of society, particularly on children. Research shows that 60% of overweight 5- to 10-year-old children already have at least one risk factor for heart disease, including hyperlipidemia and elevated blood pressure or insulin levels.

According to CDC research published in the October 13, 1999, issue of *JAMA*, more than two-thirds of American adults are trying to lose weight or keep from gaining weight but many do not follow guidelines recommending a combination of fewer calories and more physical activity. The 1996 Surgeon General's Report on Physical Activity and Health shows that more than 60% of adults are not participating in the recommended 30 minutes a day of moderate physical activity most days of the week. The Report stresses that physical activity need not be strenuous to achieve health benefits.

The October 27 *JAMA* contains two articles and an editorial on obesity by CDC authors: "The Spread of Obesity in the United States"; "Are Health-Care Professionals Advising Obese Patients to Lose Weight?"; and an editorial, "Caloric Imbalance and Public Health Policy."

Chapter 3

Do You Know the Health Risks of Being Overweight?

If you are overweight, you are more likely to develop health problems, such as heart disease, stroke, diabetes, certain types of cancer, gout (joint pain caused by excess uric acid), and gallbladder disease. Being overweight can also cause problems such as sleep apnea (interrupted breathing during sleep) and osteoarthritis (wearing away of the joints). The more overweight you are, the more likely you are to have health problems. Weight loss can help improve the harmful effects of being overweight. However, many overweight people have difficulty reaching their healthy body weight. Studies show that you can improve your health by losing as little as 10 to 20 pounds.

Are You Overweight?

Use the weight-for-height chart below to see if you are overweight. Find your height in the left-hand column and move across the row to find your weight. If your weight falls within the moderate to severe overweight range on the chart, you are more likely to have health problems. Weights above the healthy weight range are less healthy for most people.

Excerpted from "Do You Know the Health Risks of Being Overweight?" Weight-Control Information Network (WIN), National Institute of Diabetes and Digestive and Kidney Diseases (NIDDK), National Institutes of Health (NIH), NIH Pub. No. 98-4098, http://www.niddk.nih.gov/health/nutrit/pubs/health.htm, May 1998, e-text posted June 25, 1998.

What Is Your Waist Measurement?

If you are a woman and your waist measures more than 35 inches, or if you are a man and your waist measures more than 40 inches, you are more likely to develop heart disease, high blood pressure, diabetes, and certain cancers. You may want to talk to your doctor or other health professional about the health risks of your weight.

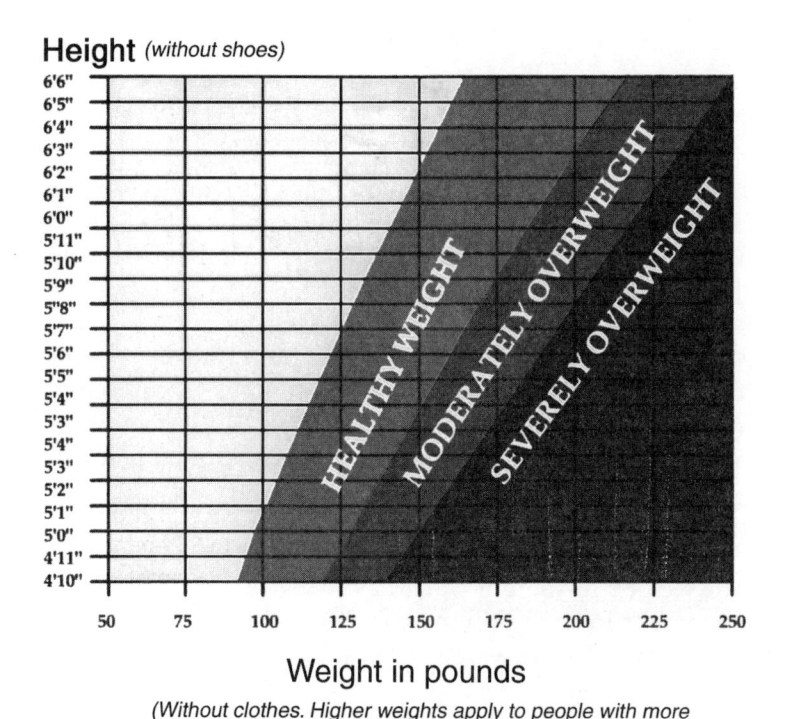

Height *(without shoes)*

Weight in pounds

(Without clothes. Higher weights apply to people with more muscle and bone, such as many men.)

Figure 3.1. Weight-for-Height Chart. Source: "Report of the Dietary Guidelines Advisory Committee on the Dietary Guidelines for Americans," 1995, pgs. 23–24.

Do You Know the Health Risks of Being Overweight?

What Are the Risks to Your Health of Being Overweight?

Heart Disease and Stroke

Heart disease and stroke are the leading causes of death and disability for both men and women in the United States. Overweight people are more likely to have high blood pressure, a major risk factor for heart disease and stroke, than people who are not overweight.

Very high blood levels of cholesterol and triglycerides (blood fats) can also lead to heart disease and often are linked to being overweight. Being overweight also contributes to angina (chest pain caused by decreased oxygen to the heart) and sudden death from heart disease or stroke without any signs or symptoms.

The good news is that losing a small amount of weight can reduce your chances of developing heart disease or a stroke. Reducing your weight by 10 percent can decrease your chance of developing heart disease by improving how your heart works, blood pressure, and levels of blood cholesterol and triglycerides.

Diabetes

Non-insulin-dependent diabetes mellitus (type 2 diabetes) is the most common type of diabetes in the United States. Type 2 diabetes reduces your body's ability to control your blood sugar. It is a major cause of early death, heart disease, kidney disease, stroke, and blindness. Overweight people are twice as likely to develop type 2 diabetes as people who are not overweight. You can reduce your risk of developing this type of diabetes by losing weight and by increasing your physical activity.

If you have type 2 diabetes, losing weight and becoming more physically active can help control your blood sugar levels. If you use medicine to control your blood sugar, weight loss and physical activity may make it possible for your doctor to decrease the amount of medication you need.

Cancer

Several types of cancer are associated with being overweight. In women, these include cancer of the uterus, gallbladder, cervix, ovary, breast, and colon. Overweight men are at greater risk for developing cancer of the colon, rectum, and prostate. For some types of cancer, such as colon or breast, it is not clear whether the increased risk is due to the extra weight or to a high-fat and high-calorie diet.

Sleep Apnea

Sleep apnea is a serious condition that is closely associated with being overweight. Sleep apnea can cause a person to stop breathing for short periods during sleep and to snore heavily. Sleep apnea may cause daytime sleepiness and even heart failure. The risk for sleep apnea increases with higher body weights. Weight loss usually improves sleep apnea.

Osteoarthritis

Osteoarthritis is a common joint disorder that most often affects the joints in your knees, hips, and lower back. Extra weight appears to increase the risk of osteoarthritis by placing extra pressure on these joints and wearing away the cartilage (tissue that cushions the joints) that normally protects them. Weight loss can decrease stress on the knees, hips, and lower back and may improve the symptoms of osteoarthritis.

Gout

Gout is a joint disease caused by high levels of uric acid in the blood. Uric acid sometimes forms into solid stone or crystal masses that become deposited in the joints. Gout is more common in overweight people and the risk of developing the disorder increases with higher body weights.

Over the short term, some diets may lead to an attack of gout in people who have high levels of uric acid or who have had gout before. If you have a history of gout, check with your doctor or other health professional before trying to lose weight.

Gallbladder Disease

Gallbladder disease and gallstones are more common if you are overweight. Your risk of disease increases as your weight increases. It is not clear how being overweight may cause gallbladder disease.

Weight loss itself, particularly rapid weight loss or loss of a large amount of weight, can actually increase your chances of developing gallstones. Modest, slow weight loss of about 1 pound a week is less likely to cause gallstones.

Do You Know the Health Risks of Being Overweight?

How You Can Lower Your Health Risks

If you are overweight, losing as little as 5 to 10% of your body weight may improve many of the problems linked to being overweight, such as high blood pressure and diabetes. For example, if you weigh 200 pounds and are considered overweight on the weight-for-height chart, you would need to lose 10 to 20 pounds. Even a small weight loss can improve your health.

Slow and steady weight loss of no more than 1 pound per week is the safest way to lose weight. Very rapid weight loss can cause you to lose muscle rather than fat. It also increases your chances of developing other problems, such as gallstones, gout, and nutrient deficiencies. Making long-term changes in your eating and physical activity habits is the best way to lose weight and keep it off over time.

Eat Better

Whether you are trying to lose weight or maintain your weight, you should take a look at your eating habits and try to improve them.

Try to eat a variety of foods, especially pasta, rice, bread, and other whole-grain foods. You should also eat plenty of fruits and vegetables. These foods will fill you up and are lower in calories than foods full of oils or fats.

Increase Physical Activity

Making physical activity a part of your daily life is an important way to help control your weight and lower your risk for health problems.

Spend less time in activities that use little energy like watching television and playing video games and more time in physical activities. Try to do at least 30 minutes of physical activity a day on most days of the week. The activity does not have to be done all at once. It can be done in short spurts—10 minutes here, 20 minutes there—as long as it adds up to 30 minutes a day. Simple ways to become more physically active include walking to the store or taking the stairs instead of the elevator.

If you are not overweight but health problems related to being overweight run in your family, it is important that you try to keep your weight steady. If you have family members with weight-related health problems, you are more likely to develop them yourself. If you are not sure of your risk of developing a weight-related health problem, you should talk to your health care provider.

Chapter 4

Understanding Adult Obesity

How Is Obesity Measured?

Everyone needs a certain amount of body fat for stored energy, heat insulation, shock absorption, and other functions. As a rule, women have more fat than men. Doctors generally agree that men with more than 25% body fat and women with more than 30% body fat are obese. Precisely measuring a person's body fat, however, is not easy. The most accurate method is to weigh a person underwater—a procedure limited to laboratories with sophisticated equipment.

There are two simpler methods for estimating body fat, but they can yield inaccurate results if done by an inexperienced person or if done on someone with severe obesity. One is to measure skin-fold thickness in several parts of the body. The second involves sending a harmless amount of electric current through a person's body (bioelectric impedance analysis). Both methods are commonly used in health clubs and in commercial weight-loss programs, but results should be viewed skeptically.

Because measuring a person's body fat is tricky, doctors often rely on other means to diagnose obesity. Two widely used measurements are weight-for-height tables and body mass index. While both

---

Excerpted from "Understanding Adult Obesity," Weight-Control Information Network (WIN), National Institute of Diabetes and Digestive and Kidney Diseases (NIDDK), National Institutes of Health (NIH), NIH Pub. No. 94-3680, http://www.niddk.nih.gov/health/nutrit/pubs/unders.htm, November 1993, e-text updated February 9, 1998.

measurements have their limitations, they are reliable indicators that someone may have a weight problem. They are easy to calculate and require no special equipment.

Weight-for-Height Tables

Most people are familiar with weight-for-height tables. Doctors have used these tables for decades to determine whether a person is overweight. The tables usually have a range of acceptable weights for a person of a given height.

One problem with using weight-for-height tables is that doctors disagree over which is the best table to use. Many versions are available, all with different weight ranges. Some tables take a person's frame size, age, and sex into account; others do not. A limitation of all weight-for-height tables is that they do not distinguish excess fat from muscle. A very muscular person may appear obese, according to the tables, when he or she is not. Still, weight-for-height tables can be used as general guidelines. [A good example of a weight-for-height table is in the chapter titled "Do You Know the Health Risks of Being Overweight" in this Sourcebook.]

Body Mass Index (BMI)

Body mass index, or BMI, is a new term to most people. However, it is the measurement of choice for many physicians and researchers studying obesity. BMI uses a mathematical formula that takes into account both a person's height and weight. BMI equals a person's weight in kilograms divided by height in meters squared. (BMI = kg/m2). [There is a BMI table in the chapter titled "Practical Dietary Therapy Information" in this Sourcebook.] To use the table, find the appropriate height in the left-hand column. Move across the row to the given weight. The number at the top of the column is the BMI for that height and weight.

In general, a person age 35 or older is obese if he or she has a BMI of 27 or more. For people age 34 or younger, a BMI of 25 or more indicates obesity. A BMI of more than 30 usually is considered a sign of moderate to severe obesity.

The BMI measurement poses some of the same problems as the weight-for-height tables. Doctors don't agree on the cutoff points for "healthy" versus "unhealthy" BMI ranges. BMI also does not provide information on a person's percentage of body fat. However, like the weight-for-height table, BMI is a useful general guideline.

Body Fat Distribution: "Pears" vs. "Apples"

Doctors are concerned with not only how much fat a person has but where the fat is on the body.

Women typically collect fat in their hips and buttocks, giving their figures a "pear" shape. Men, on the other hand, usually build up fat around their bellies, giving them more of an "apple" shape. This is not a hard and fast rule, though. Some men are pear-shaped and some women become apple-shaped, especially after menopause.

People whose fat is concentrated mostly in the abdomen are more likely to develop many of the health problems associated with obesity.

Doctors have developed a simple way to measure whether someone is an apple or a pear. The measurement is called waist-to-hip ratio.

Waist-to-Hip Ratio

To find out someone's waist-to-hip ratio, measure the waist at its narrowest point, then measure the hips at the widest point. Divide the waist measurement by the hip measurement. A woman with a 35-inch waist and 46-inch hips would do the following calculation:

$$35 \div 46 = 0.76$$

Women with waist-to-hip ratios of more than 0.8 or men with waist-to-hip ratios of more than 1.0 are "apples." They are at increased health risk because of their fat distribution.

What Causes Obesity?

In scientific terms, obesity occurs when a person's calorie intake exceeds the amount of energy he or she burns. What causes this imbalance between consuming and burning calories is unclear. Evidence suggests that obesity often has more than one cause. Genetic, environmental, psychological, and other factors all may play a part.

Genetic Factors

Obesity tends to run in families, suggesting that it may have a genetic cause. However, family members share not only genes but also diet and lifestyle habits that may contribute to obesity. Separating these lifestyle factors from genetic ones is often difficult. Still, growing evidence points to heredity as a strong determining factor of obesity. In one study of adults who were adopted as children, researchers found that the subjects' adult weights were closer to their biological parents' weights than their adoptive parents'. The environment provided by the adoptive family apparently had less influence on the development of obesity than the person's genetic makeup.

Nevertheless, people who feel that their genes have doomed them to a lifetime of obesity should take heart. As discussed in the next section, many people genetically predisposed to obesity do not become obese or manage to lose weight and keep it off.

Environmental Factors

Although genes are an important factor in many cases of obesity, a person's environment also plays a significant part. Environment includes lifestyle behaviors such as what a person eats and how active he or she is. Americans tend to have high-fat diets, often putting taste and convenience ahead of nutritional content when choosing meals. Most Americans also don't get enough exercise.

People can't change their genetic makeup, of course, but they can change what they eat and how active they are. Some people have been able to lose weight and keep it off by:

- learning how to choose more nutritious meals that are lower in fat
- learning to recognize environmental cues (such as enticing smells) that may make them want to eat when they are not hungry
- becoming more physically active

Psychological Factors

Psychological factors also may influence eating habits. Many people eat in response to negative emotions such as boredom, sadness, or anger.

While most overweight people have no more psychological disturbance than normal weight people, about 30% of the people who seek treatment for serious weight problems have difficulties with binge eating. During a binge eating episode, people eat large amounts of food while feeling they can't control how much they are eating. Those with the most severe binge eating problems are considered to have binge eating disorder. These people may have more difficulty losing weight and keeping the weight off than people without binge eating problems. Some will need special help, such as counseling or medication, to control their binge eating before they can successfully manage their weight.

Understanding Adult Obesity

Other Causes of Obesity

Some rare illnesses can cause obesity. These include hypothyroidism, Cushing's syndrome, depression, and certain neurologic problems that can lead to overeating. Certain drugs, such as steroids and some antidepressants, may cause excessive weight gain. A doctor can determine if a patient has any of these conditions, which are believed to be responsible for only about 1% of all cases of obesity.

What Are the Consequences of Obesity?

Health Risks

Obesity is not just a cosmetic problem. It's a health hazard. Someone who is 40% overweight is twice as likely to die prematurely as an average-weight person. (This effect is seen after 10 to 30 years of being obese.)

Obesity has been linked to several serious medical conditions, including diabetes, heart disease, high blood pressure, and stroke. It is also associated with higher rates of certain types of cancer. Obese men are more likely than non-obese men to die from cancer of the colon, rectum, and prostate. Obese women are more likely than non-obese women to die from cancer of the gallbladder, breast, uterus, cervix, and ovaries.

Other diseases and health problems linked to obesity include:

- gallbladder disease and gallstones

- osteoarthritis, a disease in which the joints deteriorate, possibly as a result of excess weight on the joints

- gout, another disease affecting the joints

- pulmonary (breathing) problems, including sleep apnea, in which a person can stop breathing for a short time during sleep

Doctors generally agree that the more obese a person is, the more likely he or she is to have health problems.

Psychological and Social Effects

One of the most painful aspects of obesity may be the emotional suffering it causes. American society places great emphasis on physical appearance, often equating attractiveness with slimness, especially in women. The messages, intended or not, make overweight people feel unattractive. Many people assume that obese people are gluttonous, lazy, or both. However, more and more evidence contradicts this assumption. Obese people often face prejudice or discrimination at work, at school, while looking for a job, and in social situations. Feelings of rejection, shame, or depression are common.

Who Should Lose Weight?

Doctors generally agree that people who are 20% or more overweight, especially the severely obese person, can gain significant health benefits from weight loss.

Many obesity experts believe that people who are less than 20% above their healthy weight should try to lose weight if they have any of the following risk factors.

Risk Factors

Family history of certain chronic diseases. People with close relatives who have had heart disease or diabetes are more likely to develop these problems if they are obese.

Pre-existing medical conditions. High blood pressure, high cholesterol levels, or high blood sugar levels are all warning signs of some obesity-associated diseases.

"Apple" shape. People whose weight is concentrated around their abdomens may be at greater risk of heart disease, diabetes, or cancer than people of the same weight who are pear-shaped.

Fortunately, even a modest weight loss of 10 to 20 pounds can bring significant health improvements, such as lowering one's blood pressure and cholesterol levels.

How is Obesity Treated?

The method of treatment will depend on how obese a person is. Factors such as an individual's overall health and motivation to lose weight are also important considerations. Treatment may include a combination of diet, exercise, and behavior modification. In some cases of severe obesity, gastrointestinal surgery may be recommended.

Research on Obesity

The National Institute of Diabetes and Digestive eases (NIDDK) is the part of the National Institutes responsible for obesity research. NIDDK supports sity in its own labs and clinics and at universities, search centers across the United States. NIDDK-fu helped scientists learn more about the role of genes obesity. Other NIDDK-supported studies have examin between obesity and various medical conditions. O search efforts include better ways to define and trea of obesity and understanding how the body stores an

NIDDK also oversees the National Task Force Treatment of Obesity. The task force comprises le nutrition experts who gather and assess the late obesity treatment and prevention. The task force basic and clinical research on obesity. Scientific pa interest brochures and pamphlets approved by the t able from the NIDDK's Obesity Resource Informat

In addition to NIDDK, other sections of the Nat Health (NIH) sponsor obesity research. They inclu

- The National Heart, Lung, and Blood Institute
- The National Center for Research Resources (
- The National Institute of Child Health and Hu ment (NICHD)
- The National Institute on Mental Health (NIN
- The National Cancer Institute (NCI)
- The National Institute on Aging (NIA)
- The National Institute of Nursing Research (N
- The National Institute of Arthritis and Muscu Skin Diseases (NIAMS)
- The National Institute of Neurological Disease (NINDS)
- The National Institute of Environmental and (NIEHS)

Chapter 5

Bariatric Medicine and Obesity

What Is a Bariatrician?

A bariatrician is a licensed physician (Doctor of Medicine [M.D.] or Doctor of Osteopathy [D.O.]) who, as a member of the American Society of Bariatric Physicians (ASBP), has received special training in bariatric medicine, the medical treatment of overweight and obesity and its associated conditions. Bariatricians address the obese patient with a comprehensive program of diet and nutrition, exercise, lifestyle changes and, when indicated, the prescription of appetite suppressants and other appropriate medications. (The word bariatric stems from the Greek word barros, which translates as heavy or large.)

While any licensed physician can offer a medical weight loss program to patients, members of the ASBP have been exposed, through an extensive continuing medical education program, to specialized knowledge, tools and techniques to enable them to design specialized medical weight loss programs tailored to the needs of individual patients and modify the programs, if needed, as the treatment progresses. ASBP members are uniquely equipped to treat overweight and obesity and associated conditions.

This chapter contains text from the undated pages "What is a Bariatrician?" and "Frequently Asked Questions about Bariatric Medicine and Obesity" from the American Society of Bariatric Physicians (ASBP) website. Reprinted with permission of the American Society of Bariatric Physicians, tel: 303-779-4833, website: www.asbp.org.

What Is the American Society of Bariatric Physicians?

The American Society of Bariatric Physicians (ASBP) is a national professional medical society which was formed in 1950 to establish and maintain practice guidelines and to provide education to members, the health-care community, and the public. ASBP is accredited by the Accreditation Council for Continuing Medical Education to sponsor continuing medical education (CME) programs. ASBP's CME courses have been accredited by the American Medical Association, the American Osteopathic Association, the American Academy of Family Physicians, and the American Dietetic Association.

Other than maintaining Bariatric Practice Guidelines, the ASBP does not endorse or promote any weight loss products, services or medications, either over-the-counter or prescription. Through its continuing medical education program and publications, ASBP exposes its members to cutting edge technology in the medical weight loss field to enable member physicians to design effective treatment programs for their patients.

Medical Weight Loss

According to the ASBP, a comprehensive medical weight loss program should include the following:

- an initial patient work-up to include medical history, physical examination, appropriate laboratory studies and an electrocardiogram if there is past or present evidence of cardiac disease or if the patient has coronary risk factors.

- appropriate counseling on:
  - diet and nutrition, including reduced calorie diets and very low calories diets (VLCD) and dietary supplements when needed
  - exercise, tailored to the capabilities and limitations of the overweight patient to ensure safe and effective exercise
  - behavior modification (lifestyle changes), to include discussions of proper eating habits, dealing with stress-related eating, family meal planning changes, healthful snacking, etc.
  - prescription appetite suppressants, if indicated, as an adjunct to a comprehensive medical weight loss program, and other medications

- If the use of appetite suppressants or other medications is indicated, the patient should be informed about the potential risks of such medication and the physician and patient should weigh the risks of the medication against the benefits, i.e., do the small risks of the medications outweigh the health risk of the patient remaining obese. (The use of appetite suppressants is not indicated for patients with only a small amount of weight to lose.) Often, the loss of only 5 to 10 percent of a patient's initial weight can lead to significant improvements in health status.

- adequate periodic follow-up and counseling, to include a program to help the patient maintain the weight loss that has been achieved

Frequently Asked Questions about Bariatric Medicine and Obesity

What Is Obesity?

Obesity is a chronic, debilitating and potentially fatal disease that requires treatment by a physician trained in bariatric medicine. It is marked by an excess accumulation of body fat sufficient to endanger health.

Obesity results from a complex interaction of genetic, behavioral and environmental factors causing an imbalance between energy intake and energy expenditure.

Obesity has been recognized since 1985 as a chronic disease and is the second leading cause of preventable death, exceeded only by cigarette smoking.

How Prevalent Is Obesity?

An estimated 97 million adults in the United States are overweight or obese (National Health and Nutrition Examination Survey [NHANES] III, 1988-1994).

The combined prevalence of overweight and obesity in the U.S. has increased from 46 percent of the adult population (NHANES II, 1976 to 1980) to 54.9 percent of the adult population (NHANES III, 1988 to 1991).

Increases in obesity and overweight have occurred across virtually all ethnic, racial and socioeconomic populations and all age groups (NHANES III).

Adult men and women are nearly 8 pounds heavier than they were 15 years ago (NHANES III).

What about Childhood Obesity? Is It a Problem?

Approximately one in five children in the U.S. between the ages of 6 and 17 is overweight. The number of overweight children in the U.S. has more than doubled in the past 30 years (NHANES III).

The second National Children and Youth Fitness Study found 6-9 year olds to have thicker skinfolds that their counterparts in the 1960s (*Journal of Physical Education, Recreation and Dance* 1987, 58(9), 51-56).

There is a greater likelihood that obesity beginning even in early childhood will persist through the life span (*Journal of Consulting and Clinical Psychology* 1987, 55(1), 91-95).

The risk of becoming obese is greatest among children who have two obese parents. This may be due to genetic factors or to parental modeling of both eating and exercise behaviors, indirectly affecting the child's energy balance (*Journal of Pediatrics* 1983, 103(5), 676-686).

Physical inactivity (a 1996 U.S. Surgeon General's report on fitness says that nearly half of young people ages 12 to 21 are not vigorously active), "junk" food diets (including high calorie soft drinks and fruit beverages), increased television watching accompanied by snacking, and increased time playing video and computer games all contribute to increased obesity among the young.

When we think of the major problems facing pediatrics in the next millennium, the disturbing trend toward obesity has to be among the most serious, with all the adverse health implications that obesity carries (*Pediatric Alert*, March 27, 1997).

What about Costs Related to Obesity?

Approximately 52.6 million work days a year are lost in illnesses and disabilities directly related to obesity and inactivity (Shape Up America! May 1996).

Over $68 billion is spent on excess medical expenses and loss of income in the U.S. each year. This figure does not include the $30 billion spent each year by persons trying to shed excess weight (*JAMA* 1996; 276: 1907-1915).

More than $22 billion is spent each year on health-care costs related to the cardiovascular complications of obesity (*American Family Physician*, 1997; 55(2): 551-558).

What about Medications and Special Diets?

Prescription anti-obesity medications can be a useful adjunct to a medical weight loss program, when used as part of a comprehensive program including diet and nutrition changes, exercise, and lifestyle modification. Medications alone will not lead to successful weight loss and maintenance. These medications are intended for patients who have a great deal of weight to lose, not for someone who wants to lose 5 or 10 pounds or drop a dress size. Many of the appetite suppressants and other medications available today have a long history of safe and successful use. New medications are being researched and will be available soon after clinical testing.

Just as there are some risks and side effects with almost any medication, including aspirin, acetaminophen, and birth control pills, so are there side effects and risks with anti-obesity medications. For most people, the side effects are minimal and of short duration. Bariatricians are trained to know how to prescribe the drugs properly and monitor patients taking these medications. Obese patients, particularly those with comorbid conditions, such as diabetes and cardiovascular disease, may be at greater risk from remaining obese than the risk they might incur by taking the medications. The decision to prescribe anti-obesity medications must be made by the bariatric physician and the patient after carefully weighing the risks of the medications vs. the risks of remaining obese.

Fenfluramine (the "fen" in the fen-phen combination) and dexfenfluramine (marketed as Redux) were two popular appetite suppressants which were withdrawn from the market by the manufacturer in September 1997 and are no longer available. The medications have been suspected of causing heart valve problems and primary pulmonary hypertension in some patients. Studies to determine if these suspicions are valid are currently being conducted; conclusive results of the studies have not been released as of this writing (Spring 1999).

Bariatricians frequently prescribe low calorie diets or very low calorie diets (VLCD) along with vitamins and nutritional supplements, together with exercise and lifestyle changes, to bring about a relatively rapid loss of weight. The VLCD especially should only be used under the careful supervision and monitoring of a physician and other health-care personnel trained in its use.

How Does One Maintain Weight Loss?

Learning how to keep weight off through a maintenance program is just as important as losing weight. If you want to lose weight permanently, evidence suggests it is important to make lifelong changes in how you eat and exercise (Federal Trade Commission, October 1993).

Characteristics of people who maintained their weight loss are maintaining a low-fat diet, exercising at least three times a week for 30 minutes, and cognitive-behavioral techniques (coping with relapse and stress, monitoring food intake, etc. (*Heart Disease & Stroke*, Sept.-Oct. 1994; *Journal of the American Dietetic Association*, April 1997).

Chapter 6

Why Aren't Obesity Treatments Tax Deductible?

The Internal Revenue Service (IRS) has declared that treatments for obesity are not eligible for a tax deduction. Why should they be? A tax code authorized by Congress ruled that medical care costs are deductible.

"Medical care," as defined by Congress, includes costs for the "diagnosis, cure, mitigation, treatment or prevention of disease or for the purpose of affecting any structure or function of the body." The deduction is available for persons whose medical expenses exceed 7.5% of adjusted gross income.

Deductibility is already allowed for preventable causes of death such as alcoholism treatment and drug addiction treatment. In addition, a recent IRS ruling now allows individuals to deduct costs of smoking cessation programs. Obesity is a complex, multi-factorial chronic disease involving genetic, metabolic, psychological, behavioral and environmental factors. The behavioral and environmental components, involving poor diet and inactivity, have made obesity the second leading cause of preventable death.

Obesity and the IRS

- In 1979, the IRS issued a revenue ruling stating that the cost of a physician-prescribed weight loss program was not tax deductible.

"Obesity as a Medical Deduction," from the American Obesity Association website, http://www.obesity.org/Obesity_asa_Medical_Deduction.htm, September 1999, copyright 1999 American Obesity Association. Reprinted with permission of the American Obesity Association.

- Most recently, the IRS ruled that the cost of a weight loss program for general health, even if prescribed by a doctor, could not be included as a deduction for 1998 tax returns.
- Non-deductibility of obesity treatment on individual tax returns also affects the coverage of a medical savings account (MSA). MSAs, authorized by Congress in 1996, allow employees to reduce their taxable income by setting aside an amount, through their employer, to be used for unreimbursed medical services.

Deduction for Obesity Justified

- Weight loss of as little as 5% to 10% of body weight is beneficial to the health of persons with overweight or obesity by reducing the risk or delaying the onset of a number of well-recognized medical conditions. Due to the significant impact of obesity on the health of the nation, Americans should be encouraged to achieve and maintain a healthy weight.
- Obesity can be treated with behavioral, pharmacological or surgical interventions either singly or in combination. The cost of:
  - behavioral modification programs, including diet and lifestyle changes, can cost between three to six thousand dollars ($3000 to $6000) a year. Prescription medications can range between $40 and $160 dollars per month.
  - obesity surgery, which can provide very good long-term results, can begin around fifteen thousand dollars ($15,000).
- The intent of Congress' medical care tax deduction code is to provide relief for the taxpayer that suffers from extraordinary costs in treating an illness. The decision of Congress to deny deductibility for expenses related to weight loss products and programs contradicts its intent, and:
  - fails to recognize obesity as a disease and a serious public health threat
  - is inconsistent with the statutory definition of medical care
  - is inconsistent with policies allowing for the deduction of smoking cessation products and programs, alcohol treatment and drug treatment

Why Aren't Obesity Treatments Tax Deductible?

- discourages taxpayers from obtaining necessary treatment for their obesity, thereby jeopardizing their health and increasing health care costs
- The American Obesity Association is organizing a coalition to petition the IRS to promptly issue a revenue ruling allowing for the deductibility of obesity treatments in the same manner as smoking cessation products and programs.

Chapter 7

Obesity as a Disability

Disable—to weaken, incapacitate, cripple or immobilize. The dictionary definition clearly describes the pain of persons with disabilities and the negative impact on their quality of life. Persons with severe obesity report bodily pain that affects normal daily activities. Obesity would be considered a disability when applying the dictionary definition. Legal definitions of disability, and obesity as a disability are much more complex. The Social Security Administration (SSA) and the Department of Justice (DOJ), which handles legal cases involving the American with Disabilities Act (ADA), use legal definitions to define disability. In addition, each agency interprets "disability" differently. This fact sheet will explain how the SSA and ADA interpret obesity as a disability.

Social Security Disability and Obesity

Social Security Disability provides two important safety nets to persons who qualify. First, the program provides income support. Second, after a two-year waiting period, the individual is eligible for Medicare.

Under SSA procedures, an individual undergoes a five-step application process to determine if the applicant can engage in "substantial gainful activity." They are:

From the American Obesity Association website, http://www.obesity.org/Obesity_asa_Disability.htm, September 1999, copyright 1999 American Obesity Association. Reprinted with permission of the American Obesity Association.

- Is the individual engaged in substantial gainful activity?
- Does the individual have an impairment or combination that is severe?
- Does the applicant's impairment meet or equal the criteria of a listed impairment?
- Does the individual's impairment prevent him or her from doing his or her past work?
- Does the individual's impairment prevent him or her from performing other work?

If an impairment is "listed," steps four and five are skipped and the person is considered qualified for disability determination.

Previous SSA Criteria

Since 1979 until recently, obesity has been a listed impairment. To meet the criteria, a person needed to be approximately 100% over ideal body weight—Body Mass Index was not used—and have one of the following conditions:

1. History of pain and limitation of motion in any weight bearing joints or the lower spine associated with arthritis.
2. Hypertension (with diastolic blood pressure persistently higher than 100mm Hg).
3. History of congestive heart failure.
4. Chronic venous insufficiency.
5. Respiratory disease.

- Overall, only 137,000 persons have qualified under this listing. They receive approximately $77 million per month in payments.
- Less than 3% of all disability claims use obesity as the primary impairment.
- During a year and a half-long period, initial disability determinations with a primary diagnosis of obesity were made in 59,541 cases. Nearly 40% of those were denied after review.

Social Security Proposed Rule and Response

- On March 11, 1998, SSA proposed deleting obesity as a listed impairment stating: "Current medical and vocational research demonstrates that, while many individuals with obesity are disabled, obesity, in and of itself, is not necessarily determinative of an individual"s inability to engage in any gainful activity."

- A Freedom of Information Act request, for the research studies so referenced by the SSA, was issued by the American Obesity Association (AOA). Thee SSA identified no studies supporting this decision.

- In response to SSA's proposal, AOA requested additional time for public comment, which was granted. AOA organized a coalition of organizations, which submitted extensive comments rebutting the allegations of support in the medical literature, and organized a meeting of the coalition with SSA officials in the summer of 1998.

Final Regulation

- The SSA issued a Final Regulation on August 24, 1999, in the Federal Register, which is effective on October 25, 1999. The obesity listing is revoked.

- In the Federal Register, the SSA acknowledges that it did not engage in research on the topic as they had indicated. The real reason for the change, explained SSA, was that, "our program and adjudicative experience helped to convince us that the listing was difficult to administer, subject to misinterpretation, and required findings of disability in some cases in which the claimants were clearly not disabled."

- The SSA claims that, even though they did not disclose the real reasons behind their proposal, this did not affect the validity of public comment, as required by the Administrative Procedures Act.

- Under the Final Regulation, obesity is no longer a listed impairment.

- Under the Final Regulation, an applicant with obesity will have to establish eligibility under other listings or go through the full five stages.

- Going through the full five stages exposes the applicant to the possibility of dealing with an adjudicator who is biased against persons with obesity. This is not a speculative concern.

- Legal cases and the public record in this rulemaking demonstrate such prejudice. Even without such prejudice, the application period will be lengthier, postponing the time at which the individual is eligible for Medicare—the only health insurance for which he or she may be eligible.

- In other listings for musculoskeletal, respiratory and cardiovascular body systems, boilerplate language is added to the effect that obesity is considered, "a medically determinable impairment that can be the basis for a finding of disability, and that obesity in combination with other impairments must be considered when evaluating disability at the listings step and other steps of the sequential evaluation process."

Americans with Disabilities Act (ADA)

The ADA prohibits discrimination on the basis of disability in employment; programs and services provided by state and local governments; goods and services provided by private companies; and in commercial facilities.

- The ADA requires accessibility to new and existing buildings and facilities, effective communication with people with disabilities, and reasonable modifications of policies and practices that may be discriminatory.

- Employment discrimination is prohibited against "qualified individuals with disabilities," which includes persons who meet legitimate skill, experience, education, or other requirements of an employment position that they hold or seek, and who can perform the "essential functions" of the position with or without reasonable accommodation.

ADA, Obesity, and Disability

The ADA does not protect persons who are overweight. Modifications in policies only must be made if they are reasonable and do not fundamentally alter the nature of the program or service provided. According to the DOJ, they have received only a handful of complaints about obesity.

Obesity as a Disability

According to the ADA, a person with a disability has:

- a physical or mental impairment that substantially limits one or more major life activities such as seeing, hearing, speaking, walking, breathing, performing manual tasks, learning, caring for oneself, and working. An individual with a minor, nonchronic condition of short duration, such as a sprain, broken limb, or the flu, generally would not be covered.

- a record of a physical or mental impairment, or is regarded as having such an impairment, for example, a person who has recovered from cancer or mental illness.

The ADA also protects individuals who are regarded as having a substantially limiting impairment, even though they may not have such an impairment. For example, this protects a qualified individual with a severe facial disfigurement from being denied employment because an employer feared the "negative reactions" of customers or co-workers.

Chapter 8

Obesity and Health Insurance

Many insurance plans do not provide reimbursement for weight loss treatment. According to many practitioners, few private insurance indemnity plans or managed care organizations appear to cover the costs of obesity treatment regardless of whether the service is a medically supervised program of weight reduction or maintenance, nutrition counseling, surgery, or a pharmaceutical product. The countless number of available insurance plans and ever changing policies have made it difficult to assess the extent to which obesity treatment and prevention services are covered by third party insurers. More data and better tracking is necessary to determine the health needs of persons with obesity.

Insurance Coverage Trends

A typical employer insurance plan could be similar to that of Wal-Mart. Benefits listed in their employee benefits booklet as "not payable for treatment or services" include charges from:

- medications and diet supplements which result from diet programs
- appetite control

From the American Obesity Association website, http://www.obesity.org/Obesity_Health_Insurance.htm, September 1999, copyright 1999 by American Obesity Association. Reprinted with permission of the American Obesity Association.

- weight control
- treatment of obesity or morbid obesity, including gastric bypasses and stapling procedures even if the participant has other health conditions which might be helped by the reduction of weight

The Pharmacy Benefit Management Institute reports that appetite suppression products have been excluded by more than 80% of employers, according to a sample of 375 companies representing almost 12 million beneficiaries in 1998. This represented the third straight year that the exclusion rate was above 80%. Decisions to exclude these products increased after the 1996 introduction of Redux™ by Wyeth-Ayerst.

Legislation to require health insurance coverage for weight loss programs is under consideration in at least five states—Georgia, Hawaii, Maryland, Montana and Virginia.

The American Obesity Association (AOA) receives many calls and letters from persons with obesity seeking help with denied insurance claims for obesity treatment. AOA's brochure, "Weight Management and Health Insurance," offers suggestions on requesting reimbursement for weight loss treatment from health insurance companies or employers, and appealing denials for coverage. The brochure can be obtained free of charge in single copies by contacting AOA.

Chapter 9

Courts Weigh in on Obesity

Title I of the Americans with Disabilities Act (ADA) is designed to protect people with physical or mental impairments from discrimination in the work world. It extends that protection to anyone with a perceived disability. Still, determining whether a particular condition comes under the protective umbrella of the federal law or state anti-discrimination measures is not always easy, particularly when the condition is based on weight.

In December, the New York State Court of Appeals ruled that the use of weight standards as part of an employer's hiring criteria is not necessarily discriminatory. Ironically, the employer in question, Delta Air Lines, is part of an industry once known for basing employment decisions on looks, age and marital status as well as weight in the pre-ADA, pre-Civil Rights Act days.

The case, Delta Air Lines v. New York State Division of Human Rights, was brought by 10 former Pan Am flight attendants who had hoped to work for Delta when it acquired Pan Am in 1991. Among their claims: Delta's weight standards were discriminatory and its pre-employment questions about age, physical impairments and other sensitive issues were illegal.

Not so, New York's highest court unanimously ruled. "Merely establishing that a particular question was asked, even one that might be viewed as objectionable, out of context or in the abstract, is insufficient"

Reprinted with permission from *Business & Health,* Vol. 16, No. 2. Medical Economics Co., Montvale, NJ.

to establish a claim for discrimination in the absence of a "causal consequence or relevant relationship," the court declared.

"Weight, in and of itself, does not constitute a disability for discrimination qualification purposes," according to the ruling, which offered two reasons why Delta's weight standards were not discriminatory: First, the flight attendants failed to prove that they were "medically impaired members of a protected class." Second, they were not medically incapable of meeting the standards.

The case was heard in state court and the charges based on New York's Human Rights Law, rather than the ADA. But its outcome is consistent with the federal law's view of obesity, say attorneys for the Chicago-based law firm of Goldberg, Kohn. With an estimated one in three Americans being overweight, simply weighing too much does not give an employee or prospective employee protected status, attorney David Morrison notes. On the other hand, morbid obesity—quite rare and generally defined as being twice your optimal weight or more than 100 pounds overweight—may do so.

Thus, the November finding by a Florida appellate court that a morbidly obese employee may indeed have a disabilities discrimination claim. The plaintiff charged that he had been denied promotions and subjected to harassment because of his weight.

In issuing the decision in Greene v. Seminole Electric Cooperative Inc., and sending the case back to trial court, the appeals court found that Greene may have been the victim of a perceived disability: An individual may not be substantially limited because of his condition, Morrison explains, but may still face discriminatory treatment if an employer believes him to be impaired. While Florida's Civil Rights Act does not cover perceived disabilities, the appeals court said the state law has to conform to the ADA.

What all this means for employers, says Adele Waller, a specialist in health law at Goldberg, Kohn, is that it's permissible—and safe—to ask about something that is clearly not a disability: "If a job candidate has a scruffy beard and you need a worker with a conservative, clean cut appearance, you could ask the guy whether he would shave," for example. On weightier matters, Waller jokes: "If the applicant or employee is a little chubby, it's probably OK to talk about weight. If the individual is very fat, play it safe and don't mention weight at all." Still, she and others point out that these are murky issues and that it's better to be safe than sorry. If your goal is to avoid liability, adds Judy Bauserman, a consultant at benefits firm William Mercer, better steer clear of sensitive subjects.

Part Two

Diseases Linked to Obesity

Chapter 10

Health Effects of Obesity

Persons with obesity are at risk of developing one or more serious medical conditions, which can cause poor health and premature death. Obesity is associated with more than 30 medical conditions. Scientific evidence has established a strong relationship between obesity and at least 15 conditions, and preliminary data show the impact of obesity on numerous other conditions. Weight loss of at least 5% to 10% of body weight, for persons with overweight or obesity, can improve various obesity-related medical conditions including diabetes and hypertension.

Obesity-Related Medical Conditions

Arthritis

Osteoarthritis (OA)

- Obesity is associated with the development of OA of the hand, hip, back, and especially the knee.
- At a Body Mass Index (BMI) of 25 [information about BMI can be found in the "Practical Dietary Therapy Information" chapter of this sourcebook], the incidence of OA has been shown to increase. Modest weight loss of 10 to 15 pounds is likely to relieve symptoms and delay disease progression of knee OA.

From the American Obesity Association website, http://www.obesity.org/Health_Effects.htm, September 1999, copyright 1999 American Obesity Association. Reprinted with permission of the American Obesity Association.

Rheumatoid Arthritis (RA)

- Obesity has been found related to RA in both men and women.

Birth Defects

- Maternal obesity (BMI greater than 29) has been associated with an increased incidence of neural tube defects (NTD) in several studies, although variable results have been found in this area.

- Folate intake, which decreases the risk of NTDs, was found in one study to have a reduced effect with higher pre-pregnancy weight.

Cancers

Breast Cancer

- Postmenopausal women with obesity have a higher risk of developing breast cancer. In addition, weight gain after menopause may also increase breast cancer risk.

- Women who gain nearly 45 pounds or more after age 18 are twice as likely to develop breast cancer after menopause than those who remain weight stable.

- High BMI has been associated with a decreased risk of breast cancer before menopause. However, a recent study found an increased risk of the most lethal form of breast cancer, called inflammatory breast cancer (IBC), in women with BMI as low as 26.7 regardless of menopausal status. Premenopausal women diagnosed with breast cancer who are overweight appear to have a shorter life span than women with lower BMI.

- The risk of breast cancer in men is also increased by obesity.

Cancers of the Esophagus and Gastric Cardia

- Obesity is strongly associated with cancer of the esophagus and the risk becomes higher with increasing BMI.

- The risk for gastric cardia cancer rises moderately with increasing BMI.

Health Effects of Obesity

Colorectal Cancer

- High BMI, high calorie intake, and low physical activity are independent risk factors of colorectal cancer.
- Larger waist size (abdominal obesity) is associated with colorectal cancer.

Renal Cell Cancer

- Consistent evidence has been found to associate obesity with renal cell cancer, especially in women.
- Excess weight was reported in one study to account for 21% of renal cell cancer cases.

Cardiovascular Disease (CVD)

- Obesity increases CVD risk due to its effect on blood lipid levels.
- Weight loss improves blood lipid levels by lowering triglycerides and LDL ("bad") cholesterol and increasing HDL ("good") cholesterol.
- Weight loss of 5% to 10% can reduce total blood cholesterol.
- The effects of obesity on cardiovascular health can begin in childhood, which increases the risk of developing CVD as an adult.
- Overweight and obesity increase the risk of illness and death associated with coronary heart disease.
- Obesity is a major risk factor for heart attack, and is now recognized as such by the American Heart Association.

Carpal Tunnel Syndrome (CTS)

- Obesity has been established as a risk factor for CTS.
- The odds of an obese patient having CTS were found in one study to be almost four times greater than that of a non-obese patient.
- Obesity was found in one study to be a stronger risk factor for CTS than workplace activity that requires repetitive and forceful hand use.

- Seventy percent of persons in a recent CTS study were overweight or obese.

Chronic Venous Insufficiency (CVI)

- Patients with CVI, inadequate blood flow through the veins, tend to be older, male, and have obesity.

Daytime Sleepiness

- People with obesity frequently complain of daytime sleepiness and fatigue, two probable causes of mass transportation accidents.
- Severe obesity has been associated with increased daytime sleepiness even in the absence of sleep apnea or other breathing disorders.

Deep Vein Thrombosis (DVT)

- Obesity increases the risk of DVT, a condition that disrupts the normal process of blood clotting.
- Patients with obesity have an increased risk of DVT after surgery.

Diabetes (Type 2)

- As many as 90% of individuals with type 2 diabetes are reported to be overweight or obese.
- Obesity has been found to be the largest environmental influence on the prevalence of diabetes in a population.
- Obesity complicates the management of type 2 diabetes by increasing insulin resistance and glucose intolerance, which makes drug treatment for type 2 diabetes less effective.
- A weight loss of as little as 5% can reduce high blood sugar.

End-Stage Renal Disease (ESRD)

- Obesity may be a direct or indirect factor in the initiation or progression of renal disease, as suggested in preliminary data.

Health Effects of Obesity

Gallbladder Disease

- Obesity is an established predictor of gallbladder disease.

- Obesity and rapid weight loss in obese persons are known risk factors for gallstones.

- Gallstones are common among overweight and obese persons. Gallstones appear in persons with obesity at a rate of 30% versus 10% in non-obese.

Gout

- Obesity contributes to the cause of gout—the deposit of uric acid crystals in joints and tissue.

- Obesity is associated with increased production of uric acid and decreased elimination from the body.

Heat Disorders

- Obesity has been found to be a risk factor for heat injury and heat disorders.

- Poor heat tolerance is often associated with obesity.

Hypertension

- Over 75% of hypertension cases are reported to be directly attributed to obesity.

- Weight or BMI in association with age is the strongest indicator of blood pressure in humans.

- The association between obesity and high blood pressure has been observed in virtually all societies, ages, ethnic groups, and in both genders.

- The risk of developing hypertension is five to six times greater in obese adult Americans, age 20 to 45, compared to non-obese individuals of the same age.

- Persons who are 20% overweight have shown an 8-fold greater incidence of hypertension.

Impaired Immune Response

- Obesity has been found to decrease the body's resistance to harmful organisms.

- A decrease in the activity of scavenger cells that destroy bacteria and foreign organisms in the body has been observed in patients with obesity.

Impaired Respiratory Function

- Obesity is associated with impairment in respiratory function.

- Obesity has been found to increase respiratory resistance, which in turn may cause breathlessness.

- Decreases in lung volume with increasing obesity have been reported.

Infections Following Wounds

- Obesity is associated with the increased incidence of wound infection.

- Burn patients with obesity are reported to develop pneumonia and wound infection with twice the frequency of non-obese.

Infertility

- Obesity increases the risk for several reproductive disorders, negatively affecting normal menstrual function and fertility.

- Weight loss of about 10% of initial weight is effective in improving menstrual regularity, ovulation, hormonal profiles, and pregnancy rates.

Liver Disease

- Excess weight is reported to be an independent risk factor for the development of alcohol related liver diseases including cirrhosis and acute hepatitis.

- Obesity is the most common factor of nonalcoholic steatohepatitis, a major cause of progressive liver disease.

Health Effects of Obesity

Low Back Pain

- Obesity may play a part in aggravating a simple low back problem, and contribute to a long-lasting or recurring condition.

- Women who are overweight or have a large waist size are reported to be particularly at risk for low back pain.

Obstetric and Gynecologic Complications

- Women with severe obesity have a menstrual disturbance rate three times higher than that of women with normal weight.

- High pre-pregnancy weight is associated with an increased risk during pregnancy of hypertension, gestational diabetes, urinary infection, Cesarean section and toxemia.

- Obesity is reportedly associated with the increased incidence of overdue births, induced labor and longer labors.

- Women with maternal obesity have more cesarean deliveries and higher incidence of blood loss during delivery as well as infection and wound complication after surgery.

- Complications after childbirth associated with obesity include an increased risk of endometrial infection and inflammation, urinary tract infection and urinary incontinence.

Pain

- Bodily pain is a prevalent problem among persons with obesity.

- Greater disability, due to bodily pain, has been reported by persons with obesity compared to persons with other chronic medical conditions.

- Obesity is known to be associated with musculoskeletal or joint-related pain.

- Foot pain located at the heel, known as Sever's disease is commonly associated with obesity.

Pancreatitis

- Obesity is a predictive factor of outcome in acute pancreatitis.

- Obese patients with acute pancreatitis are reported to develop significantly more complications, including respiratory failure, than nonobese.

- Patients with severe pancreatitis have been found to have a higher body-fat percentage and larger waist size than patients with mild pancreatitis.

Sleep Apnea

- Obesity, particularly upper body obesity, is the most significant risk factor for obstructive sleep apnea.

- There is a 12- to 30-fold higher incidence of obstructive sleep apnea among morbidly obese patients compared to the general population.

- Among patients with obstructive sleep apnea, at least 60% to 70% are obese.

Stroke

- Elevated BMI is reported to increase the risk of ischemic stroke independent of other risk factors including age and systolic blood pressure.

- Abdominal obesity appears to predict the risk of stroke in men.

- Obesity and weight gain are risk factors for ischemic and total stroke in women.

Surgical Complications

- Obesity is a risk factor for complications after a surgery.

- Surgical patients with obesity demonstrate a higher number and incidence of hospital acquired infections compared to normal weight patients.

Urinary Stress Incontinence

- Obesity is a well-documented risk factor for urinary stress incontinence, involuntary urine loss, as well as urge incontinence and urgency among women.

- Obesity is reported to be a strong symptoms after pregnancy and d 6 to 18 months after childbirth.

Other

- Several other obesity-related cond various researchers including abd nigricans, endocrine abnormalitie capnia, dermatological effects, dep sophageal reflux, heel spurs, hirsu mammegaly (causing considerable pain, skin damage, cervical pain, c the skin folds under the breasts, e wall masses (abdominal panniculit impeding walking, causing frequen difficulties, low back pain), muscul cancer, pseudo tumor cerebri (or be sion), and sliding hiatal hernia.

Readers should note that researche same criteria to identify overweight an American Obesity Association (AOA) h erally accepted definitions for overweigh of 25–29.9 and obesity as a BMI of 30 or fort to identify studies which have used well as other scientifically accepted mea cumference and waist to hip ratio.

Chapter 11

Lifetime Risks and Costs of Heart Disease Are Much Higher for Obese People

The expected lifetime risks and costs of heart disease are much higher for individuals who are obese, according to a study presented at the American Heart Association's 71st Scientific Sessions in Dallas, Texas.

"Compared to individuals who are not overweight, individuals who are obese have elevated risks of heart disease and can expect to incur higher medical-care costs as a result," says the study's lead author David Thompson, Ph.D., senior economist, Policy Analysis, Inc., Brookline, Mass.

The study found that men, 45 to 54 years of age who are not obese, faced a 35 percent chance of developing coronary heart disease during their lifetimes; risks increased to 38 percent for those who were mildly obese, 42 percent for those who were moderately obese, and 46 percent for those who were severely obese. Risks increased from 25 percent for the women who are not obese, to 29 percent, 32 percent, and 37 percent, depending the level of obesity.

Obesity is frequently measured using the body mass index (BMI), a method of estimating a person's body fat. BMI is calculated by dividing weight in kilograms by the square of height in meters. Based on National Institutes of Health guidelines, individuals with BMIs of 30 or greater are considered obese, while those with BMIs of 25–29

From the undated webpage "Lifetime Risks and Costs of Heart Disease Are Much Higher for Obese," from the American Society of Bariatric Physicians (ASBP) website. Reprinted with permission of the American Society of Bariatric Physician, tel: 303-779-4833, website: www.asbp.org.

are considered overweight. In this study, a BMI of 22.5 was considered to represent individuals who are not obese while BMIs of 27.5, 32.5, and 37.5 were chosen to represent mild, moderate, and severe obesity respectively.

As a result of these increased risks, average expected lifetime medical-care costs for the treatment of heart disease are as much as $6,000 higher for severely obese individuals compared to those individuals who are not obese. For men, expected lifetime costs of heart disease increased from $10,500 for the individuals who are not obese, to $12,000 for those mildly obese, $14,000 for those moderately obese, and $16,400 for those severely obese. For women, expected lifetime heart-disease costs increased from $5,800 for the individuals who are not obese, to $6,700 for those mildly obese, $7,900 for those moderately obese and $9,400 for the severely obese.

"Our findings indicate that obesity imposes a significant health and economic burden on individuals who are obese," says Thompson. "Clearly, efforts to reduce the prevalence of obesity can have important benefits in terms of reduction in the risks and costs of coronary heart disease."

The American Heart Association recently designated obesity as a major modifiable risk factor for heart disease. While health-care expenditures in the U.S. attributable to obesity have been estimated to total over $50 billion, this is the first study that pinpoints the expected lifetime costs of obesity from the perspective of an individual person, says Thompson. The study also reported that individuals who are obese are likely to live a greater portion of their lives with heart disease. The expected number of years of life with heart disease increased from 2.7 among men, age 45 to 54, who are not obese, to 3.1 for those mildly obese, 3.7 for those moderately obese, and 4.5 years for those severely obese. Expected years with heart disease for women of the same age ranged from 2.2 for those of normal weight to 3.7 for the severely obese.

The study was based on data from the Framingham Heart Study and the Third National Health and Nutrition Examination Survey. Thompson says he and his colleagues conducted the study to increase awareness of the health and economic consequences of excess body weight. "The problem of obesity is reaching epidemic proportions," he says. "In the past 15 years alone, obesity has increased from one-quarter to one-third of the U.S. population. Any increase in weight is placing a person at an increased health risk."

Chapter 12

How to Prevent High Blood Pressure

It's Important to Know about High Blood Pressure

High blood pressure, also called hypertension, is a risk factor for heart and kidney diseases and stroke. This means that having high blood pressure increases your chance (or risk) of getting heart or kidney disease, or of having a stroke. This is serious business: heart disease is the number one killer in the United States, and stroke is the third most common cause of death.

About one in every four American adults has high blood pressure. High blood pressure is especially dangerous because it often gives no warning signs or symptoms. Fortunately, though, you can find out if you have high blood pressure by having your blood pressure checked regularly. If it is high, you can take steps to lower it. Just as important, if your blood pressure is normal, you can learn how to keep it from becoming high. This chapter will tell you how.

What Is Blood Pressure, and What Happens When It Is High?

Since blood is carried from the heart to all of your body's tissue and organs in vessels called arteries, blood pressure is the force of

---

Excerpted from an undated pamphlet by the National Heart, Lung, and Blood Institute (NHLBI), NHLBI Obesity Education Initiative, National Institutes of Health (NIH), http://www.nhlbi.nih.gov/health/public/heart/hbp/prevhbp/index.htm.

the blood pushing against the walls of those arteries. In fact, each time the heart beats (about 60–70 times a minute at rest), it pumps out blood into the arteries. Your blood pressure is at its greatest when the heart contracts and is pumping the blood. This is called systolic pressure. When the heart is at rest, in between beats, your blood pressure falls. This is the diastolic pressure.

Blood pressure is always given as these two numbers, systolic and diastolic pressures. Both are important. Usually they are written one above or before the other, such as 120/80, with the top number the systolic, and the bottom the diastolic.

Different actions make your blood pressure go up or down. For example, if you run for a bus, your blood pressure goes up. When you sleep at night, your blood pressure goes down. These changes in blood pressure are normal.

Some people have blood pressure that stays up all or most of the time. Their blood pushes against the walls of their arteries with higher-than-normal force. If untreated this can lead to serious medical problems like these:

Arteriosclerosis ("hardening of the arteries"). High blood pressure harms the arteries by making them thick and stiff. This speeds the build up of cholesterol and fats in the blood vessels like rust in a pipe, which prevents the blood from flowing through the body, and in time can lead to a heart attack or stroke.

Heart attack. Blood carries oxygen to the body. When the arteries that bring blood to the heart muscle become blocked, the heart cannot get enough oxygen. Reduced blood flow can cause chest pain (angina). Eventually, the flow may be stopped completely, causing a heart attack.

Enlarged heart. High blood pressure causes the heart to work harder. Over time, this causes the heart to thicken and stretch. Eventually the heart fails to function normally causing fluids to back up into the lungs. Controlling high blood pressure can prevent this from happening.

Kidney damage. The kidney acts as a filter to rid the body of wastes. Over a number of years, high blood pressure can narrow and thicken the blood vessels of the kidney. The kidney filters less fluid, and waste builds up in the blood. The kidneys may fail altogether. When this happens, medical treatment (dialysis) or a kidney transplant may be needed.

How to Prevent High Blood Pressure

Stroke. High blood pressure can harm the arteries, causing them to narrow faster. So, less blood can get to the brain. If a blood clot blocks one of the narrowed arteries, a stroke (thrombotic stroke) may occur. A stroke can also occur when very high pressure causes a break in a weakened blood vessel in the brain (hemorrhagic stroke).

Who's Likely to Develop High Blood Pressure?

Anyone can develop high blood pressure, but some people are more likely to develop it than others. For example, high blood pressure is more common—it develops earlier and is more severe—in African-Americans than in whites.

In the early and middle adult years, men have high blood pressure more often than women. But as men and women age, the reverse is true. More women after menopause have high blood pressure than men of the same age. And the number of both men and women with high blood pressure increases rapidly in older age groups. More than half of all Americans over age 65 have high blood pressure. And older African-American women who live in the Southeast are more likely to have high blood pressure than those in other regions of the United States.

In fact, the southeastern states have some of the highest rates of death from stroke. High blood pressure is the key risk factor for stroke. Other risk factors include cigarette smoking and overweight. These 11 states—Alabama, Arkansas, Georgia, Indiana, Kentucky, Louisiana, Mississippi, North Carolina, South Carolina, Tennessee, and Virginia—have such high rates of stroke among persons of all races and in both sexes that they are called the "Stroke Belt States."

Finally, heredity can make some families more likely than others to get high blood pressure. If your parents or grandparents had high blood pressure, your risk may be increased. While it is mainly a disease of adults, high blood pressure can occur in children as well. Even if everyone is healthy, be sure you and your family get your blood pressure checked. Remember, high blood pressure has no signs or symptoms.

How Is Blood Pressure Checked?

Having your blood pressure checked is quick, easy, and painless. Your blood pressure is measured with an instrument called a sphygmomanometer (sfig-mo-ma-nom-e-ter).

It works like this: A blood pressure cuff is wrapped around your upper arm and inflated to stop the blood flow in your artery for a few seconds. A valve is opened and air is then released from the cuff and the sounds of your blood rushing through an artery are heard through a stethoscope. The first sound heard and registered on the gauge or mercury column is called the systolic blood pressure. It represents the maximum pressure in the artery produced as the heart contracts and the blood begins to flow. The last sound heard as more air is released from the cuff is the diastolic blood pressure. It represents the lowest pressure that remains within the artery when the heart is at rest.

What Do the Numbers Mean?

Blood pressure is always expressed in two numbers that represent the systolic and diastolic pressures. These numbers are measurements of millimeters (mm) of mercury (Hg). The measurement is written one above or before the other, with the systolic number on the top and the diastolic number on the bottom. For example, a blood pressure measurement of 120/80 mm Hg is expressed verbally as "120 over 80." See Table 12.1 which shows categories for blood pressure levels in adults.

If your blood pressure is less than 140/90 mm Hg, it is considered normal. However, a blood pressure below 120/80 mm Hg is even better for your heart and blood vessels. People use to think that low blood pressure (for example, 105/65 mm Hg in an adult) was unhealthy. Except

Table 12.1. Categories for Blood Pressure Levels in Adults (Age 18 Years and Older). For those not taking medicine for high blood pressure and not having a short term serious illness. These categories are from the National High Blood Pressure Education Program.

Category	Blood Pressure Level (mm Hg) Systolic	Diastolic
Normal	less than 130	less than 85
High Normal	130-139	85-89
High Blood Pressure		
Stage 1	140-159	90-99
Stage 2	160-179	100-109
Stage 3	greater than or equal to 180	greater than or equal to 110

How to Prevent High Blood Pressure

for rare cases, this is not true. High blood pressure or "hypertension" is classified by stages and is more serious as the numbers get higher.

What Causes High Blood Pressure?

For most people, there is no single known cause of high blood pressure. This type of high blood pressure is called "primary" or "essential" hypertension. This type of blood pressure can't be cured, although in most cases it can be controlled. That's why it's so important for everyone to take steps to reduce their chances of developing high blood pressure.

In a few people, high blood pressure can be traced to a known cause like tumors of the adrenal gland, chronic kidney disease, hormone abnormalities, use of birth control pills, or pregnancy. This is called "secondary hypertension." Secondary hypertension is usually cured if its cause passes or is corrected.

How Can You Prevent High Blood Pressure?

Everyone—regardless of race, age, sex, or heredity—can help lower their chance of developing high blood pressure. Here's how:

1. Maintain a healthy weight, lose weight if you are overweight,
2. Be more physically active,
3. Choose foods lower in salt and sodium, and
4. If you drink alcoholic beverages, do so in moderation.

These rules are also recommended for treating high blood pressure, although medicine is often added as part of the treatment. It is far better to keep your blood pressure from getting high in the first place.

Another important measure for your health is to not smoke: while cigarette smoking is not directly related to high blood pressure, it increases your risk of heart attack and stroke.

Let's look more closely at the four rules to prevent high blood pressure and for keeping a healthy heart:

Maintain a Health Weight, Lose Weight If You Are Overweight

As your body weight increases, your blood pressure rises. In fact, being overweight can make you two to six times more likely to develop high blood pressure than if you are at your desirable weight. Keeping your weight in the desirable range is not only important to prevent high blood pressure but also for your overall health and well being.

It's not just how much you weigh that's important: it also matters where your body stores extra fat. Your shape is inherited from your parents just like the color of your eyes or hair. Some people tend to gain weight around their belly; others, around the hips and thighs. "Apple-shaped" people who have a pot belly (that is, extra fat at the waist) appear to have higher health risks than "pear-shaped" people with heavy hips and thighs.

No matter where the extra weight is, you can reduce your risk of high blood pressure by losing weight. Even small amounts of weight loss can make a big difference in helping to prevent high blood pressure. Losing weight, if you are overweight and already have high blood pressure, can also help lower your pressure.

To lose weight, you need to eat fewer calories than you burn. But don't go on a crash diet to see how quickly you can lose those pounds. The healthiest and longest-lasting weight loss happens when you do it slowly, losing 1/2 to 1 pound a week. By cutting back by 500 calories a day by eating less and being more physically active, you can lose about 1 pound (which equals 3,500 calories) in a week.

Losing weight and keeping it off involves a new way of eating and increasing physical activity for life. Here's how to eat and get on your way to a lower weight:

Choose foods low in calories and fat. Naturally, choosing low-calorie foods cuts calories. But did you know that choosing foods low in fat also cuts calories? Fat is a concentrated source of calories, so eating fewer fatty foods will reduce calorie intake. Some examples of fatty foods to cut down on are: butter, margarine, regular salad dressings, fatty meats, skin of poultry, whole milk dairy foods like cheese, fried foods, and many cookies, cakes, pastries and snacks.

Choose foods high in starch and fiber. Foods high in starch and fiber (fruits, vegetables, whole-grain cereals, pasta and rice, whole-grain breads, dry peas and beans) are excellent substitutes for foods high in fat. They are lower in calories than foods high in fat. These foods are also good sources of vitamins and minerals.

Limit serving sizes. To lose weight, it's not just the type of foods you eat that's important, but also the amount. To take in fewer calories, you need to limit your portion sizes. Try especially to take smaller helpings of high calorie foods like high fat meats and cheeses. And try not to go back for seconds.

How to Prevent High Blood Pressure

Increase physical activity. There's more to weight loss than just eating less. Another important ingredient is increasing physical activity, which burns calories. Cutting down on fat and calories combined with regular physical activity can help you lose more weight and keep it off longer than either way by itself.

Be More Physically Active.

Besides losing weight, there are other reasons to be more active: being physically active can reduce your risk for heart disease, help lower your total cholesterol level and raise HDL-cholesterol (the "good" cholesterol that does not build up in the arteries), and help lower high blood pressure. And people who are physically active have a lower risk of getting high blood pressure—20 to 50 percent lower—than people who are not active. You don't have to be a marathon runner to benefit from physical activity. Even light activities, if done daily, can help lower your risk of heart disease. So you can fit physical activity into your daily routine in small but important ways.

More vigorous exercise has added benefits. It helps improve the fitness of the heart and lungs. And that in turn protects you more against heart disease. Activities like swimming, brisk walking, running, and jumping rope are called "aerobic." This means that the body uses oxygen to make the energy it needs for the activity. Aerobic activities can condition your heart and lungs if done at the right intensity for at least 30 minutes, three to four times a week. But if you don't have 30 minutes for a break, try to find two 15-minute periods or even three 10-minute periods. Try to do some type of aerobic activity in the course of a week.

Most people don't need to see a doctor before they start exercising, since a gradual, sensible exercise program has few health risks. But if you have a health problem like high blood pressure; if you have pains or pressure in the chest or shoulder area; if you tend to feel dizzy or faint; if you get very breathless after a mild workout; or are middle-age or older and have not been active, and you are planning a vigorous exercise program, you should check with your doctor first. Otherwise, get out, get active, and get fit—and help prevent high blood pressure.

Choose Foods Lower in Salt and Sodium

Americans eat more salt (sodium chloride) and other forms of sodium than they need. And guess what? They also have higher rates of high blood pressure than people in other countries who eat less salt.

Often, if people with high blood pressure cut back on salt and sodium, their blood pressure falls. Cutting back on salt and sodium also prevents blood pressure from rising. Some people like African-Americans and the elderly are more affected by sodium than others. Since there's really no practical way to predict exactly who will be affected by sodium, it makes sense to limit intake of salt and sodium to help prevent high blood pressure.

All Americans, especially people with high blood pressure, should eat no more than about 6 grams of salt a day, which equals about 2,400 milligrams of sodium. That's about 1 teaspoon of table salt. But remember to keep track of ALL salt eaten—including that in processed foods and added during cooking or at the table. Americans eat 4,000 to 6,000 milligrams of sodium a day, so most people need to cut back on salt and sodium.

You can teach your taste buds to enjoy less salty foods. Here are a few tips:

Check food labels for the amount of sodium in foods. Choose those lower in sodium most of the time. Look for products that say "sodium free," "very low sodium," "low sodium," "light in sodium," "reduced or less sodium," or "unsalted," especially on cans, boxes, bottles, and bags.

Buy fresh, plain frozen, or canned with "no salt added " vegetables. Use fresh poultry, fish and lean meat, rather than canned or processed types.

Use herbs, spices, and salt-free seasoning blends in cooking and at the table instead of salt:

- spices to add to meat, poultry, and fish
    - beef—bay leaf, marjoram, nutmeg, onion, pepper, sage, thyme
    - lamb—curry powder, garlic, rosemary, mint
    - pork—garlic, onion, sage, pepper, oregano
    - veal—bay leaf, curry powder, ginger, marjoram, oregano
    - chicken—ginger, marjoram, oregano, paprika, poultry seasoning, rosemary, sage, tarragon, thyme
    - fish—curry powder, dill, dry mustard, lemon juice, marjoram, paprika, pepper

How to Prevent High Blood Pressure

- spices to add to vegetables
  - carrots—cinnamon, cloves, marjoram, nutmeg, rosemary, sage
  - corn—cumin, curry powder, onion, paprika, parsley
  - green beans—dill, curry powder, lemon juice, marjoram, oregano, tarragon, thyme
  - greens—onion, pepper
  - peas—ginger, marjoram, onion, parsley, sage
  - potatoes—dill, garlic, onion, paprika, parsley, sage
  - summer squash—cloves, curry powder, marjoram, nutmeg, rosemary, sage
  - winter squash—cinnamon, ginger, nutmeg, onion
  - tomatoes—basil, bay leaf, dill, marjoram, onion, oregano, parsley, pepper

Cook rice, pasta, and hot cereals without salt. Cut back on instant or flavored rice, pasta, and cereal mixes because they usually have added salt.

Choose "convenience" foods that are lower in sodium. Cut back on frozen dinners, mixed dishes like pizza, packaged mixes, canned soups or broths, and salad dressings which often have a lot of sodium.

If You Drink Alcoholic Beverages, Do So in Moderation.

Drinking too much alcohol can raise your blood pressure. It may also lead to the development of high blood pressure. So to help prevent high blood pressure, if you drink alcohol, limit how much you drink to no more than 2 drinks a day. The "Dietary Guidelines for Americans" recommend that for overall health women should limit their alcohol to no more than 1 drink a day.

You may have heard that some alcohol is good for your heart health. Some news reports suggest that people who consume a drink or two a day have lower blood pressure and live longer than those who consume excessive amounts of alcohol. Others note that wine raises the "good" blood cholesterol that prevents the build up of fats in the arteries. While these news stories may be correct they don't tell the whole story: too much alcohol contributes to a host of other health problems, such as motor vehicle accidents, diseases of the liver and pancreas, damage to the brain and heart, an increased risk of many cancers, and fetal alcohol syndrome. Alcohol is also high in calories. So you should limit how much you drink.

Here's a Recap

After going through all the things that may affect blood pressure, it's worth noting again the things that are sure to help you prevent high blood pressure:

1. maintaining a healthy weight—losing weight if you are overweight

2. being more physically active

3. choosing foods low in salt and sodium

4. if you drink alcoholic beverages, doing so in moderation

5. By following these guidelines, you can help reduce or prevent high blood pressure for life—and, in turn, lower your risk for heart disease and stroke.

Chapter 13

Obesity and Sleep Apnea

Obstructive sleep apnea is defined as an absence of breathing during sleep. Currently, it is recognized that sleep apnea is part of a continuum from health to disease. Apnea is currently defined as cessation of airflow for at least 10 seconds and is characterized as either central (if no respiratory effort occurs), obstructive (if continued effort is noted), or mixed (if both central and obstructive components are present). Apnea is associated with either a fall in oxyhemoglobin desaturation or an arousal from sleep. Hypopneas, which are defined as partial reductions in airflow associated with falls in oxygen saturation or arousals from sleep, are also recorded.

The sleep apnea syndrome has been clinically defined as recurrent apnea or hypopnea associated with clinical impairment usually manifested as increased daytime sleepiness or altered cardiopulmonary function. In general, the average number of episodes of apnea and hypopnea per hour are reported as an index (AHI) or as a respiratory disturbance index (RDI). Classically, an AHI of greater than five episodes per hour has been the definition of the presence of the sleep apnea syndrome. Other commonly used cutoff points are an AHI of 10 or 15 episodes per hour or an overnight total of 30 apneichypopneic episodes.

Excerpted from *Clinical Guidelines on the Identification, Evaluation, and Treatment of Overweight and Obesity in Adults*, Appendix IV, pp. 137-138, National Heart, Lung, and Blood Institute (NHLBI), National Institutes of Health (NIH), June 1998.

There are several correlates of sleep apnea. It is well recognized that it is more prevalent in males, although the difference is less pronounced in population-based studies than in laboratory-based studies. Some studies have suggested that the prevalence of sleep apnea in women increases after menopause. Snoring also correlates with sleep apnea, increasing up to late middle age and decreasing thereafter. The other major correlate of sleep apnea is obesity in both men and women. In general, women have to be significantly more obese than men for the clinical syndrome to be apparent. At present, no published epidemiologic studies have examined the relationship between race and sleep apnea. Given the high prevalence of obesity among specific populations and minorities, sleep apnea may be highly prevalent in these groups.

The major pathophysiologic consequences of severe sleep apnea include severe arterial hypoxemia, recurrent arousals from sleep, increased sympathetic tone, pulmonary and systemic hypertension, and cardiac arrhythmias. These phenomena may result in acute hemodynamic and chronic structural change in the coronary arteries, possibly associated with relative myocardial ischemia, rupture of atheromatous plaques, and increased risk for thrombosis at the site of any unstable plaque. Similar mechanisms acting in the cerebrovascular system may be involved in an increased risk of stroke. Finally, the sympathetic tone may be associated with hypertension as well as increased platelet aggregability.

The primary goal for treatment of individuals with sleep apnea is to reduce the severity of the respiratory events that are associated with oxyhemoglobin desaturation and arousal from sleep. There are only two cohort studies in clinic-based populations that demonstrate a significant reduction in cardiovascular mortality among sleep apnea patients who are treated progressively compared to those who are treated conservatively. However, both of these studies were retrospective and suffered from a significant bias of ascertainment.

The evidence that treatment of obesity ameliorates obstructive sleep apnea is reasonably well established. Although the studies are small, both surgical and medical approaches to weight loss have been associated with a consistent but variable reduction in the number of respiratory events, as well as improvement in oxygenation. In general, surgical interventions, which have included a gastric bypass or jejunoileostomy, have been reserved for people who are severely obese. While this approach to weight reduction was commonly used in patients with severe obstructive sleep apnea, they recently have been abandoned because of complications and side effects. However, the use of surgical gastric procedures has been successful in improving sleep apnea in a number of studies. On the other hand, weight reduction has been associated with comparable reduction in the severity of sleep apnea, as well as improved evidence of renal function and hypertension. Both medical and surgical studies have demonstrated that as little as 10-percent weight reduction is associated with a more than 50-percent reduction in the severity of sleep apnea. Moreover, more recent data suggest a possible "threshold" effect that is directly related to the collapsibility of the upper airway. Those individuals who demonstrate a minimally collapsible upper airway apparently achieve a greater effect for the same percentage of weight reduction.

Finally, there is evidence that standard treatments for sleep apnea do reduce specific cardiovascular risk factors. Specifically, the most commonly employed treatment, continuous positive airway pressure, has been shown to reduce waking arresting carbon dioxide and reduced heart rate, and pulmonary artery pressure decreased hematocrit and improved ventricular ejection fraction. Other standard surgical approaches that have been employed to widen the upper airway have been shown to reduce the severity of the apnea, but there are no data examining the associated cardiovascular risk factors. No studies have specifically examined the effects of treatment of sleep apnea on obesity, but it generally has been noted that all non-weight loss treatments of sleep apnea have not been associated with any significant weight loss other than might be accrued from surgical interventions that temporarily reduce the ability to eat in the immediate postoperative period.

Chapter 14

Obesity and Diabetes

Obesity Associated with High Rates of Diabetes in the Pima Indians

National Institute of Diabetes and Digestive and Kidney Diseases (NIDDK) research conducted on the Pima Indians for the past 30 years has helped scientists prove that obesity is a major risk factor in the development of diabetes. One-half of adult Pima Indians have diabetes and 95% of those with diabetes are overweight.

These studies, carried out with the help of the Pima Indians, have shown that before gaining weight, overweight people have a slower metabolic rate compared to people of the same weight. This slower metabolic rate, combined with a high fat diet and a genetic tendency to retain fat may cause the epidemic overweight seen in the Pima Indians, scientists believe.

Scientists use the "thrifty gene" theory proposed in 1962 by geneticist James Neel to help explain why many Pima Indians are overweight. Neel's theory is based on the fact that for thousands of years populations who relied on farming, hunting and fishing for food, such as the Pima Indians, experienced alternating periods of feast and famine. Neel said that to adapt to these extreme changes in caloric needs,

---

This chapter contains text from "Obesity and Diabetes" and "Donna Young: Losing Weight to Avoid Diabetes" from *The Pima Indians, Pathfinders for Health*, on the National Institute of Diabetes and Digestive and Kidney Diseases (NIDDK) website, National Institutes of Health (NIH), http://www.niddk.nih.gov/health/diabetes/pima/index.htm, 1995.

these people developed a thrifty gene that allowed them to store fat during times of plenty so that they would not starve during times of famine.

This gene was helpful as long as there were periods of famine. But once these populations adopted the typical Western lifestyle, with less physical activity, a high fat diet, and access to a constant supply of calories, this gene began to work against them, continuing to store calories in preparation for famine. Scientists think that the thrifty gene that once protected people from starvation might also contribute to their retaining unhealthy amounts of fat.

Dr. Eric Ravussin, a visiting scientist at the Phoenix Epidemiology and Clinical Research Branch at NIDDK, has studied obesity in the Pima Indians since 1984. He believes the thrifty gene theory applies to the Pimas.

The Pima Indians maintained much of their traditional way of life and economy until the late 19th century, when their water supply was diverted by American farmers settling upstream, according to Ravussin. At that time, their 2,000-year-old tradition of irrigation and agriculture was disrupted, causing poverty, malnutrition and even starvation. The Pima community had to fall back on the lard, sugar and white flour the U.S. government gave them to survive, says Ravussin.

However, World War II brought great social and economic change for American Indians. Those who entered military service joined Caucasian units. Many other American Indians migrated from reservations to cities for factory employment and their estimated cash income more than doubled from 1940 to 1944.

When the war and the economic boom ended, most Native Americans returned to the reservations, but contact with the larger society had profoundly affected the Pimas' way of life. Ravussin says it is no surprise that the increase in unhealthy weight among the Pima Indians occurred in those born post-World War II.

During this century people world-wide experienced more prosperity and leisure time, and less physical work. Since the 1920s, all Americans have consumed more fat and sugar and less starch and fiber. The greatest changes have occurred in consumption of fat. In the 1890s, the traditional Pima Indian diet consisted of only about 15 percent fat and was high in starch and fiber, but currently almost 40 percent of the calories in the Pima diet are derived from fat. As the typical American diet became more available on the reservation after the war, people became more overweight.

"The only way to correct obesity is to eat less fat and exercise regularly," Ravussin says.

Obesity and Diabetes

Recently, Ravussin visited a Pima community living as their ancestors did in a remote area of the Sierra Madre mountains of Mexico. These Mexican Pimas are genetically the same as the Pima Indians of Arizona. Out of 35 Mexican Pimas studied, only three had diabetes and the population as a whole was not overweight, according to Ravussin.

"We've learned from this study of the Mexican Pimas that if the Pima Indians of Arizona could return to some of their traditions, including a high degree of physical activity and a diet with less fat and more starch, we might be able to reduce the rate, and surely the severity, of unhealthy weight in most of the population," Ravussin says.

"However, this is not as easy as it sounds because of factors such as genetic influences that are difficult to change. Our research focuses on determining the most effective way to bring about permanent weight loss in light of these factors," Ravussin adds.

Losing Weight to Avoid Diabetes

At 25, Donna Young has warm eyes, and a confident, lovely smile. She seems too young to worry about her health, much less about getting diabetes.

But in an interview at the Indian Health Service Hospital in Phoenix where she is a research volunteer, Donna says she has to think about it. Grandparents on both sides of the family had diabetes. "My dad and my mom have it, so there are lots of points against me." Although lots of her family members are aware that diabetes is in the family, Donna says, they think it won't affect them.

"That's how I was," she adds, until her aunt, also aged 25, was diagnosed as diabetic a year ago. "I did the oral glucose test and my blood sugar was 143 and that's borderline." She and a friend started walking two miles every morning. She exercised and watched her diet. Three months later, Donna's oral glucose tolerance test was 93. "I was all excited," she recounts. "I lost 5 centimeters off my thigh, and 4 off my waist." Mike Milner, an NIDDK physician's assistant who works closely with patients, said it really showed, she adds with pleasure.

"My mom was always telling me to watch my weight because she's diabetic, but I always just brushed it off. Then when I saw the results, I was all surprised and it made me happy. When I told my mom, she goes, 'Oh, I've been telling you all this time,'" Donna laughs. Her recently diagnosed aunt has been walking with her, too. "She's lost a lot of weight, and her blood sugar's gone down. She goes for regular check-ups, and she feels better. Before it didn't seem like she had too much energy. She has three young boys, and now she has a lot more energy to play with them," Donna adds.

Having seen how diabetes affects family members, Donna admits she was scared by her high blood sugar a year ago. Now, she's pleased to think she can prevent getting diabetes for a while. "I'm slowing it down with my weight loss and everything. It made such a big difference."

Chapter 15

Dieting and Gallstones

As most people know, there are significant health benefits to be gained from losing excess pounds. For example many people can reduce high blood pressure and cholesterol levels through weight loss. Overweight people are at greater risk of developing gallstones than people of average weight. However, people who are considering a diet program requiring very low intake of calories each day should be aware that during rapid or substantial weight loss, a person's risk of developing gallstones is increased.

What Are Gallstones?

Gallstones are clumps of solid material that form in the gallbladder. They may occur as a single, large stone or many small ones. Gallstones are a mixture of compounds, but typically they are mostly cholesterol.

One in ten Americans has gallstones. However, most people with gallstones don't know they have them and experience no symptoms. Painless gallstones are called silent gallstones. For an unfortunate minority, however, gallstones can cause painful attacks. Painful gallstones are called symptomatic gallstones, because they cause symptoms.

Weight-Control Information Network (WIN), National Institute of Diabetes and Digestive and Kidney Diseases (NIDDK), National Institutes of Health (NIH), NIH Pub. No. 94-3677, http://www.niddk.nih.gov/health/nutrit/pubs/dietgall.htm, November 1993, e-text posted February 20, 1998.

In rare cases gallstones can cause life-threatening complications. Symptomatic gallstones result in 600,000 hospitalizations and more than 500,000 operations each year in the United States.

What Causes Gallstones?

Gallstones develop in the gallbladder, a pear-shaped organ beneath the liver on the right side of the abdomen. It's about 3 inches long and an inch wide at its thickest part. The gallbladder stores and releases bile into the intestine to aid digestion.

Bile is a fluid made by the liver that helps in digestion. Bile contains substances called bile salts that act like natural detergents to break down fats in the food we eat. As food passes from the stomach into the small intestine, the gallbladder releases bile into the bile ducts. These ducts, or tubes, run from the liver to the intestine. Bile also helps eliminate excess cholesterol from the body. The liver secretes cholesterol into the bile, which is then eliminated from the body via the digestive system.

Most researchers believe three conditions are necessary to form gallstones. First, the bile becomes supersaturated with cholesterol, which means the bile contains more cholesterol than the bile salts can dissolve. Second, an imbalance of proteins or other substances in the bile causes the cholesterol to start to crystallize. Third, the gallbladder does not contract enough to empty its bile regularly.

Are Obese People More Likely to Develop Gallstones?

Yes. Obesity is a strong risk factor for gallstones.

Scientists often use a mathematical formula called body mass index (BMI) to define obesity (BMI = weight in kilograms divided by height in meters squared. [The BMI table is located in the "Practical Dietary Therapy Information" chapter of this sourcebook]). For example, an obese woman who is 5 ft. 4 in. tall (64 in.) and weighs 174 pounds has a BMI of 30. The more obese a person is, the greater his or her risk is of developing gallstones. Several studies have shown that women with a BMI of 30 or higher have at least double the risk of developing gallstones than women with a BMI of less than 25.

Why obesity is a risk factor for gallstones is unclear. But researchers believe that in obese people, the liver produces too much cholesterol. The excess cholesterol leads to supersaturation in the gallbladder.

Are People on a Diet to Lose Weight More at Risk for Developing Gallstones?

Yes. People who lose a lot of weight rapidly are at greater risk for developing gallstones. Gallstones are one of the most medically important complications of voluntary weight loss. The relationship of dieting to gallstones has only recently received attention.

One major study found that women who lost from 9 to 22 pounds (over a 2-year period) were 44 percent more likely to develop gallstones than women who did not lose weight. Women who lost more than 22 pounds were almost twice as likely to develop gallstones.

Other studies have shown that 10 to 25 percent of obese people develop gallstones while on a very-low-calorie diet. (Very-low-calorie diets are usually defined as diets containing 800 calories a day or less. The food is often in liquid form and taken for a prolonged period, typically 12 to 16 weeks.) The gallstones that developed in people on very-low-calorie diets were usually silent and did not produce any symptoms. However, about a third of the dieters who developed gallstones did have symptoms, and a proportion of these required gallbladder surgery.

In short, the likelihood of a person developing symptomatic gallstones during or shortly after rapid weight loss is about 4 to 6 percent. This estimate is based on reviewing just a few clinical studies, however, and is not conclusive.

Why Does Weight Loss Cause Gallstones?

Researchers believe dieting may cause a shift in the balance of bile salts and cholesterol in the gallbladder. The cholesterol level is increased and the amount of bile salts is decreased. Going for long periods without eating (skipping breakfast, for example), a common practice among dieters, also may decrease gallbladder contractions. If the gallbladder does not contract often enough to empty out the bile, gallstones may form.

Are Some Weight Loss Methods Better Than Others in Preventing Gallstones?

Possibly. If substantial or rapid weight loss increases the risk of developing gallstones, more gradual weight loss would seem to lessen the risk of getting gallstones. However, studies are needed to test this theory.

Some very low calorie-diets may not contain enough fat to cause the gallbladder to contract enough to empty its bile. A meal or snack containing approximately 10 grams (one-third of an ounce) of fat is necessary for the gallbladder to contract normally. But again, no studies have directly linked a diet's nutrient composition to the risk of gallstones.

Also, no studies have been conducted on the effects of repeated dieting on gallstone formation.

Are People Who Have Surgery to Lose Weight Also at Risk for Gallstones?

You bet. Gallstones are common among obese patients who lose weight rapidly after gastric bypass surgery. (In gastric bypass surgery, the size of the stomach is reduced, preventing the person from overeating.)

One study found that more than a third (38 percent) of patients who had gastric bypass surgery developed gallstones afterward. Gallstones are most likely to occur within the first few months after surgery.

Should People Who Already Have Gallstones Try to Lose Weight?

Scientists know that weight loss increases the risk of gallstone formation. However, they don't know whether weight loss increases the risk of silent gallstones becoming symptomatic gallstones or of other complications developing. In addition to painful gallstone attacks, complications include inflammation of the gallbladder, liver, or pancreas. These are usually caused by a gallstone getting lodged in a bile duct.

Although excluding people with pre-existing gallstones from a weight-loss program seems prudent, there is no evidence to support this action. If people have had their gallbladders removed, there is little risk of them having gallstones or bile problems while participating in a weight-loss program.

What Is the Treatment for Gallstones?

Silent gallstones are usually left alone and occasionally disappear on their own. Usually only patients with symptomatic gallstones are treated.

The most common treatment for gallstones is surgery to remove the gallbladder. This operation is called a cholecystectomy. In rare cases, drugs are used to dissolve the gallstones. Other non-surgical methods are still considered experimental.

The drug ursodeoxycholic acid prevented gallstones from forming in one clinical trial of patients on very-low-calorie diets. However, the drug is costly. Given the small proportion of patients who develop symptomatic gallstones on very-low-calorie diets, it is not known if ursodeoxycholic acid would be a cost-effective drug to recommend for all patients undergoing such diets, though people with pre-existing gallstones may benefit from this drug.

Are the Benefits of Weight Loss Greater Than the Risk of Getting Gallstones?

There's no question that obesity poses serious health risks. Obesity has been linked to heart disease, stroke, high blood pressure, high cholesterol levels, and diabetes. Obesity has also been associated with higher rates of certain types of cancer, such as gallbladder, colon, prostate, breast, cervical, and ovarian cancers.

Weight loss also reduces the risk of heart disease by lowering cholesterol levels. Even a modest weight loss of 10 to 20 pounds can bring positive changes. And the psychological boost from losing weight, such as improved self-image and greater social interaction, should not be ignored.

Patients who are thinking about beginning a commercial diet program to lose a significant amount of weight should talk with their doctors. A physician can evaluate a patient's medical history, individual circumstances, and the proposed weight-loss program. Doctor and patient can then discuss the potential benefits and risks of dieting, including the risks of developing gallstones.

Chapter 16

Cushing's Syndrome

Introduction

Cushing's syndrome is a hormonal disorder caused by prolonged exposure of the body's tissues to high levels of the hormone cortisol. Sometimes called "hypercortisolism," it is relatively rare and most commonly affects adults aged 20 to 50. An estimated 10 to 15 of every million people are affected each year.

What Are the Symptoms?

Symptoms vary, but most people have upper body obesity, rounded face, increased fat around the neck, and thinning arms and legs. Children tend to be obese with slowed growth rates.

Other symptoms appear in the skin, which becomes fragile and thin. It bruises easily and heals poorly. Purplish pink stretch marks may appear on the abdomen, thighs, buttocks, arms and breasts. The bones are weakened, and routine activities such as bending, lifting, or rising from a chair may lead to backaches and rib and spinal column fractures.

Most people have severe fatigue, weak muscles, high blood pressure and high blood sugar. Irritability, anxiety and depression are common.

Women usually have excess hair growth on their faces, necks, chests, abdomens, and thighs. Their menstrual periods may become

---

National Institute of Diabetes, Digestive, and Kidney Diseases (NIDDK), National Institutes of Health (NIH), Pub. No. 96-3007, http://www.niddk.nih.gov/health/endo/pubs/cushings/cushings.htm, June 1996, e-text posted February 20, 1998.

irregular or stop. Men have decreased fertility with diminished or absent desire for sex.

What Causes Cushing's Syndrome?

Cushing's syndrome occurs when the body's tissues are exposed to excessive levels of cortisol for long periods of time. Many people suffer the symptoms of Cushing's syndrome because they take glucocorticoid hormones such as prednisone for asthma, rheumatoid arthritis, lupus, or other inflammatory diseases.

Others develop Cushing's syndrome because of overproduction of cortisol by the body. Normally, the production of cortisol follows a precise chain of events. First, the hypothalamus, a part of the brain which is about the size of a small sugar cube, sends corticotropin releasing hormone (CRH) to the pituitary gland. CRH causes the pituitary to secrete adrenocorticotropin (ACTH), a hormone that stimulates the adrenal glands. When the adrenals, which are located just above the kidneys, receive the ACTH, they respond by releasing cortisol into the bloodstream.

Cortisol performs vital tasks in the body. It helps maintain blood pressure and cardiovascular function, reduces the immune system's inflammatory response, balances the effects of insulin in breaking down sugar for energy, and regulates the metabolism of proteins, carbohydrates, and fats. One of cortisol's most important jobs is to help the body respond to stress. For this reason, women in their last 3 months of pregnancy and highly trained athletes normally have high levels of the hormone. People suffering from depression, alcoholism, malnutrition and panic disorders also have increased cortisol levels.

When the amount of cortisol in the blood is adequate, the hypothalamus and pituitary release less CRH and ACTH. This ensures that the amount of cortisol released by the adrenal glands is precisely balanced to meet the body's daily needs. However, if something goes wrong with the adrenals or their regulating switches in the pituitary gland or the hypothalamus, cortisol production can go awry.

Pituitary Adenomas

Pituitary adenomas cause most cases of Cushing's syndrome. They are benign, or non-cancerous, tumors of the pituitary gland which secrete increased amounts of ACTH. Most patients have a single adenoma. This form of the syndrome, known as "Cushing's disease," affects women five times more frequently than men.

Cushing's Syndrome

Ectopic ACTH Syndrome

Some benign or malignant (cancerous) tumors that arise outside the pituitary can produce ACTH. This condition is known as ectopic ACTH syndrome. Lung tumors cause over 50 percent of these cases. Men are affected 3 times more frequently than women. The most common forms of ACTH-producing tumors are oat cell, or small cell lung cancer, which accounts for about 25 percent of all lung cancer cases, and carcinoid tumors. Other less common types of tumors that can produce ACTH are thymomas, pancreatic islet cell tumors, and medullary carcinomas of the thyroid.

Adrenal Tumors

Sometimes, an abnormality of the adrenal glands, most often an adrenal tumor, causes Cushing's syndrome. The average age of onset is about 40 years. Most of these cases involve non-cancerous tumors of adrenal tissue, called adrenal adenomas, which release excess cortisol into the blood.

Adrenocortical carcinomas, or adrenal cancers, are the least common cause of Cushing's syndrome. Cancer cells secrete excess levels of several adrenal cortical hormones, including cortisol and adrenal androgens. Adrenocortical carcinomas usually cause very high hormone levels and rapid development of symptoms.

Familial Cushing's Syndrome

Most cases of Cushing's syndrome are not inherited. Rarely, however, some individuals have special causes of Cushing's syndrome due to an inherited tendency to develop tumors of one or more endocrine glands. In Primary Pigmented Micronodular Adrenal Disease, children or young adults develop small cortisol-producing tumors of the adrenal glands. In Multiple Endocrine Neoplasia Type I (MEN I), hormone secreting tumors of the parathyroid glands, pancreas and pituitary occur. Cushing's syndrome in MEN I may be due to pituitary, ectopic or adrenal tumors.

How Is Cushing's Syndrome Diagnosed?

Diagnosis is based on a review of the patient's medical history, physical examination and laboratory tests. Often x-ray exams of the adrenal or pituitary glands are useful for locating tumors. These tests help to determine if excess levels of cortisol are present and why.

24-Hour Urinary Free Cortisol Level

This is the most specific diagnostic test. The patient's urine is collected over a 24-hour period and tested for the amount of cortisol. Levels higher than 50–100 micrograms a day for an adult suggest Cushing's syndrome. The normal upper limit varies in different laboratories, depending on which measurement technique is used.

Once Cushing's syndrome has been diagnosed, other tests are used to find the exact location of the abnormality that leads to excess cortisol production. The choice of test depends, in part, on the preference of the endocrinologist or the center where the test is performed.

Dexamethasone Suppression Test

This test helps to distinguish patients with excess production of ACTH due to pituitary adenomas from those with ectopic ACTH-producing tumors. Patients are given dexamethasone, a synthetic glucocorticoid, by mouth every 6 hours for 4 days. For the first 2 days, low doses of dexamethasone are given, and for the last 2 days, higher doses are given. Twenty-four hour urine collections are made before dexamethasone is administered and on each day of the test. Since cortisol and other glucocorticoids signal the pituitary to lower secretion of ACTH, the normal response after taking dexamethasone is a drop in blood and urine cortisol levels. Different responses of cortisol to dexamethasone are obtained depending on whether the cause of Cushing's syndrome is a pituitary adenoma or an ectopic ACTH-producing tumor.

The dexamethasone suppression test can produce false-positive results in patients with depression, alcohol abuse, high estrogen levels, acute illness, and stress. Conversely, drugs such as phenytoin and phenobarbital may cause false-negative results in response to dexamethasone suppression. For this reason, patients are usually advised by their physicians to stop taking these drugs at least one week before the test.

CRH Stimulation Test

This test helps to distinguish between patients with pituitary adenomas and those with ectopic ACTH syndrome or cortisol-secreting adrenal tumors. Patients are given an injection of CRH, the corticotropin-releasing hormone which causes the pituitary to secrete ACTH. Patients with pituitary adenomas usually experience a rise in blood levels of ACTH and cortisol. This response is rarely seen in patients

Cushing's Syndrome

with ectopic ACTH syndrome and practically never in patients with cortisol-secreting adrenal tumors.

Direct Visualization of the Endocrine Glands (Radiologic Imaging)

Imaging tests reveal the size and shape of the pituitary and adrenal glands and help determine if a tumor is present. The most common are the computerized tomography (CT) scan and magnetic resonance imaging (MRI). A CT scan produces a series of x-ray pictures giving a cross-sectional image of a body part. MRI also produces images of the internal organs of the body but without exposing the patient to ionizing radiation.

Imaging procedures are used to find a tumor after a diagnosis has been established. Imaging is not used to make the diagnosis of Cushing's syndrome because benign tumors, sometimes called "incidentalomas," are commonly found in the pituitary and adrenal glands. These tumors do not produce hormones detrimental to health and are not removed unless blood tests show they are a cause of symptoms or they are unusually large. Conversely, pituitary tumors are not detected by imaging in almost 50 percent of patients who ultimately require pituitary surgery for Cushing's syndrome.

Petrosal Sinus Sampling

This test is not always required, but in many cases, it is the best way to separate pituitary from ectopic causes of Cushing's syndrome. Samples of blood are drawn from the petrosal sinuses, veins which drain the pituitary, by introducing catheters through a vein in the upper thigh/groin region, with local anesthesia and mild sedation. X-rays are used to confirm the correct position of the catheters. Often CRH, the hormone which causes the pituitary to secrete ACTH, is given during this test to improve diagnostic accuracy. Levels of ACTH in the petrosal sinuses are measured and compared with ACTH levels in a forearm vein. ACTH levels higher in the petrosal sinuses than in the forearm vein indicate the presence of a pituitary adenoma; similar levels suggest ectopic ACTH syndrome.

The Dexamethasone-CRH Test

Some individuals have high cortisol levels, but do not develop the progressive effects of Cushing's syndrome, such as muscle weakness, fractures, and thinning of the skin. These individuals may have Pseudo

Cushing's syndrome, which was originally described in people who were depressed or drank excess alcohol, but is now known to be more common. Pseudo Cushing's does not have the same long-term effects on health as Cushing's syndrome and does not require treatment directed at the endocrine glands. Although observation over months to years will distinguish Pseudo Cushing's from Cushing's, the dexamethasone-CRH test was developed to distinguish between the conditions rapidly, so that Cushing's patients can receive prompt treatment. This test combines the dexamethasone suppression and the CRH stimulation tests. Elevations of cortisol during this test suggest Cushing's syndrome.

Some patients may have sustained high cortisol levels without the effects of Cushing's syndrome. These high cortisol levels may be compensating for the body's resistance to cortisol's effects. This rare syndrome of cortisol resistance is a genetic condition that causes hypertension and chronic androgen excess.

Sometimes other conditions may be associated with many of the symptoms of Cushing's syndrome. These include polycystic ovarian syndrome, which may cause menstrual disturbances, weight gain from adolescence, excess hair growth and sometimes impaired insulin action and diabetes. Commonly, weight gain, high blood pressure, and abnormal levels of cholesterol and triglycerides in the blood are associated with resistance to insulin action and diabetes; this has been described as the "Metabolic Syndrome-X." Patients with these disorders do not have abnormally elevated cortisol levels.

How Is Cushing's Syndrome Treated?

Treatment depends on the specific reason for cortisol excess and may include surgery, radiation, chemotherapy or the use of cortisol-inhibiting drugs. If the cause is long-term use of glucocorticoid hormones to treat another disorder, the doctor will gradually reduce the dosage to the lowest dose adequate for control of that disorder. Once control is established, the daily dose of glucocorticoid hormones may be doubled and given on alternate days to lessen side effects.

Pituitary Adenomas

Several therapies are available to treat the ACTH-secreting pituitary adenomas of Cushing's disease. The most widely used treatment is surgical removal of the tumor, known as transsphenoidal adenomectomy. Using a special microscope and very fine instruments, the surgeon approaches the pituitary gland through a nostril or an

Cushing's Syndrome

opening made below the upper lip. Because this is an extremely delicate procedure, patients are often referred to centers specializing in this type of surgery. The success, or cure, rate of this procedure is over 80 percent when performed by a surgeon with extensive experience. If surgery fails, or only produces a temporary cure, surgery can be repeated, often with good results. After curative pituitary surgery, the production of ACTH drops two levels below normal. This is a natural, but temporary, drop in ACTH production, and patients are given a synthetic form of cortisol (such as hydrocortisone or prednisone). Most patients can stop this replacement therapy in less than a year.

For patients in whom transsphenoidal surgery has failed or who are not suitable candidates for surgery, radiotherapy is another possible treatment. Radiation to the pituitary gland is given over a 6-week period, with improvement occurring in 40 to 50 percent of adults and up to 80 percent of children. It may take several months or years before patients feel better from radiation treatment alone. However, the combination of radiation and the drug mitotane (Lysodren®) can help speed recovery. Mitotane suppresses cortisol production and lowers plasma and urine hormone levels. Treatment with mitotane alone can be successful in 30 to 40 percent of patients. Other drugs used alone or in combination to control the production of excess cortisol are aminoglutethimide, metyrapone, trilostane, and ketoconazole. Each has its own side effects that doctors consider when prescribing therapy for individual patients.

Ectopic ACTH Syndrome

To cure the overproduction of cortisol caused by ectopic ACTH syndrome, it is necessary to eliminate all of the cancerous tissue that is secreting ACTH. The choice of cancer treatment—surgery, radiotherapy, chemotherapy, immunotherapy, or a combination of these treatments—depends on the type of cancer and how far it has spread. Since ACTH-secreting tumors (for example, small cell lung cancer) may be very small or widespread at the time of diagnosis, cortisol-inhibiting drugs, like mitotane, are an important part of treatment. In some cases, if pituitary surgery is not successful, surgical removal of the adrenal glands (bilateral adrenalectomy) may take the place of drug therapy.

Adrenal Tumors

Surgery is the mainstay of treatment for benign as well as cancerous tumors of the adrenal glands. In Primary Pigmented Micronodular

Adrenal Disease and the familial Carney's complex, surgical removal of the adrenal glands is required.

What Research Is Being Done on Cushing's Syndrome?

The National Institutes of Health (NIH) is the biomedical research component of the Federal Government. It is one of the health agencies of the Public Health Service, which is part of the U.S. Department of Health and Human Services. Several components of the NIH conduct and support research on Cushing's syndrome and other disorders of the endocrine system, including the National Institute of Diabetes and Digestive and Kidney Diseases (NIDDK), the National Institute of Child Health and Human Development (NICHD), the National Institute of Neurological Disorders and Stroke (NINDS), and the National Cancer Institute (NCI).

NIH-supported scientists are conducting intensive research into the normal and abnormal function of the major endocrine glands and the many hormones of the endocrine system. Identification of the corticotropin releasing hormone (CRH), which instructs the pituitary gland to release ACTH, enabled researchers to develop the CRH stimulation test, which is increasingly being used to identify the cause of Cushing's syndrome.

Improved techniques for measuring ACTH permit distinction of ACTH-dependent forms of Cushing's syndrome from adrenal tumors. NIH studies have shown that petrosal sinus sampling is a very accurate test to diagnose the cause of Cushing's syndrome in those who have excess ACTH production. The recently described dexamethasone suppression-CRH test is able to differentiate most cases of Cushing's from Pseudo Cushing's.

As a result of this research, doctors are much better able to diagnose Cushing's syndrome and distinguish among the causes of this disorder. Since accurate diagnosis is still a problem for some patients, new tests are under study to further refine the diagnostic process.

Many studies are underway to understand the causes of formation of benign endocrine tumors, such as those which cause most cases of Cushing's syndrome. In a few pituitary adenomas, specific gene defects have been identified and may provide important clues to understanding tumor formation. Endocrine factors may also play a role. There is increasing evidence that tumor formation is a multi-step process. Understanding the basis of Cushing's syndrome will yield new approaches to therapy.

Cushing's Syndrome

NIH supports research related to Cushing's syndrome at medical centers throughout the United States. Scientists are also treating patients with Cushing's syndrome at the NIH Warren Grant Magnuson Clinical Center in Bethesda, Maryland. Physicians who are interested in referring a patient may contact Developmental Endocrinology Branch, NICHD, Building 10, Room 10N262, Bethesda, Maryland 20892, telephone (301) 496-4686.

[See the "Additional Help and Information" section of this sourcebook for further resources and reading material on Cushing's Syndrome.]

Chapter 17

Obesity before Pregnancy Is a Risk Factor for Cesarean Delivery

A retrospective chart review of patients delivering in a rural hospital between January 1990 and June 1997 indicates that women who are obese before they become pregnant are at increased risk for cesarean delivery. The charts were reviewed for method of delivery, associated risk factors and incidence of cesarean section. Obesity was defined as a body mass index greater than 29 [See the "Practical Dietary Therapy Information" chapter of this sourcebook for more information about body mass index]. The mean body mass index among women who had primary and repeat cesarean sections was 31.9 and 32.5, respectively; the mean body mass in patients who delivered vaginally and patients who had a vaginal delivery after cesarean section was 28.3 and 26.5, respectively. However, the women who delivered vaginally had gained significantly more weight than the women who received repeat cesarean sections (28.9 lb versus 27.6 lb). Other risk factors associated with an increase in cesarean sections included older age, diabetes mellitus, gestational hypertension and previous delivery of an infant over 4,000 g (8 lb, 13 oz). The investigators believe that the possible relationship between obesity and cesarean section is very complex and will require continued investigations. (North American Primary Care Research Group)

Excerpted from Verna L. Rose, "Obesity before Pregnancy Is a Risk Factor for Cesarean Delivery." Used with permission from the March 15, 1999, issue of *American Family Physician*. Copyright © The American Academy of Family Physicians. All rights reserved.

Chapter 18

Extra Weight Could Complicate Surgery Recovery

Obesity has long been considered a potential risk factor for poor outcome following surgical procedures. However, controversy exists regarding the clinical impact of this problem because of a paucity of data regarding the incidence and risk of nosocomial infections in obese surgical patients. A retrospective study was undertaken to compare the nosocomial infection rate in obese and normal weight surgical patients. All patients undergoing general, urologic, vascular, thoracic, or gynecologic surgical procedures between October 1 and December 31, 1991, were reviewed. Nosocomial infection data were obtained from the Department of Hospital Epidemiology. A total of 849 patients were evaluated, of which 536 (63%) were normal weight (Body Mass Index, or BMI less than 27 kg/m^2), 175 (21%) were obese (BMI 27–31 kg/m^2), and 138 (16%) were severely obese (BMI greater than 31 kg/m^2). Age, mortality and American Society of Anesthesiologists (ASA) risk scores did not differ among the three groups. There were significant increases in the number and percent of nosocomial infections in the obese populations, with rates of 0.05 per cent in normal weight, compared to 2.8 per cent and 4.0 per cent in obese and severely obese groups. Infections consisted of seven wound infections, five *C. difficile* infections, one pneumonia, and three bacteremias. No differences in distribution between groups were evident. Mortality was similar

---

Excerpted from Patricia S. Choban, M.D., F.A.C.S. Rachel Heckler, B.S. Jean C. Burge, PhD., Louis Flancbaum, M.D. F.A.C.S., "Increased Incidence of Nosocomial Infections in Obese Surgical Patients," in *The American Surgeon*, November 1995, Vol. 61, pp. 1001–1005. Reprinted with permission.

among the groups. These data support the hypothesis that obesity is a significant risk factor for clinically relevant nosocomial infections in surgical patients.

Obesity is currently the most prevalent chronic disease in the United States. A review by the National Center for Health Statistics (NCHS) found 26 percent of the adult population in the United States to be overweight. Between 1976 and 1980 this group included 34 million people, 13 million of whom were severely overweight by the NCHS criteria using Body Mass Index (BMI), defined as {weight (Kg)/ [Height (m)]^2}. More recently, a follow-up study, reviewing the four National Health and Nutrition Examination Surveys (NHANES) between 1960 and 1991, demonstrated an increase in the prevalence of overweight in U.S. adults to 34.8 per cent of the population.

Because obesity is so prevalent, obese patients with problems requiring surgical intervention are common in most clinical practices. In fact, obese patients are known to be at increased risk for the development of several disorders, or "comorbid" conditions, that frequently require surgical intervention, including gallstones, reflux esophagitis, osteoarthritis, and certain malignancies, such as breast, endometrial, colon, and prostate cancer. Also of concern in this population is a growing body of information that suggests obesity is associated with or causes impaired immune function.

Obesity has long been considered a potential risk factor for poor outcome following surgical procedures. Many standard textbooks of anesthesiology, obstetrics and gynecology, orthopedics, and general surgery contain broad general statements concerning the increased morbidity and mortality associated with surgery in the obese patient. These statements appear to be based on theoretical considerations and clinical anecdotes. In reality, there have been few studies to accurately determine the magnitude of surgical risk posed by obesity. This study was undertaken to determine the risk of hospital acquired infectious complications and death in patients with increasing degrees of obesity, and to ascertain what, if any, difference was due to the severity of the patient's underlying disease, as estimated by the American Society of Anesthesiologists (ASA) Physical Status Classification.

Discussion

Hospital-acquired or nosocomial infections pose significant risks for all hospitalized patients. The consequences of nosocomial infections can range from minor inconveniences to the patient to life-threatening events that substantially increase the cost of care and

Extra Weight Could Complicate Surgery Recovery

lengthen hospital stay. The costs of nosocomial infections and their contribution to the total cost of health care are also significant. Haley et al. estimated that nosocomial infections accounted for 7.5 million additional hospital days and $1 billion in extra costs in 1976. By 1992, these were estimated to affect over 2 million patients per year at a cost in excess of 4.5 billion dollars. As medical care reimbursement moves to prospective payment, capitation, and managed care systems, these expenditures will become more critical, as it appears that most of the additional costs incurred by hospitals are not recovered under these arrangements.

Obese patients are perceived to be, and in fact may be, at an increased risk for a variety of perioperative complications, but infectious complications have been addressed in only a cursory fashion to date. Jackson found that obesity increased the risk of infectious and noninfectious perioperative pulmonary complications. Postlethwait and Johnson noted an increased rate of atelectasis in their series of patients treated for duodenal ulcer disease, but this did not result in an increase in postoperative pneumonias. In a review of risk factors for postoperative pneumonia in 520 patients undergoing elective thoracic and upper or lower abdominal surgery, Garibaldi et al. did not find massive obesity to be a risk factor when the data were controlled for duration and site of surgery.

Wound infection is the most common cause of morbidity in obese patients following gastric bypass or gastroplasty. The incidence of wound complications is also significantly greater in obese patients undergoing cholecystectomy, surgery for duodenal ulcer disease, hysterectomy, cesarean section, coronary artery bypass grafting, and renal transplantation. These wound problems may be accounted for by local changes in the surrounding tissues, such as an increase in adipose tissue which, as a relatively avascular mass, has poor resistance to infection, and an increase in local tissue trauma related to retraction of the largo abdominal wall. The increase in operative time due to the size of the patients may also contribute to the development of wound problems.

Independent of the systemic factors relating to glucose homeostasis, which contribute to impaired wound healing and immune system dysfunction, obesity is associated with change in cell mediated and humoral immunity. Many of these changes return to normal with weight reduction. Whether these abnormalities are related to the mass of adipose tissue itself or to the types of dietary lipids ingested remains to be determined.

In this study, both the number and incidence of nosocomial infections in obese and severely obese surgical patients were increased in comparison to a comparable group of normal weight patients. This suggests that the immune dysfunction associated with obesity may have real clinical consequences. Surgical wound infections accounted for the majority of nosocomial infections, but were not the only type of infectious complication seen. The occurrence of *C. difficile* infections in hospitalized patients generally reflects the use of systemic antibiotics to treat other infectious processes. This relationship may warrant further review in obese patients to determine whether there are predisposing risk factors in addition to those accounted for by the use of antibiotics alone. There were no significant differences in the specific types of infectious complications noted, which may reflect the low overall incidence of infectious complications in the entire series.

The increased risk for nosocomial infection correlated only with the increase in obesity and was not related to an increase in preoperative risk or severity of the underlying disease state, as reflected by ASA class. The ASA classification did not differ between the different weight groups, which may reflect a number of factors, including the fact that ours is a tertiary care institution with many patients having multiple medical problems, or that a large number of patients with clinically severe obesity are treated at this institution, so that obesity alone did not prompt an increase in ASA classification by our anesthesia staff. The increase in infectious complications was not associated with an increase in patient mortality.

These data support the increasing body of literature which suggests that obese patients may be at increased risk for perioperative infectious complications, particularly wound complications. Since these complications did not impact adversely on death rates, obese patients should be offered surgical treatment for their disease when surgery constitutes the most appropriate therapy. Further studies to more accurately determine the perioperative risk for complications associated with varying degrees of obesity are needed in order to improve outcome and contain costs.

Chapter 19

Excess Pounds May Lead to Asthma

Conventional wisdom holds that if you have asthma, you're more likely to become overweight—presumably because shortness of breath, wheezing, and coughing make it difficult, if not impossible, to burn calories via exercise. But researchers at Harvard Medical School are now saying that it may be the other way around: instead of being just a by-product of asthma, extra pounds could make people more vulnerable to developing the disease.

The Harvard researchers analyzed weight and health information on almost 90,000 women followed from 1991 to 1995 in the Nurses' Health Study II. At first, none of the women had been found to have asthma by a physician—but by 1995, some 1,650 of them had been diagnosed with it. The heavier a woman was for her height, the more likely she was to develop the condition. In fact, the women who were most overweight in 1991 were three times as likely to have developed asthma as me thinnest ones.

Study leader Carlos Camargo, MD, speculates that excess weight could contribute to asthma by compressing the airways and preventing the lungs from expanding properly. Or it could be that people who are already overweight tend to sit inside more often, thereby exposing themselves to higher levels of indoor air pollutants that could contribute to asthma, including pet dander and dust.

Tufts University Health & Nutrition Letter, June 1998, Vol. 16, N. 4, pp. 2–3. Reprinted with permission, *Tufts University Health & Nutrition Letter*, tel: 1-800-274-7581.

The researchers note that obesity is on the rise in developed countries, theorizing that this could help explain why asthma rates are also increasing.

Chapter 20

Getting to Know Gout

Say the word "gout" and some people will think of a bloated king surveying the remains of a sumptuous feast, wine glass in hand, swollen foot propped on a pillow—looking for all the world like the dismal product of a grossly overindulgent life.

There are a couple of flaws in that conventional image. We know, for example, that gout doesn't afflict only the privileged classes and that women, too, are susceptible, though a lot less than men.

But still there's a good deal right with that picture. It correctly reflects that:

- About 90 percent of people afflicted with gout are men over 40.

- Obesity in general, and in particular excessive weight gain in men between ages 20 and 40, has been shown to increase the risk of gout. In fact, about half of all gout sufferers are overweight.

- Alcohol abuse and so-called "binge" drinking are associated with gout, as is eating purine-rich foods such as brains, kidneys, liver, sardines, anchovies, and dried beans and peas.

In addition, careful scientific surveys have shown that occupational exposure to lead, the use of certain drugs to control high blood pressure, some surgical procedures, family history (possibly a genetic

Ken Flieger, *FDA Consumer*, March 1995, Vol. 29, N. 2, pp. 19–23, copyright 1995 U.S. Department of Health and Human Services.

predisposition), and trauma are all linked to an increased risk of gout. Indeed, the prevalence of gout—the number of gout sufferers for each 100,000 people—is rising rapidly in the United States and other developed countries. Some authorities believe the increase is related to higher living standards.

Our fanciful image of a gouty Henry VIII (or other bloated monarch) can't show, however, the one common denominator that ties together this mixed bag of risk factors: failure of the metabolic process that controls the amount of uric acid in the blood. For most people, the process works just fine. But in some 1 million Americans, uric acid metabolism has gone seriously haywire. As a result, they suffer from gout.

And suffer they do. An Englishman, Thomas Sydenham, writing in the 17th century, left this unfortunately all-too-accurate description of a typical attack of gout: The victim goes to bed ... in good health. About two o'clock in the morning, he is awakened by a severe pain in the great toe; more rarely in the heel, ankle, or instep. The pain is like that of a dislocation. [It] becomes more intense... So exquisite and lively meanwhile is the feeling of the part affected, that it cannot bear the weight of the bedclothes nor the jar of a person walking in the room. The night is passed in torture...

A Crystal Culprit

In spite of the agony and havoc it can cause, uric acid is a normal constituent of the human body. Ordinarily about one-third of the uric acid in our system comes from food, especially foods like those noted earlier that are rich in purines. The rest we produce ourselves through ordinary metabolism.

The body converts purines to uric acid. The level of uric acid in the blood fluctuates in response to diet, fluid intake, overall health status, and other factors. Men normally have somewhat more uric acid than women do (although the difference begins to narrow after menopause), and in both sexes it tends to increase with advancing age.

Higher-than-normal amounts of uric acid in the blood, a condition called hyperuricemia, is quite common and only rarely warrants medical treatment. On the other hand, sustained hyperuricemia is the primary risk factor for gout. It's safe to say that, while not all people with hyperuricemia develop gout, virtually everyone with gout is hyperuricemic. It works this way:

At normal and even somewhat elevated levels, uric acid stays in solution in the blood. It moves through the circulation, gets filtered by the kidneys, and is excreted in the urine. When, however, blood uric acid levels rise above a certain concentration (which varies with temperature and blood acidity), it forms needle-like crystals that lodge in or around a joint.

In response to irritation caused by uric acid crystals, the skin covering the affected area rapidly becomes tight, inflamed, swollen, and red or purplish. These classical signs of inflammation, together with sudden and extreme pain (just as Thomas Sydenham described), strongly suggest an acute attack of gout. The diagnosis is confirmed by laboratory finding of uric acid crystals in fluid taken from the affected joint.

Why is the big toe the most common site for an initial gout attack? Perhaps because first, the extremities are a bit cooler than other parts of the body, and uric acid crystals form more readily at lower temperatures; and second, normal walking and standing subject the feet to considerable stress. Together, these factors might explain why the big toe, heel, instep, and Achilles tendon are among the places that gout attacks first. Other targets, especially in untreated patients who have recurrent attacks of gout, are the knee, elbow, wrist, fingers and, less often, the shoulder, pelvis, spine, and internal organs.

Gout is classified as a form of arthritis because it is initially and predominantly a disease of the joints. Other similar conditions exist; one called "pseudogout" is somewhat milder than true gout and is caused by calcium rather than uric acid crystals. Infection or trauma to the affected area can mimic gout and mislead both patients and health professionals. Accurate diagnosis is essential for appropriate treatment.

Without treatment, an initial acute attack of gout will run its painful course within several days or a few weeks, by which time all outward evidence of the disease disappears. The next acute attack—50 or more percent of gout sufferers will have a second attack—may not occur for months or years. Subsequent attacks, however, are likely to be more frequent, more severe, and more destructive to joints and other tissue unless the problem is treated. Over time, uric acid crystals accumulate in the body, causing gritty, chalky deposits called tophi that are sometimes visible under the skin, particularly around joints and in the edges of the ears. Tophi may also form inside bone near the joints, in the kidneys, and in other organs and tissues, causing permanent damage. Advances in treatment, fortunately, have made this kind of chronic gout extremely rare.

Treatment

As with most illnesses, effective treatment of gout depends on a correct diagnosis. Gout can be unequivocally diagnosed by telltale uric acid crystals in joint fluid. But appropriate treatment is often started after a "clinical" diagnosis based on painfully obvious signs and symptoms and other relevant factors, such as the patient's uric acid level, age, weight, gender, diet, and alcohol use. If this picture adds up to a strong suspicion of gout, treatment can be started with the immediate goal of arresting the acute attack.

Acute gout is treated with drugs that block the inflammatory reaction. One of the oldest agents known to be effective against acute gout is colchicine, which comes from a common European plant, the autumn crocus, and is marketed in this country primarily as a generic drug. An English clergyman, Sidney Smith, said a century and a half ago that he had only to go into his garden and hold out his gouty toe to the plant to obtain a prompt cure. This may have been an exaggeration, but a rapid response to colchicine suggests that the patient does indeed have gout.

This old, powerful remedy is now used less often than it once was because it can be quite toxic, causing nausea, vomiting, diarrhea, and stomach cramps when taken by mouth and severe (even fatal) blood disorders when taken intravenously. Moreover, modern agents, specifically non-steroidal anti-inflammatory drugs (NSAIDs) are highly effective against acute gout and less toxic than colchicine. To treat an acute case of gout, the first choice of many physicians is the NSAID Indocin (and other brands of indomethacin). Naprosyn (naproxen) is another NSAID commonly used in acute gout.

Steroid drugs, such as Deltasone (and other brands of prednisone) and Acthar (and other brands of adrenocorticotropic hormone), may be used if NSAIDs fail to control an acute attack. Steroids may be taken by mouth or by injection into the bloodstream or muscle.

Drug treatment usually relieves the symptoms of acute gout within 48 hours. Subsequent treatment, which may well be lifelong, is aimed at preventing further attacks by controlling uric acid in the blood—keeping it below concentrations at which crystals can form. Two main treatment approaches are used, in some cases simultaneously.

One approach is to slow the rate at which the body produces uric acid. Zyloprim (allopurinol) has been approved for the treatment of gout and is frequently prescribed for gout patients who have uric acid kidney stones or other kidney problems. Side effects include skin rash and upset stomach, both of which usually subside as the body becomes used to the drug. Zyloprim makes some patients drowsy, so they need to be cautious about driving or using machinery.

The other approach to controlling gout following an initial acute attack is to increase the amount of uric acid excreted in urine. Two so-called uricosuric drugs commonly used for this are Benemid

Getting to Know Gout

(probenecid) and Anturane (sulfinpyrazone), both approved by the Food and Drug Administration (FDA) for gout treatment. In addition to lowering blood uric acid levels, these drugs help dissolve deposits of uric acid crystals around joints and in other tissue. Zyloprim is also used to dissolve tophaceous gout in uric acid over-producers. Uricosurics can cause nausea, stomach upset, headache, and a potentially serious skin rash.

Drugs to control uric acid levels may, paradoxically, prolong an acute attack. For this reason, Benemid, Anturane and Zyloprim are not used during the acute stage of gout. They may, in fact, induce gout flare-ups during the early part of long-term use. Accordingly, colchicine in a dose low enough to avoid toxic side effects is sometimes prescribed to prevent acute attacks during this phase of treatment.

Common-Sense Measures

Better understanding of what gout is, what causes it, and how to treat it has perhaps dispelled some of the traditional myths about what has been erroneously called "the disease of kings." Then, too, folk wisdom about gout, coupled with good science and medicine, points to measures that prudent people can take to prevent or at least lessen the severity of the condition.

Many authorities and the Arthritis Foundation, which supports research and public service programs relating to gout, advocate weight control as a logical aid to gout prevention. They point out, however, that people who are overweight should get professional guidance in planning a weight-reduction program, because fasting or severe dieting can actually increase uric acid levels.

Experts generally agree that people with gout can eat pretty much what they want, within limits. People who have kidney stones caused by uric acid may need to avoid purine-rich foods. But this problem can usually be handled effectively with drug treatment.

Curbing alcohol use and avoiding "binge" drinking can reduce the likelihood of acute attacks. So can drinking six or eight glasses of water a day, which dilutes uric acid and aids its removal by the kidneys. Some medicines—in particular the thiazide diuretics ("water pills") used to control high blood pressure—tend to increase uric acid levels. A gout patient taking one of these drugs may have to switch to another type of diuretic or blood pressure medicine.

Finally, although uncommon, it might be helpful to find out if an environmental or occupational exposure to lead is playing a role in a patient's problem with gout.

While a cure for gout—a treatment that gets rid of the condition once and for all—isn't on the horizon, reliable and effective ways of diagnosing gout and keeping it under control constitute one of the more impressive success stories of modern medical science.

There may be no sure-fire way to keep a person from having that first agonizing attack, but prompt treatment can minimize the risk of further attacks and virtually rule out the damaging and crippling effects of chronic gouty arthritis.

Part Three

Managing Obesity

Chapter 21

Setting Goals for Weight Loss

There are lots of reasons for people who are overweight or obese to lose weight. To be healthier. To look better. To feel better. To have more energy.

No matter what the reason, successful weight loss and healthy weight management depend on sensible goals and expectations. If you set sensible goals for yourself, chances are you'll be more likely to meet them and have a better chance of keeping the weight off. In fact, losing even five to 10 percent of your weight is the kind of goal that can help improve your health.

Most overweight people should lose weight gradually. For safe and healthy weight loss, try not to exceed a rate of two pounds per week. Sometimes, people with serious health problems associated with obesity may have legitimate reasons for losing weight rapidly. If so, a physician's supervision is required.

What you weigh is the result of several factors:

- how much and what kinds of food you eat
- whether your lifestyle includes regular physical activity
- whether you use food to respond to stress and other situations in your life

---

"Setting Goals for Weight Loss," a pamphlet by Partnership for Healthy Weight Management, www.consumer.gov/weightloss/setgoals.htm, February 1999.

- your physiologic and genetic make-up
- your age and health status

Successful weight loss and weight management should address all of these factors. And that's the reason to ignore products and programs that promise quick and easy results, or that promise permanent results without permanent changes in your lifestyle. Any ad that says you can lose weight without lowering the calories you take in and/or increasing your physical activity is selling fantasy and false hope. In fact, some people would call it fraud. Furthermore, the use of some products may not be safe.

A Realistic Approach

Many people who are overweight or obese have decided not to diet per se, but to concentrate on engaging in regular physical activity and maintaining healthy eating habits in accordance with the Dietary Guidelines for Americans, emphasizing lowered fat consumption, and an increase in vegetables, fruits and whole grains. Others—who try to diet— report needing help to achieve their weight management goals.

Fad diets that ignore the principles of the Dietary Guidelines may result in short term weight loss, but may do so at the risk of your health. How you go about managing your weight has a lot to do with your long-term success. Unless your health is seriously at risk due to complications from being overweight or obese, gradual weight loss should be your rule—and your goal. Here's how to do it:

- Check with your doctor. Make sure that your health status allows lowering your caloric intake and increasing your physical activity.

- Follow a calorie-reduced, but balanced diet that provides for as little as one or two pounds of weight loss a week. Be sure to include at least five servings a day of fruits and vegetables, along with whole grains, lean meat and low fat dairy products. It may not produce headlines, but it can reduce waistlines. It's not "miracle" science—just common sense. Most important, it's prudent and healthy.

- Make time in your day for some form of physical activity. Start by taking the stairs at work, walking up or down an escalator, parking at the far end of a lot instead of cruising around for the closest spot. Then, assuming your physician gives the okay,

Setting Goals for Weight Loss

gradually add some form of regular physical activity that you enjoy. Walking is an excellent form of physical activity that almost everyone can do.

- Consider the benefits of moderate weight loss. There's scientific evidence that losing five to 10 percent of your weight and keeping it off can benefit your health—lower your blood pressure, for example. If you are 5 feet 6 inches tall and weigh 180 pounds, and your goal weight is 150, losing five to 10 percent (nine to 18 pounds) is beneficial. When it comes to successful weight loss and weight management, steady and slow can be the way to go.

For many people who are overweight or obese, long-term—and healthy—weight management generally requires sensible goals and a commitment to make realistic changes in their lifestyle and improve their health. A lifestyle based on healthy eating and regular physical activity can be a real lifesaver.

Determining Your Weight/Health Profile

Overweight and obesity have been associated with increased risk of developing such conditions as high blood pressure, type 2 diabetes and coronary artery disease. For most people, determining the circumference of your waist and your body mass index (BMI) are reliable ways to estimate your body fat and the health risks associated with being overweight, overfat, or obese. BMI is reliable for most people between 19 and 70 years of age except women who are pregnant or breast feeding, competitive athletes, body builders, and chronically ill patients. Generally, the higher your BMI, the higher your health risk, and the risk increases even further if your waist size is greater than 40 inches for men or 35 inches for women. There are other ways, besides BMI, to determine your body fat composition, and your doctor can tell you about them, but the method recommended here will help you decide if you are at risk. Use the chart in the "Practical Dietary Therapy Information" chapter of this sourcebook to determine your BMI. Then, measure your waist size. Now, with your BMI and waist size determined, use the table below to determine your health risk relative to normal weight.

Body Mass Index

Body mass index, or BMI, is a new term to most people. However, it is the measurement of choice for many physicians and researchers studying obesity. BMI uses a mathematical formula that takes into account both a person's height and weight. BMI equals a person's weight in kilograms divided by height in meters squared (BMI = kg/m^2).

Several other factors, including your medical history, can increase your health risk. See your doctor for advice about your overall health risk and the weight loss options that are best for you. Together, decide whether you should go on a moderate diet (1200 calories daily for women, 1400 calories daily for men), or whether other options might be appropriate.

Once you and your doctor have determined the type of diet that makes the most sense for you, you may want to choose a product or a plan to help you reach your goal. Consider:

- If your doctor prescribes a medication, ask about complications or side effects, and tell the doctor what other medications you take, including over-the-counter drug products and dietary supplements, and other conditions you're being treated for. After you start taking the medication, tell the doctor about changes you experience, if any.

Table 21.1. Risk of Associated Disease According to BMI and Waist Size

BMI		Waist less than or equal to 40 in. (men) or 35 in. (women)	Waist greater than 40 in. (men) or 35 in. (women)
18.5 or less	Underweight	—	N/A
18.5–24.9	Normal	—	N/A
25.0–29.9	Overweight	Increased	High
30.0–34.9	Obese	High	Very High
35.0–39.9	Obese	Very High	Very High
40 or greater	Extremely Obese	Extremely High	Extremely High

Setting Goals for Weight Loss

- If your treatment includes periodic monitoring, counseling, or other activities that require your attendance, make sure the location is easy to get to and the appointment times are convenient.

- Some methods for losing weight have more risks and complications than others. Ask for details about the side effects, complications, or risks of any product or service that promotes weight loss and how to deal with problems should they occur.

- Where appropriate to the program, ask about the credentials and training of the program staff.

- Ask for an itemized price list for all the costs of the plan you're considering, including membership fees, fees for weekly visits, the costs of any diagnostic tests, costs for meal replacements, foods, nutritional supplements, or other products that are part of the weight loss program or plan.

Where to Get More Help

The Partnership for Healthy Weight Management is a coalition of representatives from science, academia, the health-care professions, government, commercial enterprises, and organizations whose mission is to promote sound guidance on strategies for achieving and maintaining a healthy weight.

Partners with information that can help you with issues about overweight and obesity or design your own healthy weight management plan are listed below. [See the "Additional Help and Information" section of this Sourcebook for contact information for these organizations:]

- American Dietetic Association

- American Obesity Association

- The Council on Size and Weight Discrimination

- Department of Nutrition Sciences, University of Alabama at Birmingham

- National Institute of Diabetes and Digestive and Kidney Diseases

- North American Association for the Study of Obesity

For access to helpful information from our commercial partners, write:

Federal Trade Commission
Consumer and Business Education Office
600 Pennsylvania Avenue, NW
Washington, DC 20580

Chapter 22

Weight Loss for Life

How We Lose Weight

Your body weight is controlled by the number of calories you eat and the number of calories you use each day. So, to lose weight you need to take in fewer calories than you use. You can do this by becoming more physically active or by eating less. Following a weight-loss program that helps you to become more physically active and decrease the amount of calories that you eat is most likely to lead to successful weight loss. The weight-loss program should also help you keep the weight off by making changes in your physical activity and eating habits that you will be able to follow for the rest of your life.

Types of Weight-Loss Programs

To lose weight and keep it off, you should be aware of the different types of programs available and the important parts of a good program. Knowing this information should help you select or design a weight-loss program that will work for you. The three types of weight-loss programs include: do-it-yourself programs, non-clinical programs, and clinical programs.

Excerpted from "Weight Loss for Life," Weight-Control Information Network (WIN), National Institute of Diabetes and Digestive and Kidney Diseases (NIDDK), National Institutes of Health (NIH), NIH Pub. No. 98-3700, http://www.niddk.nih.gov/health/nutrit/pubs/wtloss/wtloss.htm, January 1998, e-text posted April 9, 1998.

Do-It-Yourself Programs

Any effort to lose weight by yourself or with a group of like-minded others through support groups or worksite or community-based programs fits in the "do-it-yourself" category. Individuals using a do-it-yourself program rely on their own judgment, group support, and products such as diet books for advice (Note: Not all diet books are reliable sources of weight-loss information).

Non-Clinical Programs

These programs may or may not be commercially operated, such as through a privately-owned, weight-loss chain. They often use books and pamphlets that are prepared by health-care providers. These programs use counselors (who usually are not health-care providers and may or may not have training) to provide services to you. Some programs require participants to use the program's food or supplements.

Clinical Programs

This type of program may or may not be commercially owned. Services are provided in a health-care setting, such as a hospital, by licensed health professionals, such as physicians, nurses, dietitians, and/or psychologists. In some clinical programs, a health professional works alone; in others, a group of health professionals works together to provide services to patients. Clinical programs may offer you services such as nutrition education, medical care, behavior change therapy, and physical activity.

Clinical programs may also use other weight-loss methods, such as very low-calorie diets, prescription weight-loss drugs, and surgery, to treat severely overweight patients. These treatments are described below:

- Very low-calorie diets (VLCDs) are commercially prepared formulas that provide no more than 800 calories per day and replace all usual food intake. VLCDs help individuals lose weight more quickly than is usually possible with low-calorie diets. Because VLCDs can cause side effects, obesity experts recommend that only people who are severely overweight use these diets, and only with proper medical care. A fact sheet on VLCDs is available from the Weight-Control Information Network (WIN).

Weight Loss for Life

- Prescribed weight-loss drugs should be used only if you are likely to have health problems caused by your weight. You should not use drugs to improve your appearance. Prescribed weight-loss drugs, when combined with a healthy diet and regular physical activity, may help some obese adults lose weight. However, before these medications can be widely recommended, more research is needed to determine their long-term safety and effectiveness. Whatever the results, prescription weight-loss drugs should be used only as part of an overall program that includes long-term changes in your eating and physical activity habits. A fact sheet on prescription medications for the treatment of obesity is available from the Weight-Control Information Network (WIN) [contact information for WIN is available in the "Resources" chapter of this sourcebook].

- You may consider gastric surgery to promote weight loss if you are more than 80 pounds overweight. The surgery, sometimes called bariatric surgery, causes weight loss in one of two ways: 1) by limiting the amount of food your stomach can hold by closing off or removing parts of the stomach or 2) by causing food to be poorly digested by bypassing the stomach or part of the intestines. After surgery, patients usually lose weight quickly. While some weight is often regained, many patients are successful in keeping off most of their weight. In some cases, the surgery can lead to problems that require follow-up operations. Surgery may also reduce the amount of vitamins and minerals in your body and cause gallstones. For additional information, a fact sheet on gastric surgery is available from WIN.

If you are considering a weight-loss program and you have medical problems, or if you are severely overweight, programs run by trained health professionals may be best for you. These professionals are more likely to monitor you for possible side effects of weight loss and to talk to your doctor when necessary.

Whether you decide to use the do-it-yourself, non-clinical, or clinical approach, the program should help you lose weight and keep it off by teaching you healthy eating and physical activity habits that you will be able to follow for the rest of your life.

Diet

The word "diet" probably brings to mind meals of lettuce and cottage cheese. By definition, "diet" refers to what a person eats or drinks during the course of a day. A diet that limits portions to a very small size or that excludes certain foods entirely to promote weight loss may not be effective over the long term. Rather, you are likely to miss certain foods and find it difficult to follow this type of diet for a long time. Instead, it is often helpful to gradually change the types and amounts of food you eat and maintain these changes for the rest of your life. The ideal diet is one that takes into account your likes and dislikes and includes a wide variety of foods with enough calories and nutrients for good health.

How much you eat and what you eat play a major role in how much you weigh. So, when planning your diet, you should consider: What calorie level is appropriate? Is the diet you are considering nutritionally balanced? Will the diet be practical and easy to follow? Will you be able to maintain this eating plan for the rest of your life? The following information will help you answer these questions.

Calorie Level

Low-calorie diets. Most weight-loss diets provide 1,000 to 1,500 calories per day. However, the number of calories that is right for you depends on your weight and activity level. At these calorie levels, diets are referred to as low-calorie diets. Self-help diet books and clinical and non-clinical weight-loss programs often include low-calorie diet plans.

The calorie level of your diet should allow for a weight loss of no more than 1 pound per week (after the first week or two when weight loss may be more rapid because of initial water loss). If you can estimate how many calories you eat in a day, you can design a diet plan that will help you lose no more than 1 pound per week. You may need to work with a trained health professional, such as a registered dietitian. Or, you can use a standardized low-calorie diet plan with a fixed calorie level.

The selected calorie level, however, may not produce the recommended rate of weight loss, and you may need to eat more or less.

Good Nutrition

Make sure that your diet contains all the essential nutrients for good health. Using the Nutrition Facts Label that is found on most processed food products and the Food Guide Pyramid can help you choose a healthful diet. The Pyramid shows you the kinds and amounts of food that you need each day for good health. The Nutrition Facts

Label will help you select foods that meet your daily nutritional needs. A healthful diet should include:

Adequate vitamins and minerals. Eating a wide variety of foods from all the food groups on the Food Guide Pyramid will help you get the vitamins and minerals you need. If you eat less than 1,200 calories per day, you may benefit from taking a daily vitamin and mineral supplement.

Adequate protein. The average woman 25 years of age and older should get 50 grams of protein each day, and the average man 25 years of age and older should get 63 grams of protein each day. Adequate

Fats, Oils, & Sweets
USE SPARINGLY

KEY
☐ Fat (naturally occurring and added) ■ Sugars (added)
These symbols show that fat and added sugars come mostly from fats, oils, and sweets, but can be part of or added to foods from the other food groups as well.

Milk, Yogurt, & Cheese Group
2-3 SERVINGS

Meat, Poultry, Fish, Dry Beans, Eggs, & Nuts Group
2-3 SERVINGS

Vegetable Group
3-5 SERVINGS

Fruit Group
2-4 SERVINGS

Bread, Cereal, Rice, & Pasta Group
6-11 SERVINGS

Source: U.S. Department of Agriculture/U.S. Department of Health and Human Services

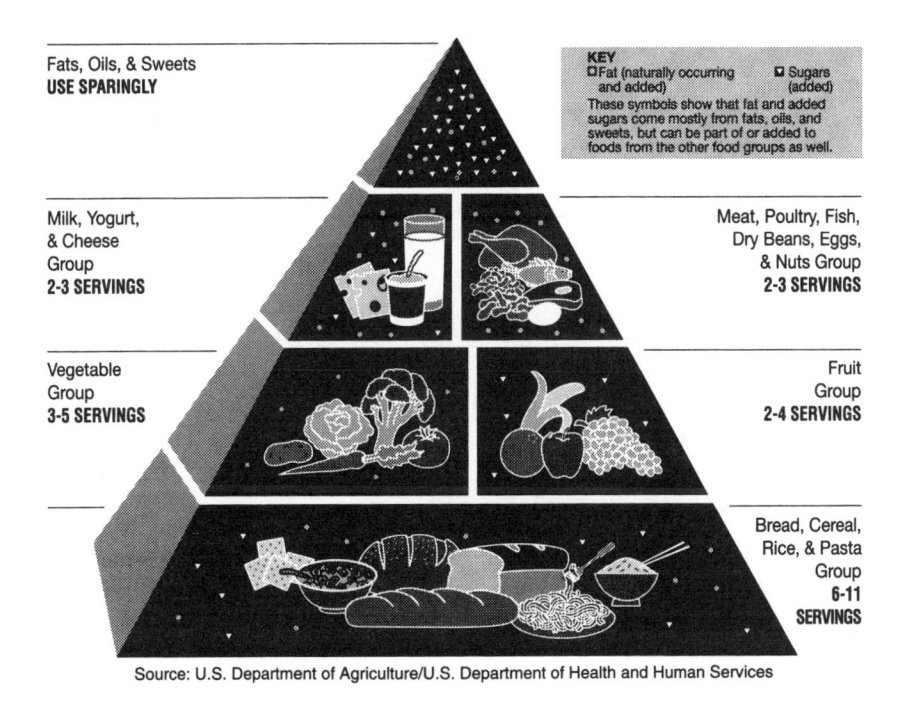

Figure 22.1. The Food Guide Pyramid. A range of servings is given for each food group. The smaller number is for people who consume about 1,600 calories a day, such as sedentary women. The larger number is for those who consume about 2,800 calories a day, such as active men. Source: U.S. Department of Agriculture/U.S. Department of Health and Human Services.

protein is important because it prevents muscle tissue from breaking down and repairs all body tissues such as skin and teeth. To get adequate protein in your diet, make sure you eat 2–3 servings (see the "serving guide" below) from the Meat, Poultry, Fish, Dry Beans, Eggs, and Nuts Group on the Food Guide Pyramid every day. These foods are all good sources of protein.

Table 22.1. Examples of the equivalent of one serving from the major food groups.

Grain Products Group (bread, cereal, rise, and pasta)

- 1 slice of bread
- 1 ounce of ready-to-eat cereal
- 1/2 cup of cooked cereal, rice, or pasta

Vegetable Group

- 1 cup of raw leafy vegetables
- 1/2 cup of other vegetables—cooked or chopped raw
- 3/4 cup of vegetable juice

Fruit Group

- 1 medium apple, banana, orange
- 1/2 cup of chopped, cooked, or canned fruit
- 3/4 cup of fruit juice

Milk Group (milk, yogurt, and cheese)

- 1 cup of milk or yogurt
- 1½ ounces of natural cheese
- 2 ounces of processed cheese

Meat and Beans Group (meat, poultry, fish, dry beans, eggs, and nuts)

- 2–3 ounces of cooked lean meat, poultry, or fish
- 1/2 cup of cooked dry beans or 1 egg counts as 1 ounce of lean meat. Two tablespoons of peanut butter or 1/3 cup of nuts count as 1 ounce of meat.

Adequate carbohydrates. At least 100 grams of carbohydrates per day are needed to prevent fatigue and dangerous fluid imbalances. To make sure you get enough carbohydrates, eat 6–11 servings (see the "serving guide") from the Bread, Cereal, Rice, and Pasta Group on the Food Guide Pyramid every day.

A daily fiber intake of 20 to 30 grams. Adequate fiber helps with proper bowel function. If you were to eat 1 cup of bran cereal, 1/2 cup of carrots, 1/2 cup of kidney beans, a medium-sized pear, and a medium-sized apple together in 1 day, you would get about 30 grams of fiber.

No more than 30 percent of calories, on average, from fat per day, with less than 10 percent of calories from saturated fat (such as fat from meat, butter, and eggs). Limiting fat to these levels reduces your risk for heart disease and may help you lose weight. In addition, you should limit the amount of cholesterol in your diet. Cholesterol is a fat-like substance found in animal products such as meat and eggs. Your diet should include no more than 300 milligrams of cholesterol per day (one egg contains about 215 milligrams of cholesterol, and 3.5 ounces of cooked hamburger contain 100 milligrams of cholesterol).

At least 8 to 10 glasses, 8 ounces each, of water or water-based beverages, per day. You need more water if you exercise a lot.

These nutrients should come from a variety of low-calorie, nutrient-rich foods. One way to get variety—and with it, an enjoyable and nutritious diet—is to choose foods each day from the Food Guide Pyramid.

Types of Diets

Fixed-menu diet. A fixed-menu diet provides a list of all the foods you will eat. This kind of diet can be easy to follow because the foods are selected for you. But, you get very few different food choices which may make the diet boring and hard to follow away from home. In addition, fixed-menu diets do not teach the food selection skills necessary for keeping weight off. If you start with a fixed-menu diet, you should switch eventually to a plan that helps you learn to make meal choices on your own, such as an exchange-type diet.

Exchange-type diet. An exchange-type diet is a meal plan with a set number of servings from each of several food groups. Within each group, foods are about equal in calories and can be interchanged as you wish. For example, the "starch" category could include one slice of bread or 1/2 cup of oatmeal; each is about equal in nutritional value and calories. If your meal plan calls for two starch choices at breakfast, you could choose to eat two slices of bread, or one slice of bread and 1/2 cup of oatmeal. With the exchange-type diet plans, you have more day-to-day variety and you can easily follow the diet away from home. The most important advantage is that exchange-type diet plans teach the food selection skills you need to keep your weight off.

Prepackaged-meal diet. These diets require you to buy prepackaged meals. Such meals may help you learn appropriate portion sizes. However, they can be costly. Before beginning this type of program, find out whether you will need to buy the meals and how much the meals cost. You should also find out whether the program will teach you how to select and prepare food, skills that are needed to sustain weight loss.

Formula diet. Formula diets are weight-loss plans that replace one or more meals with a liquid formula. Most formula diets are balanced diets containing a mix of protein, carbohydrate, and usually a small amount of fat. Formula diets are usually sold as liquid or a powder to be mixed with liquid. Although formula diets are easy to use and do promote short-term weight loss, most people regain the weight as soon as they stop using the formula. In addition, formula diets do not teach you how to make healthy food choices, a necessary skill for keeping your weight off.

Questionable diets. You should avoid any diet that suggests you eat a certain nutrient, food, or combination of foods to promote easy weight loss. Some of these diets may work in the short term because they are low in calories. However, they are often not well balanced and may cause nutrient deficiencies. In addition, they do not teach eating habits that are important for long-term weight management.

Flexible diets. Some programs or books suggest monitoring fat only, calories only, or a combination of the two, with the individual making the choice of both the type and amount of food eaten. This flexible type of approach works well for many people, and teaches them how to control what they eat. One drawback of flexible diets is that some don't consider the total diet. For example, programs that monitor fat only often allow people to take in unlimited amounts of excess calories from sugars, and therefore don't lead to weight loss.

Weight Loss for Life

It is important to choose an eating plan that you can live with. The plan should also teach you how to select and prepare healthy foods, as well as how to maintain your new weight. Remember that many people tend to regain lost weight. Eating a healthful and nutritious diet to maintain your new weight, combined with regular physical activity, helps to prevent weight regain.

Physical Activity

Regular physical activity is important to help you lose weight and build an overall healthy lifestyle. Physical activity increases the number of calories your body uses and promotes the loss of body fat instead of muscle and other nonfat tissue. Research shows that people who include physical activity in their weight-loss programs are more likely to keep their weight off than people who only change their diet. In addition to promoting weight control, physical activity improves your strength and flexibility, lowers your risk of heart disease, helps control blood pressure and diabetes, can promote a sense of well-being, and can decrease stress.

Any type of physical activity you choose to do—vigorous activities such as running or aerobic dancing or moderate-intensity activities such as walking or household work—will increase the number of calories your body uses. The key to successful weight control and improved overall health is making physical activity a part of your daily life.

For the greatest overall health benefits, experts recommend that you do 20 to 30 minutes of vigorous physical activity (see the following list of activities) three or more times a week and some type of muscle strengthening activity, such as weight resistance, and stretching at least twice a week. However, if you are unable to do this level of activity, you can improve your health by performing 30 minutes or more of moderate-intensity physical activity (see the list of activities below) over the course of a day, at least five times a week. When including physical activity in your weight-loss program, you should choose a variety of activities that can be done regularly and are enjoyable for you. Also, if you have not been physically active, you should see your doctor before you start, especially if you are older than 40 years of age, very overweight, or have medical problems. A fact sheet on physical activity and weight control is available from WIN.

Vigorous Activities

- aerobic dancing
- running

- brisk walking
- cycling
- swimming

Moderate-Intensity Activities

- walking up the stairs instead of taking the elevator
- walking part or all of the way to work
- using a push mower to cut the grass
- playing actively with children

Behavior Change

Behavior change focuses on learning eating and physical activity behaviors that will help you lose weight and keep it off. The first step is to look at your eating and physical activity habits, thus uncovering behaviors (such as television watching) that lead you to overeat or be inactive. Next you'll need to learn how to change those behaviors.

Getting support from others is a good way to help you maintain your new eating and physical activity habits. Changing your eating and physical activity behaviors increases your chances of losing weight and keeping it off. For additional information on behavior change, you may wish to ask a weight-loss counselor or refer to books on this topic, which are available in local libraries.

What Works for You?

A variety of options exist to help you lose weight and keep it off. The key to successful weight loss is making changes in your eating and physical activity habits that you will be able to maintain for the rest of your life. [See the "Additional Help and Information" section of this sourcebook for additional reading and resources on weight loss.]

Chapter 23

Choosing a Safe and Successful Weight-Loss Program

Introduction

Almost any of the commercial weight-loss programs can work, but only if they motivate you sufficiently to decrease the amount of calories you eat or increase the amount of calories you burn each day (or both). What elements of a weight-loss program should an intelligent consumer look for in judging its potential for safe and successful weight loss?

A Responsible and Safe Weight-Loss Program

A responsible and safe weight-loss program should be able to document for you the five following features:

The diet should be safe. It should include all of the Recommended Daily Allowances (RDAs) for vitamins, minerals, and protein. The weight-loss diet should be low in calories (energy) only, not in essential foodstuffs.

The weight-loss program should be directed towards a slow, steady weight loss unless your doctor feels your health condition would benefit from more rapid weight loss. Expect to lose only about a pound a week after the first week or two. With many calorie-restricted diets

---

Weight-Control Information Network (WIN), National Institute of Diabetes and Digestive and Kidney Diseases (NIDDK), National Institutes of Health (NIH), NIH Pub. No. 94-3700, http://www.niddk.nih.gov/health/nutrit/pubs/choose.htm, December 1993, e-text posted February 19, 1998.

there is an initial rapid weight loss during the first 1 to 2 weeks, but this loss is largely fluid. The initial rapid loss of fluid also is regained rapidly when you return to a normal-calorie diet. Thus, a reasonable goal of weight loss must be expected.

If you plan to lose more than 15 to 20 pounds, have any health problems, or take medication on a regular basis, you should be evaluated by your doctor before beginning your weight-loss program. A doctor can assess your general health and medical conditions that might be affected by dieting and weight loss. Also, a physician should be able to advise you on the need for weight loss, the appropriateness of the weight-loss program, and a sensible goal of weight loss for you. If you plan to use a very-low-calorie diet (a special liquid formula diet that replaces all food intake for 1 to 4 months), you definitely should be examined and monitored by a doctor.

Your program should include plans for weight maintenance after the weight loss phase is over. It is of little benefit to lose a large amount of weight only to regain it. Weight maintenance is the most difficult part of controlling weight and is not consistently implemented in weight-loss programs. The program you select should include help in permanently changing your dietary habits and level of physical activity, to alter a lifestyle that may have contributed to weight gain in the past. Your program should provide behavior modification help, including education in healthy eating habits and long-term plans to deal with weight problems. One of the most important factors in maintaining weight loss appears to be increasing daily physical activity, often by sensible increases in daily activity, as well as incorporating an individually tailored exercise program.

A commercial weight-loss program should provide a detailed statement of fees and costs of additional items such as dietary supplements.

Weight Control Must Be Considered a Life-Long Effort

Obesity is a chronic condition. Too often it is viewed as a temporary problem that can be treated for a few months with a strenuous diet. However, as most overweight people know, weight control must be considered a life-long effort. To be safe and effective, any weight-loss program must address the long-term approach or else the program is largely a waste of money and effort.

Obesity affects about one in four adult Americans, and during any one year, over half of Americans go on a weight-loss diet or are trying to maintain their weight. For many people who try to lose weight, it is difficult to lose more than a few pounds, and few succeed in

Choosing a Safe and Successful Weight-Loss Program

remaining at the reduced weight. The difficulty in losing weight and keeping it off leads many people to turn to a professional or commercial weight-loss program for help. These programs are quite popular and are widely advertised in newspapers and on television. What is the evidence that any of these programs is worthwhile, that they will help you lose weight and keep it off and that they will do it safely?

This statement was developed with the advice of the National Task Force on Prevention and Treatment of Obesity, a subcommittee of the National Digestive Diseases Advisory Board.

Chapter 24

The Facts about Weight Loss Products and Programs

The Weight-Loss Industry

Looking for a quick and easy way to lose weight? You're not alone. An estimated 50 million Americans will go on diets this year. And while some will succeed in taking the weight off, very few—perhaps 5 percent—will manage to keep all of it off in the long run.

One reason for the low success rate is that many people look for quick and easy solutions to their weight problems. They find it hard to believe in this age of scientific innovations and medical miracles that an effortless weight-loss method doesn't exist.

So they succumb to quick-fix claims like "Eat All You Want and Still Lose Weight!" or "Melt Fat Away While You Sleep!" And they invest their hopes (and their money) in all manner of pills, potions, gadgets, and programs that hold the promise of a slimmer, happier future.

The weight-loss business is a booming industry. Americans spend an estimated $30 billion a year on all types of diet programs and products, including diet foods and drinks. Trying to sort out all of the competing claims-often misleading, unproven, or just plain false-can be confusing and costly.

This chapter is designed to give you the facts behind the claims, to help you avoid the outright scams, and to encourage you to consider

---

Food and Drug Administration (FDA), Federal Trade Commission (FTC), National Association of Attorneys General (NAAG), DHHS Pub. No. (FDA) 92-1189, http://www.cfsan.fda.gov/~dms/wgtloss.html, 1992, e-text updated January 6, 1997.

thoroughly the costs and consequences of the dieting decisions you make.

The Facts about Weight Loss

Being obese can have serious health consequences. These include an increased risk of heart disease, stroke, high blood pressure, diabetes, gallstones, and some forms of cancer. Losing weight can help reduce these risks. Here are some general points to keep in mind:

- Any claims that you can lose weight effortlessly are false. The only proven way to lose weight is either to reduce the number of calories you eat or to increase the number of calories you burn off through exercise. Most experts recommend a combination of both.

- Very low-calorie diets are not without risk and should be pursued only under medical supervision. Unsupervised very low-calorie diets can deprive you of important nutrients and are potentially dangerous.

- Fad diets rarely have any permanent effect. Sudden and radical changes in your eating patterns are difficult to sustain over time. In addition, so-called "crash" diets often send dieters into a cycle of quick weight loss, followed by a "rebound" weight gain once normal eating resumes, and even more difficulty reducing when the next diet is attempted.

- To lose weight safely and keep it off requires long-term changes in daily eating and exercise habits. Many experts recommend a goal of losing about a pound a week. A modest reduction of 500 calories per day will achieve this goal, since a total reduction of 3,500 calories is required to lose a pound of fat. An important way to lower your calorie intake is to learn and practice healthy eating habits.

In Search of the "Magic Bullet"

Some dieters peg their hopes on pills and capsules that promise to "burn," "block," "flush," or otherwise eliminate fat from the system. But science has yet to come up with a low-risk "magic bullet" for weight loss. Some pills may help control the appetite, but they can have serious side effects. Amphetamines, for instance, are highly addictive and can have an adverse impact on the heart and central nervous system. Other pills are utterly worthless.

The Facts about Weight Loss Products and Programs

The Federal Trade Commission (FTC) and a number of state Attorneys General have successfully brought cases against marketers of pills claiming to absorb or burn fat. The Food and Drug Administration (FDA) has banned 111 ingredients once found in over-the-counter diet products. None of these substances, which include alcohol, caffeine, dextrose, and guar gum, have proved effective in weight-loss or appetite suppression.

Beware of the following products that are touted as weight-loss wonders:

- Diet patches, which are worn on the skin, have not been proven to be safe or effective. The FDA has seized millions of these products from manufacturers and promoters.

- "Fat blockers" purport to physically absorb fat and mechanically interfere with the fat a person eats.

- "Starch blockers" promise to block or impede starch digestion. Not only is the claim unproven, but users have complained of nausea, vomiting, diarrhea, and stomach pains.

- "Magnet" diet pills allegedly "flush fat out of the body." The FTC has brought legal action against several marketers of these pills.

- Glucomannan is advertised as the "Weight Loss Secret That's Been in the Orient for Over 500 Years." There is little evidence supporting this plant root's effectiveness as a weight-loss product.

- Some bulk producers or fillers, such as fiber-based products, may absorb liquid and swell in the stomach, thereby reducing hunger. Some fillers, such as guar gum, can even prove harmful, causing obstructions in the intestines, stomach, or esophagus. The FDA has taken legal action against several promoters containing guar gum.

- Spirulina, a species of blue-green algae, has not been proven effective for losing weight.

Phony Devices and Gadgets

Phony weight-loss devices range from those that are simply ineffective to those that are truly dangerous to your health. At minimum, they are a waste of your hard-earned money. Some of the fraudulent gadgets that have been marketed to hopeful dieters over the years include:

- Electrical muscle stimulators have legitimate use in physical therapy treatment. But the FDA has taken a number of them off the market because they were promoted for weight loss and body toning. When used incorrectly, muscle stimulators can be dangerous, causing electrical shocks and burns.
- "Appetite suppressing eyeglasses" are common eyeglasses with colored lenses that claim to project an image to the retina which dampens the desire to eat. There is no evidence these work.
- "Magic weight-loss earrings" and devices custom-fitted to the purchaser's ear that purport to stimulate acupuncture points controlling hunger have not been proven effective.

Diet Programs

Approximately 8 million Americans a year enroll in some kind of structured weight-loss program involving liquid diets, special diet regimens, or medical or other supervision. In 1991, about 8,500 commercial diet centers were in operation across the country, many of them owned by a half-dozen or so well-known national companies.

Before you join such a program, you should know that according to published studies, relatively few participants succeed in keeping off weight long-term. Recently, the FTC brought action against several companies challenging weight-loss and weight-maintenance claims. Unfortunately, some other companies continue to make overblown claims.

The FTC stopped one company from claiming its diet program caused rapid weight loss through the use of tablets that would "burn fat" and a protein drink mix that would adjust metabolism. The FTC also took action against three major programs using doctor-supervised, very low-calorie liquid diets, and they agreed to stop making claims unless they could back them up with hard data.

Before you sign up with a diet program, you might ask these questions:

- What are the health risks?
- What data can you show me that proves your program actually works?
- Do customers keep off the weight after they leave the diet program?

The Facts about Weight Loss Products and Programs

- What are the costs for membership, weekly fees, food, supplements, maintenance, and counseling? What's the payment schedule? Are any costs covered under health insurance? Do you give refunds if I drop out?

- Do you have a maintenance program? Is it part of the package or does it cost extra?

- What kind of professional supervision is provided? What are the credentials of these professionals?

- What are the program's requirements? Are there special menus or foods, counseling visits, or exercise plans?

Clues to Fraud

It is important for consumers to be wary of claims that sound too good to be true. When it comes to weight-loss schemes, consumers should be particularly skeptical of claims containing words and phrases like:

- easy
- effortless
- guaranteed
- miraculous
- magical
- breakthrough
- new discovery
- mysterious
- exotic
- secret
- exclusive
- ancient

Sensible Weight Maintenance Tips

Losing weight may not be effortless, but it doesn't have to be complicated. To achieve long-term results, it's best to avoid quick-fix schemes and complex regimens. Focus instead on making modest changes to your life's daily routine. A balanced, healthy diet, and sensible, regular exercise are the keys to maintaining your ideal weight. Although nutrition science is constantly evolving, here are some generally-accepted guidelines for losing weight:

- Consult with your doctor, a dietician, or other qualified health professional to determine your ideal healthy body weight.

- Eat smaller portions and choose from a variety of foods.

- Load up on foods naturally high in fiber: fruits, vegetables, legumes, and whole grains.

- Limit portions of foods high in fat: dairy products like cheese, butter, and whole milk; red meat; cakes and pastries.
- Exercise at least three times a week.

For Help and Information

The Federal Trade Commission has jurisdiction over advertising and marketing of foods, non-prescription drugs, medical devices, and health-care services. The FTC can seek federal court injunctions to halt fraudulent claims and obtain redress for injured consumers.

The Food and Drug Administration has jurisdiction over the content and labeling of foods, drugs, and medical devices. The FDA can take law enforcement action to seize and prohibit the sale of products that are falsely labeled.

Most state Attorneys General have authority under state consumer protection statutes to investigate and prosecute unfair or deceptive acts and practices. Many have the power to seek consumer restitution, civil fines, and revocation of a company's authority to do business.

To get more information or to file complaints about weight-loss products or programs, write any of the following organizations [specific contact information is located in the "Resources" chapter of this Sourcebook]:

- Federal Trade Commission
- Food and Drug Administration
- Your State Attorney General, Office of Consumer Protection, Your State Capital

Chapter 25

Weight-Loss Aids and Dietary Changes

Introduction

Obesity is a heterogeneous disorder, the result of genetic and environmental factors, according to Artemis P. Simopoulos, M.D., president of the Center for Genetics, Nutrition and Health, Washington, D.C., in the September-October 1995 issue of *Nutrition Today*.

She maintains that studies using twins indicate that obesity is familial with strong genetic components, although specific genes, genetic markers or genetically-determined mechanisms have not yet been identified. In studies of twins by Stunkard, et al., genetic influences accounted for 70 percent of the differences in body mass index (BMI) later in life, while childhood environment had little, or no, influence.

Home Environment Affects Weight

This does not mean, she adds, that what goes on in the home environment makes no difference. However, the study measured the genetic influence in a range of particular environmental conditions.

"One of the most revealing experiences about the effects of the genes on human body fat variation occurs when humans are exposed to either a standardized chronic overfeeding treatment or a negative balance regimen," Simopoulos says.

"Weight-Loss Aids, with Dietary Changes, Help Us Reach Our Goal," *Better Nutrition*, February 1996, Vol. 58, N. 2, pp. 36–40. Copyright 1996 Argus Press.

As an example, she adds, in the overfeeding study with twins by Bouchard, et al., the variation within pairs was one third of the variation between pairs. In one result, those who gained weight had a rise in diastolic (resting) blood pressure from 66 to 70 mmHg.

Central Abdominal Obesity Is Related to Many Other Health Problems

She adds that there is conclusive evidence that obesity located in the central abdominal part of the body is statistically associated with a number of metabolic derangements, such as insulin resistance, high cholesterol levels, high blood pressure, non-insulin-dependent diabetes mellitus, etc.

"Obesity—particularly central obesity—high blood pressure, diabetes Type II and coronary artery disease cluster in some families," Simopoulos continues. "These clusters could be mediated through insulin action as has been hypothesized by Ferrannini." The key dietary component (contributing to obesity) could be a decrease in the intake of longer-chain polyunsaturated fatty acids (PUFAs), or too much trans fatty acid intake (found in some margarines), or an increase in dietary linoleic acid, as was hypothesized by Simopoulos (in a chart in the *Nutrition Today* article).

She notes that a number of anthropologic, nutritional and genetic studies indicate that humans' overall diet, including energy intake and energy expenditure, has changed over the past 10,000 years, with significant change occurring during the past 150 years in the type and amount of fat.

"Eaton and Konner have estimated higher intakes for protein, calcium, potassium and vitamin C, and lower sodium intakes for the diet of the late paleolithic period than the current U.S. and Western diet," Simopoulos adds.

Three Overall Dietary Changes Contribute to Obesity

Today, she says, industrialized societies are characterized by:

- an increase in energy intake (calories) combined with a decrease in energy expenditure
- an increase in the consumption of saturated fat, omega-6 fatty acids (vegetable oils) and trans fatty acids, and a decrease in omega-3 fatty acid intake (salmon, sardines, flax seed oil, etc.)
- a decrease in the consumption of complex carbohydrates and fiber

Weight-Loss Aids and Dietary Changes

"It has been estimated that the present Western diet is deficient in omega-3 fatty acids, with a ratio of omega-6 to omega-3 of 10 to 14:1, instead of 1:1 as is the case with wild animals and presumably humans," Simopoulos says.

She went on to say that humans evolved on a diet where there was a balance between the omega-6 and omega-3 fatty acids, which is a more physiological state in terms of the production of prostaglandins, leukotrienes, and interleukin-1 (IL-1), immune factors that, when over-produced, can lead to inflammation and even cell damage.

"The current recommendation to substitute vegetable oils (omega-6) for unsaturated fats leads to unnatural increases in IL-1, prostaglandins and leukotrienes; is not consistent with human evolution; and may lead to maladaptation in those genetically predisposed," Simopoulos adds.

She says that, genetically speaking, today we live in a nutritional environment that differs from that for which our genetic constitution was selected. Therefore, increased dietary intake in the presence of sedentary lifestyles leads to overweight and obesity, which is the most prominent and serious health problem of industrialized societies.

Obesity is also the cause of other serious health problems, such as heart disease. The current approach to the treatment of coronary heart disease with positive dietary changes and drugs aiming to lower plasma cholesterol concentrations has led to decreases in mortality rate from coronary heart disease, but not to all-cause mortality in one study, she continues.

"The general recommendation to lower saturated fat and cholesterol ignore other important aspects of diet known to influence lipid levels, fibrinogen (a protein in the blood involved with clotting) levels, and blood vessel wall interactions that are affected by a balance of omega-6 and omega-3 essential fatty acids," Simopoulos says.

She adds that saturated fats are formed in the body from excessive calorie intake, and that obesity is due either to excessive calorie intake and/or decreased energy expenditure in a genetically-predisposed individual and is an independent risk factor for coronary heart disease.

"Universal dietary recommendations have been used by nutritionists who were concerned with undernutrition," she says, "but universal dietary recommendations are not appropriate when the problem is one of overnutrition. Individual dietary recommendations taking into consideration genetic predisposition and energy expenditure are in order."

In order to achieve permanent weight loss, one must make changes in choosing what foods to eat and when to eat them, according to

Michael T. Murray, N.D., in *Natural Alternatives to Over-the-Counter and Prescription Drugs*.

In addition, he says, some people find that meal-replacement formulas can be used effectively to achieve ideal body weight. The formulas are mixed with water, juice or milk to produce a drink that is then used to replace a meal.

While these formulas can provide short-term benefit, in the long run, a successful program must incorporate more healthful food choices, Murray says. Here are his recommendations for choosing a healthful formula:

- Look for a product that contains high-quality protein from grains and legumes, whey or hydrolyzed lactalbumin. Avoid casein-based formulas, since this milk protein is often difficult for some to digest, while some are allergic to it.

- The formula should contain at least 5 g of a combination of soluble (i.e., from oats, vegetables) and insoluble (i.e., from wheat bran) dietary fibers per serving.

- Look for balanced high-quality nutrition with enhanced levels of nutrients critical to weight loss, such as chromium.

- The formula should have a low total fat content, but it should supply some essential fatty acids (EFAs).

- It should not contain sweeteners, artificial flavors or other artificial food additives. Refined sugar leads to a loss of blood sugar control, diabetes and obesity.

Since chromium picolinate is a main ingredient in some weight-loss formulas, consumers were startled by recent news reports that "reasonable" amounts of chromium picolinate can produce chromosomal damage and cancer.

In a rebuttal in the November 2, 1995 issue of *The New York Times*, the Chromium Information Bureau, Inc., (www.chromiuminfo.org) said that chromosome breakage was produced, not in living animals, but in cells grown in a test tube, using abnormally high amounts of the mineral.

"The lowest concentration of chromium picolinate that could produce chromosome damage was 6,000 times higher than the serum level of chromium that results from supplementation," the Bureau reports.

Weight-Loss Aids and Dietary Changes

The Bureau added that Dr. Richard Anderson of the U.S. Department of Agriculture, and a leading chromium research scientist, recently completed a long-term study of chromium picolinate in rats. He found no toxicity at even the extreme dosage of 10,000 times the recommended dietary intake (50 to 200 mcg/day). These findings agree with those of all previous studies examining nutritional chromium. Added the Bureau: "Chromium is one of the safest of all nutrients."

Other forms of chromium supplements, including chromium chloride and niacin-bound chromium nicotinate (or polynicotinate)—which have been used in supplements for over 10 years—have not caused any chromosome damage at non-toxic doses, according to a study recently announced by Diane Stearns and Karen Wetterhan of Dartmouth College in New Hampshire and John Wise and Steven Patierno of the George Washington University Medical Center in Washington, D.C.

Another useful addition to some weight-reducing formulas is L-carnitine, the amino acid. However, synthetic-source derived DL-carnitine is generally not recommended.

Carnitine May Be Useful for Those on a Low-Calorie Diet

"It has been hypothesized that carnitine might be a useful supplement for those who are on low-calorie diets; carnitine, by enhancing the efficiency of fatty-acid oxidation (increasing the burn rate of calories stored as fat), may make low-calorie diets easier to tolerate by reducing feelings of hunger and weakness that result from less efficient oxidation of fats," reported Sheldon Saul Hendler, M.D., Ph.D., in *The Doctors' Vitamin and Mineral Encyclopedia*.

Hendler adds that the DL form of carnitine has been shown to cause a muscular-weakness syndrome in some patients. But, he says, the L-carnitine form has not produced negative side effects, even in some individuals taking 1.6 g/day for over a year.

In addition to deciding how to change your diet in order to achieve sensible weight loss, you may find the various weight-loss formulas in your health food store beneficial. You also need to undertake an exercise program specifically designed for you.

References

"Chromium Picolinate: The Science Supports Its Safety," ad by the Chromium Information Bureau, Inc., *The New York Times*, Nov. 2, 1995, p. B13.

Hendler, Sheldon Saul, M.D., Ph.D. *The Doctors' Vitamin and Mineral Encyclopedia.* New York: Simon and Schuster, 1990, pp. 350–351.

Murray, Michael T., N.D. *Natural Alternatives to Over-the-Counter and Prescription Drugs.* New York: William Morrow & Co., Inc., 1994, pp. 239–240.

Simopoulos, Artemis P., M.D. "Genetic Variation and Nutrition. Part 2: Genetic Variation, Nutrition and Chronic Diseases," *Nutrition Today* 30(5):194–206, Sept.-Oct. 1995.

Chapter 26

Food Labels Make Good Eating Easier

Tortilla chips. Chocolate pudding. Frozen yogurt. Allison Gilliam, 16, of Gaithersburg, Md., points out some of her favorite foods at her neighborhood grocery store.

Sliced turkey. Dried fruit. The list of items goes on. They're all delicious, and you might never guess that they're also all low in or without fat. Even the chocolate pudding!

It says so right on the food label, and Gilliam, a high-school junior, spots the information right away. A front-label fat claim draws her to the product, and she finds the Nutrition Facts panel on the side or back of the package with more complete information.

Gilliam uses the food label to help her control her fat intake. "I used to be fat," she says. "I lost 45 pounds."

She knows dietary fat is the most concentrated source of calories (9 calories per gram versus 4 calories per gram for carbohydrate and protein), so she checks the label to see how much fat a food contains. If the fat content is over 5 grams per serving, she considers buying something else instead.

Like Gilliam, you can make the food label work for you—whether your concern is losing weight, gaining weight, eating enough protein, eating less fat, or simply staying in the good shape you're in.

Paula Kurtzweil, "On the Teen Scene: Food Label Makes Good Eating Easier," *FDA Consumer*, September 1995, revised December 1997, FDA Pub. No. 98-8894, http://www.fda.gov/fdac/features/795_teenfood.html.

New Label

The food label was revamped in 1994, thanks to regulations from the Food and Drug Administration (FDA) and the U.S. Department of Agriculture. As a result, you get:

- easy-to-read nutrition information required on almost every packaged food
- % Daily Values, which show how a serving of food fits into a total day's diet
- serving sizes that are closer to the amounts most people actually eat than previous labeling
- nutrition claims that mean the same on every product
- voluntary information for the most commonly eaten fresh fruits and veges, and raw fish and cuts of meat. This information may appear on posters or in brochures in the same area as the food.

Get the Facts

The main draw is the "Nutrition Facts" panel, which gives information about nutrients people are most concerned about today. For example, the panel gives the lowdown on fat, saturated fat, and cholesterol because of their link to heart disease.

You may find particularly useful information about nutrients that teenagers especially need. For instance, girls, who often eat fewer calories than boys, sometimes don't get enough calcium and iron, so they can use the label to help them choose foods that give a good supply of those nutrients. Girls also have special needs for these nutrients: consumption of milk and other products containing calcium in teen years may help prevent osteoporosis later in life; extra iron is sometimes needed to replace what's lost during menstruation.

Almost everyone wants to know about calorie content. For sports-minded teens, getting enough calories may be the concern, while those who tend to be overweight may want to reduce their calorie intake. The food label can help because it almost always will list the calories in a serving of food.

% *Daily Values*

The amount of nutrients in a food is given in one or two ways: in grams (or milligrams) or as a percentage of the Daily Value, a new label reference tool.

Food Labels Make Good Eating Easier

The % Daily Value shows how a serving of food fits in with current recommendations for a healthful daily diet. These reference numbers—called Daily Values—are based on the government's Dietary Guidelines; for example, one guideline recommends restricting fat intake to 30 percent or less of calorie intake.

The government has set 2,000 calories a day as the basis for calculating % Daily Values. Of course, not everyone eats this amount. Teen-age girls often average 2,200 calories a day, while some teenage boys may eat 2,500 or more calories a day.

Whatever your calorie intake, you still can use the % Daily Values on the label to get a general idea of how a serving of food fits into the total daily diet.

The goal is to eat about 100 percent of the Daily Value for each nutrient each day. For nutrients that may be related to health problems—such as fat, saturated fat, and sodium—100 percent should be the upper limit. For other nutrients that are often needed to maintain good health and which may be in short supply—such as fiber and calcium—the goal is to eat at least 100 percent.

A good rule of thumb: If the % Daily Value listed on the panel is 5 or less, the food contributes a small amount of that nutrient to the diet.

Nutrient Claims

Just as Gilliam does for low-fat products, you can easily spot foods offering the kind of nutritional benefits you want by looking for claims on the package.

The government has set strict definitions for 12 "core" terms:

- free
- reduced
- lean
- less
- light
- extra lean
- low
- fewer
- high
- more
- good source
- healthy

These terms can be used only if the food meets certain criteria, so when you see them, you can believe them.

Health Claims

Another type of claim, the health claim, also can alert you to nutritious foods. The Food and Drug Administration (FDA) has approved 10 claims. They show a link between:

- calcium and a lower risk of osteoporosis. The claim must state that regular exercise and a healthy diet with enough calcium helps teen and young adult white and Asian women maintain good bone health and may reduce their high risk of osteoporosis later in life.
- fat and a greater risk of cancer
- saturated fat and cholesterol and a greater risk of heart disease
- fiber-containing grain products, fruits and vegetables and a reduced risk of cancer
- fruits, vegetables and grain products that contain fiber and a reduced risk of heart disease
- sodium and a greater risk of high blood pressure
- fruits and vegetables and a reduced risk of cancer
- folic acid and a decreased risk of neural tube defects in fetuses. Neural tube malformations are serious birth defects that cause disability or death.
- dietary sugar alcohols and a reduced risk of cavities
- soluble fiber from whole oats, as part of a diet low in saturated fat and cholesterol, and a reduced risk of heart disease.

Look for the Info

The food label won't tell you what foods to eat—that's your decision—but it will help you find foods with the kinds of nutritional benefits you want.

Also, many fast-food places voluntarily offer nutrition information about their foods. The information is often available on request. Many of these restaurants now offer low-fat choices, including lettuce salads and low-fat entrees.

So, like teenage Gilliam, you, too, may soon find yourself eating a whole new way. In Gilliam's case, that's a low-fat diet that includes such foods as baked tortilla chips, fat-free pudding, nonfat frozen yogurt, and skim milk. After all, said Gilliam, "It's second nature to me now."

What Some Claims Mean

- high-protein: at least 10 grams (g) high-quality protein per serving

Food Labels Make Good Eating Easier

- good source of calcium: at least 100 milligrams (mg) calcium per serving
- more iron: at least 1.8 mg more iron per serving than reference food (label will say 10 percent more of the Daily Value for iron)
- fat-free: less than 0.5 g fat per serving
- low-fat: 3 g or less fat per serving (if the serving size is 30 g or less or 2 tablespoons or less, 3 g or less fat per 50 g of the food)
- reduced or fewer calories: at least 25 percent fewer calories per serving than the reference food
- sugar-free: less than 0.5 g sugar per serving
- light (two meanings):
  - one-third fewer calories or half the fat of the reference food (if 50 percent or more of the food's calories are from fat, the fat must be reduced by 50 percent)
  - a "low-calorie," "low-fat" food whose sodium content has been reduced by 50 percent of the reference food

For Teachers

A 50-page food label education program for 10th- through 12th-grade students is available for $5 a copy.

The New Food Label: There's Something in It for Everybody was developed by FDA and the International Food Information Council Foundation to help students learn how to use the food label to choose healthy foods. The brochure covers a range of food labeling topics—from product dating to Nutrition Facts.

It consists of five lesson plans with learner outcomes, learning strategies, handouts, charts and worksheets, and suggested activities.

To order, send check or money order payable to the International Food Information Council Foundation to IFIC Foundation, 1100 Connecticut Ave., N.W., Suite 430, Washington, DC 20036. State number of copies desired at $5 each. (D.C. residents add 6 percent sales tax.) You can also order the brochure at http://ificinfo.health.org.

—by Paula Kurtzweil

Paula Kurtzweil is a member of FDA's public affairs staff.

Chapter 27

Very Low-Calorie Diets

Introduction

Traditional weight loss methods include low-calorie diets between 800 to 1,500 calories a day and regular exercise. An alternative method sometimes considered for bringing about significant short-term weight loss in moderately to severely obese people is the very low-calorie diet (VLCD).

What Is a Very Low-Calorie Diet (VLCD)?

VLCDs are commercially prepared formulas of 800 calories or less that replace all usual food intake. VLCDs are not the same as over-the-counter meal replacements, which are meant to be substituted for one or two meals a day. VLCDs, when used under proper medical supervision, effectively produce significant short-term weight loss in moderately to severely obese patients.

Who Should Use a VLCD?

VLCDs are generally safe when used under proper medical supervision in patients with a body mass index (BMI) greater than 30. BMI

Excerpted from "Very Low-Calorie Diets," National Institute of Diabetes and Digestive and Kidney Diseases (NIDDK), National Institutes of Health (NIH), NIH Pub. No. 95-3894, http://www.niddk.nih.gov/health/nutrit/pubs/vlcd.htm, March 1995, e-text last updated February 9, 1998.

is a mathematical formula that takes into account both a person's height and weight. To calculate BMI, a person's weight in kilograms is divided by height in meters squared [a complete BMI chart is located in the "Practical Dietary Therapy Information" chapter of this sourcebook]. Use of VLCDs in patients with a BMI of 27 to 30 should be reserved for those who have medical complications resulting from their obesity. VLCDs are not recommended for pregnant women or breastfeeding women. VLCDs are not appropriate for children or adolescents, except in specialized treatment programs.

Very little information exists regarding the usage of VLCDs in older individuals. Because individuals over 50 already experience normal depletion of lean body mass, use of a VLCD may not be warranted. Additionally, persons over 50 may not tolerate the side effects associated with VLCDs because of preexisting medical conditions or need for other medications. Therefore, a physician, on a case by case basis, must evaluate increased risks and potential benefits of drastic weight loss in older individuals. Additionally, people with significant medical problems or who are on medications may be able to use a VLCD, but this too must be determined on an individual basis by a physician.

Health Benefits Associated with a VLCD

A VLCD may allow a severely to moderately obese patient to lose about 3 to 5 pounds per week, for an average total weight loss of 44 pounds over 12 weeks. Such a weight loss can improve obesity-related medical conditions, including diabetes, high blood pressure, and high cholesterol. Combining a VLCD with behavioral therapy and exercise may also increase weight loss and may slow weight regain. However, VLCDs are no more effective than more modest dietary restrictions in the long-term maintenance of reduced weight.

Adverse Effects Associated with a VLCD

Many patients on a VLCD for 4 to 16 weeks report minor side effects such as fatigue, constipation, nausea, and diarrhea, but these conditions usually improve within a few weeks and rarely prevent patients from completing the program. The most common serious side effect seen with VLCDs is gallstone formation. Gallstones, which often develop in obese people, anyway, (especially women), are even more common during rapid weight loss. Some research indicates that rapid weight loss appears to decrease the gallbladder's ability to contract bile. But, it is unclear whether VLCDs directly cause gallstones or whether the amount of weight loss is responsible for the formation of gallstones [see the "Dieting and Gallstones" chapter of this sourcebook for more complete information].

Conclusion

For most obese individuals, obesity is a long-term condition that requires a lifetime of attention even after a formal weight loss treatment ends. Although VLCDs are efficient for short-term weight loss, they are no more effective than other dietary treatments in the long-term maintenance of reduced weight. Therefore, obese patients should be encouraged to commit to a long-term treatment program that includes permanent lifestyle changes of healthier eating, regular physical activity, and an improved outlook about food because without a long-term commitment, their body weights will drift back up the scale.

Chapter 28

Weight Control through Exercise: Tips and Guidelines

Physical Activity and Weight Control

Regular physical activity is an important part of effective weight loss and weight maintenance. It also can help prevent several diseases and improve your overall health. It does not matter what type of physical activity you perform—sports, planned exercise, household chores, yard work, or work-related tasks—all are beneficial. Studies show that even the most inactive people can gain significant health benefits if they accumulate 30 minutes or more of physical activity per day. Based on these findings, the U.S. Public Health Service has identified increased physical activity as a priority in Healthy People 2000, our national objectives to improve the health of Americans by the year 2000.

Research consistently shows that regular physical activity, combined with healthy eating habits, is the most efficient and healthful way to control your weight. Whether you are trying to lose weight or maintain it, you should understand the important role of physical activity and include it in your lifestyle.

This chapter includes text from "Physical Activity and Weight Control," Weight-Control Information Network (WIN), National Institute of Diabetes and Digestive and Kidney Diseases (NIDDK), National Institutes of Health (NIH), NIH Pub. No. 96-4031, http://www.niddk.nih.gov/health/nutrit/pubs/physact.htm, April 1996, e-text posted February 20, 1998, and "Guide to Physical Activity," an undated web page from the National Heart, Lung, and Blood Institute (NHLBI), NHLBI Obesity Education Initiative, http://www.nhlbi.nih.gov/health/public/heart/obesity/lose_wt/phy_act.htm.

How Can Physical Activity Help Control My Weight?

Physical activity helps to control your weight by using excess calories that otherwise would be stored as fat. Your body weight is regulated by the number of calories you eat and use each day. Everything you eat contains calories, and everything you do uses calories, including sleeping, breathing, and digesting food. Any physical activity in addition to what you normally do will use extra calories.

Balancing the calories you use through physical activity with the calories you eat will help you achieve your desired weight. When you eat more calories than you need to perform your day's activities, your body stores the extra calories and you gain weight. When you eat fewer calories than you use, your body uses the stored calories and you lose weight. When you eat the same amount of calories as your body uses, your weight stays the same.

Any type of physical activity you choose to do—strenuous activities such as running or aerobic dancing or moderate-intensity activities such as walking or household work—will increase the number of calories your body uses. The key to successful weight control and improved overall health is making physical activity a part of your daily routine.

What Are the Health Benefits of Physical Activity?

In addition to helping to control your weight, research shows that regular physical activity can reduce your risk for several diseases and conditions and improve your overall quality of life. Regular physical activity can help protect you from the following health problems.

- *Heart disease and stroke.* Daily physical activity can help prevent heart disease and stroke by strengthening your heart muscle, lowering your blood pressure, raising your high-density lipoprotein (HDL) levels (good cholesterol) and lowering low-density lipoprotein (LDL) levels (bad cholesterol), improving blood flow, and increasing your heart's working capacity.

- *High blood pressure.* Regular physical activity can reduce blood pressure in those with high blood pressure levels. Physical activity also reduces body fatness, which is associated with high blood pressure.

- *Non-insulin-dependent diabetes.* By reducing body fatness, physical activity can help to prevent and control this type of diabetes.

Weight Control through Exercise: Tips and Guidelines

- *Obesity.* Physical activity helps to reduce body fat by building or preserving muscle mass and improving the body's ability to use calories. When physical activity is combined with proper nutrition, it can help control weight and prevent obesity, a major risk factor for many diseases.

- *Back pain.* By increasing muscle strength and endurance and improving flexibility and posture, regular exercise helps to prevent back pain.

- *Osteoporosis.* Regular weight-bearing exercise promotes bone formation and may prevent many forms of bone loss associated with aging.

Studies on the psychological effects of exercise have found that regular physical activity can improve your mood and the way you feel about yourself. Researchers also have found that exercise is likely to reduce depression and anxiety and help you to better manage stress.

Keep these health benefits in mind when deciding whether or not to exercise. And remember, any amount of physical activity you do is better than none at all.

How Much Should I Exercise?

For the greatest overall health benefits, experts recommend that you do 20 to 30 minutes of aerobic activity three or more times a week and some type of muscle strengthening activity and stretching at least twice a week. However, if you are unable to do this level of activity, you can gain substantial health benefits by accumulating 30 minutes or more of moderate-intensity physical activity a day, at least five times a week.

If you have been inactive for a while, you may want to start with less strenuous activities such as walking or swimming at a comfortable pace. Beginning at a slow pace will allow you to become physically fit without straining your body. Once you are in better shape, you can gradually do more strenuous activity.

Moderate-Intensity Activity

Moderate-intensity activities include some of the things you may already be doing during a day or week, such as gardening and housework. These activities can be done in short spurts—10 minutes here, 8 minutes there. Alone, each action does not have a great effect on your health, but regularly accumulating 30 minutes of activity over the course of the day can result in substantial health benefits.

To become more active throughout your day, take advantage of any chance to get up and move around. Here are some examples:

- take a short walk around the block
- rake leaves
- play actively with the kids
- walk up the stairs instead of taking the elevator
- mow the lawn
- take an activity break—get up and stretch or walk around
- park your car a little farther away from your destination and walk the extra distance

The point is not to make physical activity an unwelcome chore, but to make the most of the opportunities you have to be active.

Aerobic Activity

Aerobic activity is an important addition to moderate-intensity exercise. Aerobic exercise is any extended activity that makes you breathe hard while using the large muscle groups at a regular, even pace. Aerobic activities help make your heart stronger and more efficient. They also use more calories than other activities. Some examples of aerobic activities include:

- brisk walking
- jogging
- bicycling
- swimming
- aerobic dancing
- racket sports
- rowing
- ice or roller skating
- cross-country or downhill skiing
- using aerobic equipment (i.e., treadmill, stationary bike)

Weight Control through Exercise: Tips and Guidelines

To get the most health benefits from aerobic activity, you should exercise at a level strenuous enough to raise your heart rate to your target zone. Your target heart rate zone is 50 to 75 percent of your maximum heart rate (the fastest your heart can beat). To find your target zone, look for the category closest to your age in the chart below and read across the line. For example, if you are 35 years old, your target heart rate zone is 93–138 beats per minute.

To see if you are exercising within your target heart rate zone, count the number of pulse beats at your wrist or neck for 15 seconds, then multiply by four to get the beats per minute. Your heart should be beating within your target heart rate zone. If your heart is beating faster than your target heart rate, you are exercising too hard and should slow down. If your heart is beating slower than your target heart rate, you should exercise a little harder.

When you begin your exercise program, aim for the lower part of your target zone (50 percent). As you get into better shape, slowly build up to the higher part of your target zone (75 percent). If exercising within your target zone seems too hard, exercise at a pace that is comfortable for you. You will find that, with time, you will feel more comfortable exercising and can slowly increase to your target zone.

Table 28.1. Target heart rate zone.

Age	Target Heart Rate Zone 50–75%	Average Maximum Heart Rate 100%
20–30 years	98–146 beats per min.	195
31–40 years	93–138 beats per min.	185
41–50 years	88–131 beats per min.	175
51–60 years	83–123 beats per min.	165
61+ years	78–116 beats per min.	155

Stretching and Muscle Strengthening Exercises

Stretching and strengthening exercises such as weight training should also be a part of your physical activity program. In addition to using calories, these exercises strengthen your muscles and bones and help prevent injury.

Tips to a Safe and Successful Physical Activity Program

Make sure you are in good health. Answer the following questions before you begin exercising.

- Has a doctor ever said you have heart problems?
- Do you frequently suffer from chest pains?
- Do you often feel faint or have dizzy spells?
- Has a doctor ever said you have high blood pressure?
- Has a doctor ever told you that you have a bone or joint problem, such as arthritis, that has been or could be aggravated by exercise?
- Are you over the age of 65 and not accustomed to exercise?
- Are you taking prescription medications, such as those for high blood pressure?
- Is there a good medical reason, not mentioned here, why you should not exercise?

If you answered "yes" to any of these questions, you should see your doctor before you begin an exercise program.

- Follow a gradual approach to exercise to get the most benefits with the fewest risks. If you have not been exercising, start at a slow pace and as you become more fit, gradually increase the amount of time and the pace of your activity.
- Choose activities that you enjoy and that fit your personality. For example, if you like team sports or group activities, choose things such as soccer or aerobics. If you prefer individual activities, choose things such as swimming or walking. Also, plan your activities for a time of day that suits your personality. If you are a morning person, exercise before you begin the rest of your day's activities. If you have more energy in the evening, plan activities that can be done at the end of the day. You will be more likely to stick to a physical activity program if it is convenient and enjoyable.
- Exercise regularly. To gain the most health benefits it is important to exercise as regularly as possible. Make sure you choose activities that will fit into your schedule.

Weight Control through Exercise: Tips and Guidelines

- Exercise at a comfortable pace. For example, while jogging or walking briskly you should be able to hold a conversation. If you do not feel normal again within 10 minutes following exercise, you are exercising too hard. Also, if you have difficulty breathing or feel faint or weak during or after exercise, you are exercising too hard.

- Maximize your safety and comfort. Wear shoes that fit and clothes that move with you, and always exercise in a safe location. Many people walk in indoor shopping malls for exercise. Malls are climate controlled and offer protection from bad weather.

- Vary your activities. Choose a variety of activities so you don't get bored with any one thing.

- Encourage your family or friends to support you and join you in your activity. If you have children, it is best to build healthy habits when they are young. When parents are active, children are more likely to be active and stay active for the rest of their lives.

- Challenge yourself. Set short-term as well as long-term goals and celebrate every success, no matter how small.

Whether your goal is to control your weight or just to feel healthier, becoming physically active is a step in the right direction. Take advantage of the health benefits that regular exercise can offer and make physical activity a part of your lifestyle.

Guide to Physical Activity

An increase in physical activity is an important part of your weight management program. Most weight loss occurs because of decreased caloric intake. Sustained physical activity is most helpful in the prevention of weight regain. In addition, exercise has a benefit of reducing risks of cardiovascular disease and diabetes, beyond that produced by weight reduction alone. Start exercising slowly, and gradually increase the intensity. Trying too hard at first can lead to injury.

Examples of Moderate Amounts of Physical Activity

Common Chores

- washing and waxing a car for 45–60 minutes
- washing windows or floors for 45–60 minutes

- gardening for 30–45 minutes
- wheeling self in wheelchair 30–40 minutes
- pushing a stroller 1 1/2 miles in 30 minutes
- raking leaves for 30 minutes
- walking 2 miles in 30 minutes (15 min/mile)
- shoveling snow for 15 minutes
- stairwalking for 15 minutes

Sporting Activities

- playing volleyball for 45–60 minutes
- playing touch football for 45 minutes
- walking 1 3/4 miles in 35 minutes (20 min/mile)
- basketball (shooting baskets) 30 minutes
- bicycling 5 miles in 30 minutes
- dancing fast (social) for 30 minutes
- water aerobics for 30 minutes
- swimming laps for 20 minutes
- basketball (playing game) for 15–20 minutes
- bicycling 4 miles in 15 minutes
- jumping rope for 15 minutes
- running 1 1/2 miles in 15 min. (10 min/mile)

    Your exercise can be done all at one time, or intermittently over the day. Initial activities may be walking or swimming at a slow pace. You can start out by walking 30 minutes for three days a week and can build to 45 minutes of more intense walking, at least five days a week. With this regimen, you can burn 100 to 200 calories more per day. All adults should set a long-term goal to accumulate at least 30 minutes or more of moderate-intensity physical activity on most, and preferably all, days of the week. This regimen can be adapted to other forms of physical activity, but walking is particularly attractive because of its safety and accessibility. Also, try to increase "every day" activity such as taking the stairs instead of the elevator. Reducing

Weight Control through Exercise: Tips and Guidelines

sedentary time is a good strategy to increase activity by undertaking frequent, less strenuous activities. With time, you may be able to engage in more strenuous activities. Competitive sports, such as tennis and volleyball, can provide an enjoyable form of exercise for many, but care must be taken to avoid injury.

Activity Progression

For the beginner, activity level can begin at very light and would include an increase in standing activities, special chores like room painting, pushing a wheelchair, yard work, ironing, cooking, and playing a musical instrument.

The next level would be light activity such as slow walking of 24 minutes/mile, garage work, carpentry, house cleaning, child care, golf, sailing, and recreational table tennis.

The next level would be moderate activity such as walking 15 minutes/mile, weeding and hoeing a garden, carrying a load, cycling, skiing, tennis, and dancing.

High activity would include walking 10 minutes/mile or walking with load uphill, tree felling, heavy manual digging, basketball, climbing, or soccer/kick ball.

You may also want to try:

- flexibility exercise to attain full range of joint motion
- strength or resistance exercise
- aerobic conditioning

Chapter 29

Guide to Behavior Change

Behaviors That Will Help You Lose Weight and Maintain It

Set the Right Goals

Setting the right goals is an important first step. Most people trying to lose weight focus on just that one goal: weight loss. However, the most productive areas to focus on are the dietary and exercise changes that will lead to that long-term weight change. Successful weight managers are those who select two or three goals at a time that they are willing to take on, that meet the following criteria of useful goals:

Effective goals are:

1. specific
2. attainable
3. forgiving (less than perfect)

"Exercise more" is a commendable ideal, but it's not specific. "Walk five miles everyday" is specific and measurable, but is it attainable if you're just starting out? "Walk 30 minutes every day" is more attainable, but what happens if you're held up at work one day and there's a thunderstorm during your walking time another day? "Walk 30

From an undated web page from the National Heart, Lung, and Blood Institute (NHLBI), NHLBI Obesity Education Initiative, National Institutes of Health (NIH), http://www.nhlbi.nih.gov/health/public/heart/obesity/lose_wt/behavior.htm

minutes, five days each week" is specific, attainable, and forgiving. In short, a great goal!

Nothing Succeeds Like Success

Shaping is a behavioral technique in which you select a series of short-term goals that get closer and closer to the ultimate goal (e. g., an initial reduction of fat intake from 40% of calories to 35% of calories, and later to 30%). It is based on the concept that "nothing succeeds like success." Shaping uses two important behavioral principles:

1. Consecutive goals that move you ahead in small steps are the best way to reach a distant point.
2. Consecutive rewards keep the overall effort invigorated.

Reward Success (but Not with Food)

Rewards that you control can be used to encourage attainment of behavioral goals, especially those that have been difficult to reach. An effective reward is something that is desirable, timely, and contingent on meeting your goal. The rewards you administer may be tangible (e. g., a movie or music CD or a payment toward buying a more costly item) or intangible (e. g., an afternoon off from work or just an hour of quiet time away from family). Numerous small rewards, delivered for meeting smaller goals, are more effective than bigger rewards, requiring along, difficult effort.

Balance Your (Food) Checkbook

Self-monitoring refers to observing and recording some aspect of your behavior, such as calorie intake, servings of fruits and vegetables, exercise sessions, medication usage, etc., or an outcome of these behaviors, such as weight. Self-monitoring of a behavior can be used at times when you're not sure how you're doing, and at times when you want the behavior to improve. Self-monitoring of a behavior usually changes the behavior in the desired direction and can produce "real-time" records for review by you and your health-care provider. For example, keeping a record of your exercise can let you and your provider know quickly how you're doing, and when the record shows that your exercise is increasing, you'll be encouraged to keep it up. Some patients find that specific self-monitoring forms make it easier, while others prefer to use their own recording system.

While you may or may not wish to weigh yourself frequently while losing weight, regular monitoring of your weight will be essential to help you maintain your lower weight. When keeping a record of your weight, a graph may be more informative than a list of your weights. When weighing yourself and keeping a weight graph or table, however, remember that one day's diet and exercise patterns won't have a measurable effect on your fat weight the next day. Today's weight is not a true measure of how well you followed your program yesterday, because your body's water weight will change much more from day to day than will your fat weight, and water changes are often the result of things that have nothing to do with your weight-management efforts.

Avoid a Chain Reaction

Stimulus (cue) control involves learning what social or environmental cues seem to encourage undesired eating, and then changing those cues. For example, you may learn from reflection or from self-monitoring records that you're more likely to overeat while watching television, or whenever treats are on display by the office coffee pot, or when around a certain friend. You might then try to sever the association of eating with the cue (don't eat while watching television), avoid or eliminate the cue (leave coffee room immediately after pouring coffee), or change the circumstances surrounding the cue (plan to meet with friend in non-food settings). In general, visible and accessible food items are often cues for unplanned eating.

Get the Fullness Message

Changing the way you go about eating can make it easier to eat less without feeling deprived. It takes 15 or more minutes for your brain to get the message you've been fed. Slowing the rate of eating can allow satiety (fullness) signals to begin to develop by the end of the meal. Eating lots of vegetables can also make you feel fuller. Another trick is to use smaller plates so that moderate portions do not appear meager. Changing your eating schedule, or setting one, can be helpful, especially if you tend to skip, or delay, meals and overeat later.

Chapter 30

You Can Control Your Weight As You Quit Smoking

If you want to stop smoking but are worried about gaining weight, this chapter may help you. Many ex-smokers do gain a few pounds, but only a few gain a lot of weight. The best action you can take to improve your health is to quit smoking. Smoking is much more harmful to your health than gaining a few pounds. Making some simple changes, like developing healthier eating and physical activity habits, should help you control your weight gain when you quit smoking.

Will I Gain Weight If I Stop Smoking?

Not everyone gains weight when they stop smoking. On average, people who quit smoking gain only about 10 pounds. You are more likely to gain weight when you stop smoking if you have smoked for 10 to 20 years or smoked one or more packs of cigarettes a day. You can control your weight while you quit smoking by making healthy eating and physical activity a part of your life. Although you might gain a few pounds, remember you have stopped smoking and taken a big step toward a healthier life.

Excerpted from "You Can Control Your Weight As You Quit Smoking," Weight-Control Information Network (WIN), National Institute of Diabetes and Digestive and Kidney Diseases (NIDDK), National Institutes of Health (NIH), NIH Pub. No. 98-4159, http://www.niddk.nih.gov/health/nutrit/pubs/quitsmok/index.htm, July 1998, e-text posted October 7, 1998.

What Causes Weight Gain after Quitting?

When nicotine, a chemical in cigarette smoke, leaves your body, you may experience:

- short-term weight gain. The nicotine kept your body weight low, and when you quit smoking, your body returns to the weight it would have been had you never smoked.

- a gain of 3 to 5 pounds due to water retention during the first week after quitting.

- a need for fewer calories. After you stop smoking, you may use fewer calories than when you were smoking.

Will This Weight Gain Hurt My Health?

The health risks of smoking are far greater than the risks of gaining 5 to 10 pounds. Smoking causes more than 400,000 deaths each year in the United States. You would have to gain about 100 to 150 pounds after quitting to make your health risks as high as when you smoked. The health risks of smoking and the benefits of quitting are listed below.

The Health Risks of Smoking

When you smoke...

- Your heart rate increases.

- You expose yourself to some 4,000 chemicals in cigarette smoke and 40 of these chemicals cause cancer.

- You are much more likely to get lung cancer than a nonsmoker. Men are 22 times more likely to develop lung cancer, while women who smoke are 12 times more likely.

- You are twice as likely to have a heart attack as a nonsmoker.

- You increase your risk for heart disease, stroke, some types of cancer, emphysema, chronic bronchitis, and other lung diseases.

- You are hurting not only your own health, but the health of anyone who breathes the smoke, including nonsmokers.

The Benefits of Quitting

When you quit smoking...

- Your body begins to heal from the effects of the nicotine within 12 hours after your last cigarette.

- Your heart and lungs start repairing the damage caused by cigarette smoke.

- You breathe easier and your smoker's cough starts to go away.

- You lower your risk for illness and death from heart disease, stroke, chronic bronchitis, emphysema, lung cancer, and other types of cancer.

- You contribute to cleaner air, especially for children who are at risk for illnesses because they breathe others' cigarette smoke.

What Can I Do to Avoid Gaining Weight When I Quit Smoking?

To avoid gaining weight when you quit smoking, you need to become more physically active and improve your eating habits before you stop. Physical activity helps to control your weight by increasing the number of calories your body uses. Making healthy changes to your eating habits will prevent weight gain by controlling the amount of calories you eat. Try to reduce your chances of gaining weight by being more physically active and improving your eating habits before you stop smoking.

Become More Physically Active

Becoming physically active is a healthy way to control your weight and take your mind off smoking. In one study, women who stopped smoking and added 45 minutes of walking a day gained less than 3 pounds. In addition to helping control your weight, exercise increases your energy, promotes self-confidence, improves your health, and may help relieve the stress and depression caused by the lack of nicotine in your body.

You can become more physically active by spending less time doing activities that use little energy, like watching television and playing video games, and spending more time doing physical activities. Try to do at least 30 minutes of physical activity a day on most days of the week. The activity does not have to be done all at once. It can be done in short spurts—10 minutes here, 20 minute there—as long as it adds up to 30 minutes a day. Simple ways to become more physically active include gardening, housework, mowing the lawn, playing actively with children, and taking the stairs instead of the elevator.

Improve Your Eating Habits

Try to gradually improve your eating habits. Changing your eating habits too quickly can add to the stress you may feel as you try to quit smoking. Eating a variety of foods is a good way to improve your health. To make sure you get all of the nutrients needed for good health, choose a variety of foods from each group in the Food Guide Pyramid each day. The Nutrition Facts Label that is found on most processed food products can also help you select foods that meet your daily nutritional needs. For a healthy diet, use the Pyramid to guide your daily food choices and make sure you:

- Eat plenty of grain products, vegetables, and fruits.
- Choose lean and lowfat foods and low-calorie beverages most often. Choose lowfat dairy products, lean meats, fish, poultry, and dry beans to get the nutrients you need without extra calories and fat.
- Choose less often foods that are high in fat and sugars and low in nutrients.

When You Are Ready to Quit Smoking

Pick a day to quit smoking during a non-stressful period. For example, try not to quit smoking during holiday seasons when you might be tempted to eat more. Quitting during a stressful time at work or at home might cause extra snacking or a smoking relapse.

Try to focus on quitting smoking and healing your body. Your first goal should be to quit smoking and let your body heal from the effects of nicotine. After you feel better and are not smoking, work harder on improving your eating and physical activity habits to help you lose any weight that you might have gained.

After You Quit

Once you stop smoking, it is important to learn how to handle cravings for cigarettes and food. Remember, a craving only lasts about 5 minutes. Consider these actions to help deal with your cravings.

You Can Control Your Weight As You Quit Smoking

- Replace smoking with other activities. Snack on fruit or sugarless gum to satisfy any sweet cravings. Keep your hands busy. Replace the action of holding cigarettes with activities like doodling, working puzzles, knitting, twirling a straw, or holding a pen or pencil.

- Drink less caffeine. Try to avoid drinking beverages that contain caffeine, such as sodas. Nicotine withdrawal will make you feel jittery and nervous, and the caffeine may only make nicotine withdrawal worse.

- Get enough sleep. When you feel tired, you are more likely to crave cigarettes and food.

- Reduce tension. To help relieve tension, relax by meditating, taking a walk, soaking in the tub, or taking deep breaths. Find something that will help you relax and replace the urge to smoke.

- Get support and encouragement. You need a lot of support when you quit smoking. Talk to a friend when you get the urge to smoke or join a support group such as Nicotine Anonymous. You can also participate in workshops offered by health-care providers that will help you quit smoking. If you can, find a friend to quit with you for mutual support.

- Talk to your doctor about nicotine replacement. If you have significant withdrawal symptoms or are concerned about weight gain, talk to your doctor. Some nicotine replacement products, formerly available by prescription only, are now available over the counter. Using nicotine gum or a nicotine patch, along with improved eating habits and physical activity, will help you reduce your risk of a smoking relapse. Nicotine gum has been shown to delay weight gain after quitting. You may also want to talk to your doctor about prescription medications that are available to help you quit smoking.

- Try not to do things that tempt you to smoke or eat when you are not hungry. Keep a journal of where and when you feel most tempted to smoke and avoid these situations. Substitute healthy activities for smoking to help you avoid the urge to smoke or eat when you are not hungry.

Try not to panic about modest weight gain. Accept some weight gain as a normal result of the nicotine leaving your body. Know that quitting smoking is the best thing that you can do for you and those around you. If possible, before you quit, prepare a plan to quit smoking that includes simple changes in your eating and exercise habits. Improving your lifestyle as you stop smoking can help you prevent a large weight gain and become a healthy nonsmoker.

Chapter 31

Smoking Cessation and Overweight

Between 1978 and 1990, the proportion of overweight adults in the US increased by 9.6% for men and 8.0% for women. During the same time period, the prevalence of cigarette smoking decreased. It has been hypothesized that the two may be associated, since smoking is associated with lower body weight and cessation of smoking is associated with weight gain. The following study, conducted by researchers from the National Center for Health Statistics, examined the relationship between smoking status and body weight, using data from the 1988-91 Third National Health and Nutrition Examination Survey (NHANES 111).

Data on current and past weight and smoking status were collected from a national sample of 5,247 adults aged 35 or older. Of the various smoking-status groups, current smokers, both male and female, had the lowest prevalence of overweight and the lowest mean body mass index, while people who had quit smoking within the previous 10 years had the highest. Smokers who had quit within the past 10 years were significantly more likely than never-smokers to become overweight. Smoking cessation was associated with a 10-year weight gain of 4.4 kg for men and 5.0 kg for women.

Among smokers who had quit within the past 10 years, there was a large increase in the prevalence of overweight. However, because this group made up a relatively small percentage of the population,

Nutrition Research Newsletter, November-December 1995, Vol. 14, N. 11-12, pp. 129–130, copyright 1995 Lyda Associates Inc. Reprinted by permission of John Wiley & Sons, Inc.

the net effect of smoking cessation on the prevalence of overweight in the population as a whole was relatively small. Smoking cessation accounted for a quarter of the increase in the prevalence of overweight in men and a sixth of the increase in women.

The authors conclude that "although its health benefits are undeniable, smoking cessation may nevertheless be associated with a small increase in the prevalence of overweight." They note that efforts to prevent weight gain after smoking cessation have been relatively unsuccessful, perhaps because the weight gain may be a physiologic process reflecting nicotine withdrawal. Concern over weight and weight gain may be an important factor leading to the initiation and continuation of smoking. In the view of these authors, reducing concern about initial weight gain after smoking cessation may be better than trying to prevent it. However, former smokers should be encouraged to limit any further weight gain after the first few months.

"Public health efforts to discourage the initiation of smoking and to promote its cessation must continue. To the extent these efforts are successful, they are likely to lead to further increases in the proportion of the population that is overweight. Nonetheless, it is important to discourage the use of smoking as a means of weight control and to encourage the cessation of smoking, while continuing research aimed at understanding and moderating the degree of weight gain among former smokers."

This article was adapted from Katherine M Flegal, Richard P Troiano, Elsie R Pamuk, Robert J Kuczmarski, and Stephen M Campbell, "The Influence of Smoking Cessation on the Prevalence of Overweight in the United States," *New England J Medicine* 333(18): pp. 1165–1170, November 2, 1995. Reprints: Katherine M Flegal, PhD, National Center for Health Statistics, 6525 Belcrest Road, Rm 900, Hyattsville MD 207821.

Chapter 32

Prescription Medications for the Treatment of Obesity

Obesity is a chronic disease that affects many people and often requires long-term treatment to promote and sustain weight loss. As in other chronic conditions, such as diabetes or high blood pressure, long-term use of prescription medications may be appropriate for some individuals. While most side effects of prescription medications for obesity are mild, serious complications have been reported. Valvular heart disease has recently been reported to occur in association with the use of certain appetite suppressant medications. As a result of these reports, the manufacturer has voluntarily withdrawn two medications, fenfluramine (Pondimin) and dexfenfluramine (Redux) from the market. There are few long-term studies evaluating the safety or effectiveness of other currently approved appetite suppressant medications. In particular, the safety and effectiveness of combining more than one appetite suppressant medication or combining appetite suppressant medications with other medications for the purpose of weight loss is unknown. Appetite suppressant medications should be used only by patients who are at increased medical risk because of their obesity and should not be used for "cosmetic" weight loss.

Weight-Control Information Network (WIN), National Institute of Diabetes and Digestive and Kidney Diseases (NIDDK), National Institutes of Health (NIH), NIH Pub. No. 97-4191, http://www.niddk.nih.gov/health/nutrit/pubs/presmeds.htm, December 1996, e-text last updated March 16, 1998.

Medications That Promote Weight Loss

The medications most often used in the management of obesity are commonly known as "appetite suppressant" medications. Appetite suppressant medications promote weight loss by decreasing appetite or increasing the feeling of being full. These medications decrease appetite by increasing serotonin or catecholamine—two brain chemicals that affect mood and appetite.

Most currently available appetite suppressant medications are approved by the U.S. Food and Drug Administration (FDA) for short-term use, meaning a few weeks or months. Sibutramine is the only appetite suppressant medication approved for longer-term use in significantly obese patients, although the safety and effectiveness have not been established for use beyond one year (see Table 32.1 for the generic and trade names of prescription appetite suppressant medications). While the FDA regulates how a medication can be advertised or promoted by the manufacturer, these regulations do not restrict a doctor's ability to prescribe the medication for different conditions, in different doses, or for different lengths of time. The practice of prescribing medication for periods of time or for conditions not approved is known as "off-label" use. While such use often occurs in the treatment of many conditions, you should feel comfortable about asking your doctor if he or she is using a medication or combination of medications in a manner that is not approved

Table 32.1. Prescription appetite suppressant medications.

Generic Name	Trade Name(s)
Dexfenfluramine	Redux (Withdrawn)
Diethylpropion	Tenuate, Tenuate dospan
Fenfluramine	Pondimin (Withdrawn)
Mazindol	Sanorex, Mazanor
Phendimetrazine	Bontril, Plegine, Prelu-2, X-Trozine
Phentermine	Adipex-P, Fastin, Ionamin, Oby-trim
Sibutramine	Meridia

by the FDA. The use of more than one appetite suppressant medication at a time (combined drug treatment) is an example of an off-label use. Using currently approved appetite suppressant medication for more than a short period of time (i.e., more than "a few weeks") is also considered off-label use.

Single Drug Treatment

Several appetite suppressant medications are available to treat obesity. In general, these medications are modestly effective, leading to an average weight loss of 5 to 22 pounds above that expected with non-drug obesity treatments. People respond differently to appetite suppressant medications, and some people experience more weight loss than others. Some obese patients using medication lose more than 10 percent of their starting body weight—an amount of weight loss that may reduce risk factors for obesity-related diseases, such as high blood pressure or diabetes. Maximum weight loss usually occurs within 6 months of starting medication treatment. Weight then tends to level off or increase during the remainder of treatment. Studies suggest that if a patient does not lose at least 4 pounds over 4 weeks on a particular medication, then that medication is unlikely to help the patient achieve significant weight loss. Few studies have looked at how safe or effective these medications are when taken for more than 1 year.

Some antidepressant medications have been studied as appetite suppressant medications. While these medications are FDA approved for the treatment of depression, their use in weight loss is an "off-label" use. Studies of these medications generally have found that patients lost modest amounts of weight for up to 6 months. However, most studies have found that patients who lost weight while taking antidepressant medications tended to regain weight while they were still on the drug treatment. Amphetamines and closely-related compounds are not recommended for use in the treatment of obesity due to their potential for abuse and dependence.

Combined Drug Treatment

Combined drug treatment using fenfluramine and phentermine ("fen/phen") is no longer available due to the withdrawal of fenfluramine from the market. Little information is available about the safety or effectiveness of other drug combinations for weight loss, including fluoxetine/phentermine, phendimetrazine/phentermine, herbal combinations, or others. Until more information on their safety or effectiveness is available, using combinations of medications for weight loss is not recommended except as part of a research study.

Potential Benefits of Medication Treatment

Over the short term, weight loss in obese individuals may reduce a number of health risks. Studies looking at the effects of appetite suppressant medication treatment on obesity-related health risks have found that some agents lower blood pressure, blood cholesterol, triglycerides (fats), and decrease insulin resistance (the body's inability to use blood sugar) over the short term. However, long-term studies are needed to determine if weight loss from appetite suppressant medications can improve health.

Potential Risks and Areas of Concern When Considering Medication Treatment

When considering long-term appetite suppressant medication treatment for obesity, you should consider the following areas of concern and potential risks.

Potential for Abuse or Dependence

Currently, all prescription medications to treat obesity are controlled substances, meaning doctors need to follow certain restrictions when prescribing appetite suppressant medications. Although abuse and dependence are not common with non-amphetamine appetite suppressant medications, doctors should be cautious when they prescribe these medications for patients with a history of alcohol or other drug abuse.

Development of Tolerance

Most studies of appetite suppressant medications show that a patient's weight tends to level off after 4 to 6 months while still on medication treatment. While some patients and physicians may be concerned that this shows tolerance to the medications, the leveling off may mean that the medication has reached its limit of effectiveness. Based on the currently available studies, it is not clear if weight gain with continuing treatment is due to drug tolerance.

Prescription Medications for the Treatment of Obesity

Reluctance to View Obesity as a Chronic Disease

Obesity often is viewed as the result of a lack of willpower, weakness, or a lifestyle "choice"—the choice to overeat and underexercise. The belief that persons choose to be obese adds to the hesitation of health professionals and patients to accept the use of long-term appetite suppressant medication treatment to manage obesity. Obesity, however, is more appropriately considered a chronic disease than a lifestyle choice. Other chronic diseases, such as diabetes and high blood pressure, are managed by long-term drug treatment, even though these diseases also improve with changes in lifestyle, such as diet and exercise. Although this issue may concern physicians and patients, social views on obesity should not prevent patients from seeking medical treatment to prevent health risks that can cause serious illness and death. Appetite suppressant medications are not "magic bullets," or a one-shot fix. They cannot take the place of improving one's diet and becoming more physically active. The major role of medications appears to be to help a person stay on a diet and exercise plan to lose weight and keep it off.

Side Effects

Because appetite suppressant medications are used to treat a condition that affects millions of people, many of whom are basically healthy, their potential for side effects is of great concern. Most side effects of these medications are mild and usually improve with continued treatment. Rarely, serious and even fatal outcomes have been reported. Two approved appetite suppressant medications that affect serotonin release and reuptake have been withdrawn from the market (fenfluramine, dexfenfluramine). Medications that affect catecholamine levels (such as phentermine, diethylpropion, and mazindol) may cause symptoms of sleeplessness, nervousness, and euphoria (feeling of well-being). Sibutramine acts on both the serotonin and catecholamine systems, but unlike fenfluramine and dexfenfluramine, sibutramine does not cause release of serotonin from cells. The primary known side-effects of concern with sibutramine are elevations in blood pressure and pulse, which are usually small, but which may be significant in some patients. People with poorly controlled high blood pressure, heart disease, irregular heart beat, or history of stroke should not take sibutramine, and all patients taking the medication should have their blood pressure monitored on a regular basis.

Primary pulmonary hypertension (PPH) is a rare but potentially fatal disorder that affects the blood vessels in the lungs and results in death within 4 years in 45 percent of its victims. Patients who use appetite suppressant medications for more than 3 months have a greater risk for developing this condition, estimated at 1 in 22,000 to 1 in 44,000 patients per year. While the risk of developing PPH is very small, physicians and patients should be aware of this possible complication when considering the risks and benefits of using appetite suppressant medications in the long-term treatment of obesity. Patients taking appetite suppressant medications should contact their doctors if they experience any symptoms such as shortness of breath, chest pain, faintness, or swelling in lower legs and ankles. It should be noted that the vast majority of cases of PPH have occurred in patients who were taking fenfluramine or dexfenfluramine, either alone or in combination. There have been only a few case reports of PPH in patients taking phentermine alone, although the possibility that phentermine alone may be associated with PPH cannot be ruled-out. No cases of PPH have been reported with sibutramine, but because of the low incidence of this disease in the underlying population, it is not know whether or not sibutramine may cause this disease.

Some animal studies have suggested that appetite suppressant medications affecting the serotonin system, such as fenfluramine and dexfenfluramine, can lead to damage to the central nervous system. Damage to the central nervous system has not been reported in humans. Some patients have reported depression or memory loss when using some appetite suppressant medications or combinations of medications, but it is not known if these problems are caused by the medication or by other factors.

In July, 1997, researchers at the Mayo Clinic reported a case series of 24 women who developed an unusual form of disease of the heart valves. All 24 women were using the combination of fenfluramine and phentermine. The disease primarily affected the left side of the heart, and five patients required valve replacement. In cases where samples of valve tissue were obtained, there was an unusual appearance of the heart valves generally only seen with a serotonin-producing tumor called carcinoid or with excessive amounts of medications containing ergot. Following these initial case reports, the Food and Drug Administration (FDA) has continued to receive a number of reports of similar valve disease from physicians. Some of these cases involved patients who were taking fenfluramine or dexfenfluramine alone. No cases were reported in patients taking phentermine alone. In addition, physicians at five sites provided information to the FDA regarding patients, most of whom did not have signs or symptoms of valve disease. About 30% of patients at these sites showed some evidence of damaged valves, usually mild or moderate. While this was not a controlled study, and further studies are needed to determine how common the problem is in treated patients compared to the general population of overweight people, the findings were of enough concern to prompt the FDA to ask the manufacturers of fenfluramine and dexfenfluramine to voluntarily recall the drugs. This withdrawal took place on September 15th 1997. Patients who were on fenfluramine or dexfenfluramine have been advised to discontinue the drug, and to contact their physicians for an evaluation to look for signs and symptoms of heart disease and to determine the need for an echocardiogram. For more information about the withdrawal of fenfluramine and dexfenfluramine, you can access the FDA website on Questions and Answers about Withdrawal of Fenfluramine (Pondimin) and Dexfenfluramine (Redux) at http://www.fda.gov/cder/news/phen/fenphenqa2.htm. Two small studies looking at relationships between sibutramine and valvular heart disease did not find any increase in valve lesions in patients taking sibutramine compared with placebo.

Commonly Asked Questions about Appetite Suppressant Medication Treatment

Can Medications Replace Physical Activity or Changes in Eating Habits as a Way to Lose Weight?

No. The use of appetite suppressant medications to treat obesity should be combined with physical activity and improved diet to lose and maintain weight successfully over the long term.

Will I Regain Some Weight after I Stop Taking Appetite Suppressant Medications?

Probably. Most studies show that the majority of patients who stop taking appetite suppressant medications regain the weight they had lost. Maintaining healthy eating and physical activity habits will increase your likelihood of keeping weight off.

How Long Will I Need to Take Appetite Suppressant Medications to Treat Obesity?

The answer depends upon whether the medication helps you to lose and maintain weight and whether you have any side effects. Because obesity is a chronic disease, any treatment, whether drug or non-drug, may need to be continued for years, and perhaps a lifetime, to improve health and maintain a healthy weight. There is little information on how safe and effective appetite suppressant medications are for more than 1 year of use.

What Dosage of Appetite Suppressant Medication Would Be Right for Me?

There is no one correct dose for appetite suppressant medications. Your doctor will decide what works best for you based on his or her evaluation of your medical condition and response to treatment.

I Only Need to Lose Ten Pounds. Are Appetite Suppressant Medications Appropriate for Me?

Appetite suppressant medications may be appropriate for carefully selected patients who are at significant medical risk because of their obesity. They are not recommended for use by people who are only mildly overweight unless they have health problems that are made worse by their weight. These medications should not be used only to improve appearance.

What to Discuss with Your Doctor before Choosing Appetite Suppressant Medication Treatment

Before choosing appetite suppressant medication treatment for the long-term management of obesity, you should talk to your doctor about any concerns you may have. In addition, it is important that you discuss the following issues with your doctor.

How will I be evaluated to determine if I am an appropriate candidate for appetite suppressant medication treatment? Your physician will look at a number of factors to determine if you are a good candidate for prescription appetite suppressant medication treatment of obesity. He or she will determine how overweight you are and where your body fat is distributed. Your doctor may do the following:

- Take a careful medical history and perform a physical examination.
- Look at your personal weight history.
- Ask whether you have relatives with illnesses related to overweight, such as noninsulin-dependent diabetes mellitus (NIDDM) or heart disease.

Prescription Medications for the Treatment of Obesity

- Discuss the methods you have used to lose weight in the past.
- Evaluate your risk for obesity-related health problems by measuring your blood pressure and doing blood tests.

If your doctor determines that you have obesity-related health problems or are at high risk for such problems, and if you have been unable to lose weight or maintain weight loss with non-drug treatment, he or she may recommend that you use prescription appetite suppressant medications. Appetite suppressant medications may be appropriate for carefully selected patients who are at significant medical risk because of their obesity. They are not recommended for people who are only mildly overweight unless they have health problems that are made worse by their weight. These medications should not be used only to improve appearance.

What other medical conditions or medications might influence my decision to take an appetite suppressant medication? It is important that you notify your physician if you have any of the following medical conditions:

- pregnancy or breast-feeding
- history of drug or alcohol abuse
- history of an eating disorder
- history of depression or manic depressive disorder
- use of monoamine oxidase (MAO) inhibitors or antidepressant medications
- migraine headaches requiring medication
- glaucoma
- diabetes
- heart disease or heart condition, such as an irregular heart beat
- high blood pressure
- planning on surgery that requires general anesthesia

What type of program will be provided along with the medication to help me improve my eating and physical activity habits? Studies show that appetite suppressant medications work best when combined with a weight-management program that helps you improve your eating and physical activity habits. Ask your doctor any questions or concerns that you may have about good nutrition and physical activity.

Appropriate Treatment Goals for Using Prescription Appetite Suppressant Medications

If you and your doctor believe that the use of appetite suppressant medications may be helpful for you, it is important to discuss the goals of treatment. Improving your health and reducing your risk for disease should be the primary goals. For most severely obese people, achieving an "ideal body weight" is both unrealistic and unnecessary to improve their health and reduce their risk for disease. Most patients should not expect to reach an ideal body weight using the currently available medications. Even a modest weight loss of 5 to 10 percent of your starting body weight can improve your health and reduce your risk factors for disease. Use of appetite suppressant medications for cosmetic purposes is not appropriate.

Appetite suppressant medications should be used with a program of behavioral treatment and nutritional counseling, designed to help you make long-term changes in your diet and physical activity. You should see your physician regularly so that he or she can monitor how you are responding to the medication, not only in terms of weight loss, but how it effects your overall health. Again, if you experience any serious symptoms, such as chest pains or shortness of breath, contact your doctor immediately.

Long-term use of prescription appetite suppressant medications may be helpful for carefully selected individuals, but little information is available on the safety and effectiveness of these medications when used for more than 1 year. By evaluating your risk of experiencing obesity-related health problems, you and your physician can make an informed choice as to whether medication can be a useful part of your weight-management program.

Chapter 33

Orlistat for Obesity

The Food and Drug Administration has approved orlistat, a new drug to treat obesity. Orlistat is the first drug in a new class of non-systemically acting anti-obesity drugs known as lipase inhibitors.

Unlike other obesity drugs, orlistat prevents enzymes in the gastrointestinal tract from breaking down dietary fats into smaller molecules that can be absorbed by the body. Absorption of fat is decreased by about 30 percent. Since undigested triglycerides are not absorbed, the reduced caloric intake may have a positive effect on weight control.

The effects of orlistat on weight loss, weight maintenance, and weight regain and on a number of obesity-related illnesses were assessed in seven long-term multicenter, clinical trials. These studies included about 2800 patients treated with orlistat and 1400 patients treated with placebo. A well-balanced, reduced-calorie diet was recommended for all patients in the weight-loss and weight-maintenance study periods. The diet was intended to decrease caloric intake by 20 percent and to provide 30 percent of calories from fat. In addition, all patients were offered nutritional counseling.

Of the patients who completed one year of treatment, 57 percent of the patients treated with orlistat and 31 percent of the placebo-treated patients lost at least 5 percent of their baseline body weight.

The recommended dose of orlistat is one capsule with each main meal that includes fat. During treatment, the patient should be on a

"FDA Approves Orlistat for Obesity," Food and Drug Administration (FDA), FDA Talk Paper, T99-19, http://www.fda.gov/bbs/topics/answers/ans00951.html, April 26, 1999.

nutritionally balanced, reduced-calorie diet that contains no more than 30 percent of calories from fat. Orlistat is indicated for obese patients with a body mass index (BMI, a measure of weight in relation to height [see the "Practical Dietary Therapy Information" chapter of this sourcebook for a BMI chart]) of 30 or more, or for patients with a BMI of 27 or more who also have high blood pressure, high cholesterol, or diabetes. A person who is 5'5" in height and weighs 180 pounds would have a BMI of 30.

Because orlistat reduces the absorption of some fat-soluble vitamins and beta carotene, patients should take a supplement that contains fat soluble (A, D, E, and K) vitamins and beta carotene. The most common side effects of orlistat are oily spotting, gas with discharge, fecal urgency, fatty/oily stools and frequent bowel movements.

Orlistat is manufactured by Roche Laboratories Inc. under the trade name Xenical.

Chapter 34

"Fen-Phen" Update

The Food and Drug Administration (FDA), acting on new evidence about significant side-effects associated with fenfluramine and dexfenfluramine, has asked the manufacturers to voluntarily withdraw both treatments for obesity from the market. Dexfenfluramine is manufactured for Interneuron Pharmaceuticals and marketed under the name of Redux by Wyeth-Ayerst Laboratories, a subsidiary of American Home Products Corp. of Madison, NJ, which also manufactures and markets fenfluramine under the brand name Pondimin. Both companies have agreed to voluntarily withdraw their drugs. The FDA is not requesting the withdrawal of phentermine, the third widely used medication for obesity.

The action is based on new findings from doctors who have evaluated patients taking these two drugs with echocardiograms, a special procedure that can test the functioning of heart valves. These findings indicate that approximately 30 percent of patients who were evaluated had abnormal echocardiograms, even though they had no symptoms. This is a much higher than expected percentage of abnormal test results.

"These findings call for prompt action," said Michael A. Friedman, M.D., the Lead Deputy Commissioner of the FDA. "The data we have obtained indicate that fenfluramine, and the chemically closely related

---

"FDA Announces Withdrawal of Fenfluramine and Dexfenfluramine," Food and Drug Administration (FDA), http://www.fda.gov/cder/news/phen/fenphenpr81597.htm, September 15, 1997.

dexfenfluramine, present an unacceptable risk at this time to patients who take them."

FDA recommends that patients using either of these products stop taking them. Users of these two products should contact their doctors to discuss their treatment.

These new findings suggest fenfluramine and dexfenfluramine are the likely cause of heart valve problems of the type that prompted FDA's two earlier warnings concerning "fen-phen," a combination of fenfluramine and phentermine. "Fen-phen" has been widely used off-label in recent years for the long-term management of obesity.

In July, researchers at the Mayo Clinic and Mayo Foundation reported 24 cases of rare valvular disease in women who took the "fen-phen" combination therapy. FDA alerted medical doctors that it had received nine additional reports of the same type, and requested all health-care professionals to report any such cases to the agency's MedWatch program (1-800-FDA-1088) or to the respective pharmaceutical manufacturers.

Subsequently, FDA received 66 additional reports of heart valve disease associated mainly with "fen-phen." There were also reports of cases seen in patients taking only fenfluramine or dexfenfluramine. FDA requested that the manufacturers of fenfluramine and dexfenfluramine stress the potential risk to the heart in the drugs' labeling and patient package inserts. FDA continues to receive reports of cardiac valvular disease in persons who have taken these drugs.

Chapter 35

Questions and Answers about Withdrawal of Fenfluramine and Dexfenfluramine

What is "Fen-Phen"?

Fen-phen refers to the use in combination of fenfluramine and phentermine. Phentermine has also been used in combination with dexfenfluramine ("dexfen-phen"). Fenfluramine ("fen") and phentermine ("phen") are prescription medications that have been approved by the FDA for many years as appetite suppressants for the short-term (a few weeks) management of obesity. Phentermine was approved in 1959 and fenfluramine in 1973. Dexfenfluramine (Redux) was approved in 1996 for use as an appetite suppressant in the management of obesity. Recently, some physicians have prescribed fenfluramine or dexfenfluramine in combination with phentermine, often for extended periods of time, for use in weight loss programs. Use of drugs in ways other than described in the FDA-approved label is called "off-label use." In the case of fen-phen and dexfen-phen, no studies were presented to the FDA to demonstrate either the effectiveness or safety of the drugs taken in combination.

What is the difference between Fenfluramine and Dexfenfluramine?

Fenfluramine (Pondimin) contains dexfenfluramine and levofenfluramine. Levofenfluramine may have some activities not directly related to appetite suppression. Dexfenfluramine (Redux) contains only dexfenfluramine.

Food and Drug Administration (FDA), Center for Drug Evaluation and Research, http://www.fda.gov/cder/news/phen/fenphenqa2.htm, September 18, 1997.

What is the new evidence that prompted withdrawal of Fenfluramine and Dexfenfluramine?

On July 8, 1997, the Mayo Clinic reported 24 patients developed heart valve disease after taking fen-phen. In five patients who underwent valve replacement surgery, the diseased valves were found to have distinctive features similar to those seen in carcinoid syndrome. The cluster of unusual cases of valve disease in fen-phen users suggested that there might be an association between fen-phen use and valve disease.

On July 8, FDA issued a Public Health Advisory that described the Mayo findings. The Mayo findings were reported in the August 28 issue of the *New England Journal of Medicine*, along with an FDA letter to the editor describing additional cases. FDA has received over 100 reports (including the original 24 Mayo cases) of heart valve disease associated mainly with fen-phen. There were also reports of cases of heart valve disease in patients taking only fenfluramine or dexfenfluramine. No cases meeting FDA's definition of a case were reported in patients taking phentermine alone.

Within the past several weeks, additional information received by the FDA has raised more concern. Most of the cases previously brought to the FDA's attention were in patients who had symptoms of heart disease. Recently, FDA has received reports from five physicians who had performed heart studies (echocardiograms) on patients who had received fen-phen or dexfen-phen and did not have symptoms of heart disease. Of 291 asymptomatic patients screened, about 30 percent had abnormal valve findings, primarily aortic regurgitation. Based on these data, the manufacturers have agreed to withdraw the products from the market and FDA has recommended that patients stop taking the drugs.

Why isn't Phentermine being withdrawn from the market?

At the present time, no cases of heart valve disease meeting FDA's case definition have been reported with phentermine alone. Analysis of the data points to an association of heart valve disease with fenfluramine and dexfenfluramine.

Why wasn't this problem discovered earlier?

The type of valve disease that FDA believes may be associated with fenfluramine and dexfenfluramine is an extremely unusual type of

Q&A about Withdrawal of Fenfluramine and Dexfenfluramine

drug reaction. Because valve disease is not usually associated with drug use, it is not normally screened for in human clinical testing of drugs. Since valvular heart disease is not screened for in clinical trials, it would usually not be detected unless patients developed symptoms. No cases were detected in 500 patients followed for one year in a clinical trial of dexfenfluramine. Furthermore, asymptomatic heart valve disease (heart valve disease without symptoms) would not likely be detected in patients taking the drugs as part of a weight loss program. The number of patients who have been reported to have symptoms of heart valve disease associated with recent exposure to the drugs has been very small, compared to the number of recent prescriptions, although there may be a delay in the development of symptoms. And even in symptomatic patients, the link between the symptoms and drug use may not be obvious because such a reaction is not common. These factors may explain why this problem was not discovered earlier.

During the last few years, there has been a marked increase in amount and duration of use of fenfluramine, as it became widely prescribed as part of the fen-phen regimen.

In 1992, articles were published about study results suggesting that the combined use of phentermine and fenfluramine would result in significant weight loss when used over an extended period of time. The results of these studies were not reviewed by FDA, and the conclusion about long-term use of the combination of drugs has not received FDA approval. The increased magnitude and duration of use probably led to an increase in the number of cases of symptomatic heart valve disease, which may have contributed to the recent recognition of this association.

With respect to dexfenfluramine (Redux), which was approved on April 29, 1996, the labeling states that safety has not been shown for longer than one year of use. This reflects the length of the study upon which dexfenfluramine was approved. It was a one-year European study of 1,000 subjects, half of whom were treated with dexfenfluramine. The study population was 80 percent women with an average age of 41. Heart disease was not noted in the study. A follow-up study directed toward uncovering heart disease after termination of the study was not performed because there was no reason to believe at that time that the heart was affected. In addition, dexfenfluramine had been marketed in Europe for over a decade without detection of an association between dexfenfluramine and heart valve problems. FDA is currently trying to obtain such follow-up.

What is valvular heart disease?

The heart contains four major valves that regulate the flow of blood through the heart and to the lungs and general circulation. Disease may cause excessive tightness (stenosis) or leakiness (regurgitation) of the valves. In the case of valve disease associated with fenfluramine and dexfenfluramine, leakiness is the problem. Valvular damage may ultimately produce severe heart and/or lung disease.

What is the relationship of Fenfluramine and Dexfenfluramine to heart disease?

Patients who have taken those drugs may have changes in their heart valves that cause leakiness and backflow of blood. If this is severe, the heart has to work harder. This may cause problems in heart function. However, the full medical implications of this relationship, especially in the asymptomatic patients, is not fully understood.

What are the signs and symptoms of valvular heart disease?

The patient may have no symptoms. The physician may hear a new heart murmur (abnormal sound as the blood flows over a valve), or the changes may be detected with a painless, non-invasive special heart test called an echocardiogram. An echocardiogram is usually performed by a cardiologist. If the disease is severe, the patient may experience such symptoms as shortness of breath, excessive tiredness, chest pain, fainting, and swelling of the legs (edema).

Is the valve disease reversible?

It is not known at this time. One report has been submitted to FDA in which the valve disease appeared to improve. However, we encourage those people who have taken fenfluramine or dexfenfluramine to contact their physician and discuss the appropriate follow-up, even after stopping their medicine. The full medical implications of these findings are not known at this time, especially as they relate to the asymptomatic valvular changes. The FDA and other government agencies, the manufacturers, and medical researchers will aggressively follow this concern and keep patients and health-care providers informed of what is learned about the natural history of the valvular disease caused by these medications.

Q&A about Withdrawal of Fenfluramine and Dexfenfluramine

How is valvular disease treated?

It depends on the degree of damage. Medications may help the heart function. If the damage is severe, the valves may have to be replaced surgically.

Should I stop taking Fen-Phen, Fenfluramine, or Dexfenfluramine right now?

Yes, this is the FDA's recommendation. Although we believe these drugs can be stopped at once for most persons, you should consult your physician about whether he/she advises you to taper the dosage over, for example, a 1 to 2 week period. The manufacturers of these drugs are withdrawing fenfluramine and dexfenfluramine from the marketplace, effective September 15, as the concerns about the effects of these drugs on heart valves continue to grow. The drugs will no longer be available in pharmacies. Though the potential long-term medical implications are not known at this time as there are still a number of unanswered questions, the FDA and the manufacturers believe it is in the best interest of the patients that they stop taking these medications. Please be aware that at present this recommendation does not apply to phentermine taken alone.

Should I get an echocardiogram if I've been taking Fenfluramine or Dexfenfluramine?

You should consult your physician about having an echocardiogram. Your physician's recommendation will depend upon your symptoms, if any, his or her examination of you, and your history of exposure to these drugs.

Does "Herbal Fen-Phen" have the same problem?

Herbal fen-phen is a product that does not contain fenfluramine, dexfenfluramine, or phentermine. Products called "herbal fen-phen" often contain a combination of ephedra (an ephedrine containing herb) and caffeine, but may also contain other herbal ingredients. FDA has not reviewed these herbal products for safety or efficacy. Ephedrine is pharmacologically different from fenfluramine and dexfenfluramine.

Can selective serotonin reuptake inhibitor (SSRI) antidepressants such as Prozac, Zoloft, Luvox and Paxil be substituted for Fenfluramine in the Phen/Fen combination?

FDA has not reviewed the safety or efficacy of such combinations and has not approved their use. These drugs are active in serotonin metabolism but have somewhat different activity than fenfluramine and dexfenfluramine. No currently available weight-loss drugs have been studied adequately in combinations to permit a recommendation by FDA for combined use.

I have heard the FDA recently denied a citizen petition that sought to suspend the approval of Redux (dexfenfluramine). Why did the FDA deny that request?

The citizen petition did not contain any additional medical information that was not already known. The FDA had taken appropriate actions based on the knowledge at that time. Since that time, more information has been obtained that raised enough additional concerns to warrant withdrawal of Redux from the market.

Is this just a disease of women?

Though the majority of cases of which FDA is aware are women, there is no reason at present to believe that men are not also at risk. Most of the use of these products is in women, so what we have seen to date could be only a reflection of the usage patterns of the products. FDA advises that both male and female patients consult their health-care professionals.

Chapter 36

Warnings about the Drug Promotion of "Herbal Fen-Phen" for Weight Loss

The FDA is warning consumers that unapproved so-called "herbal fen-phen" products have not been shown to be safe or effective and may contain ingredients that have been associated with injuries. The FDA is taking appropriate regulatory action to remove these products from the market. This warning comes in the face of increasing promotion on the Internet and through weight loss clinics, print ads, and retail outlets of various dietary supplement-type products as "natural" herbal alternatives to the prescription drugs fenfluramine and phentermine. Herbal fen-phen contains neither of these medications.

FDA considers these products to be unapproved drugs because their names reflect that they are intended for the same use as the anti-obesity drugs, fenfluramine and phentermine. Fenfluramine (marketed as Pondimin) and dexfenfluramine (marketed as Redux) were withdrawn by the manufacturer in September.

The main ingredient of most herbal fen-phen products is ephedra, commonly known as Ma Huang. Ephedra is an amphetamine-like compound with potentially powerful stimulant effects on the nervous system and heart, according to the FDA. The agency has received and investigated more than 800 reports of adverse events associated with the use of ephedrine alkaloid-containing products since 1994. These events ranged from episodes of high blood pressure, heart rate

---

From the undated page "FDA Warns against Drug Promotion of 'Herbal Fen-Phen' for Weight Loss," from the American Society of Bariatric Physicians (ASBP) website, http://www.asbp.org. Used with permission.

irregularities, insomnia, nervousness, tremors and headaches to seizures, heart attacks, strokes and death.

Many ephedra-containing herbal fen-phen products also contain hypericum perforatum, an herb commonly known as St. John's wort and sometimes referred to as "herbal Prozac." The actions and possible side effects of St. John's wort have not been studied under carefully controlled trials either alone or in combination with ephedra.

Other herbal fen-phen products contain 5-hydroxy-tryptophan, a compound closely related to L-tryptophan, a dietary supplement widely used in the U.S. until 1990. Used primarily as a sleep aid, L-tryptophan was pulled from the market after it was found to be linked to more than 1,500 cases, including about 38 deaths, of a rare blood disorder known as eosinophilia myalgia syndrome. (From FDA Talk Paper T97-56, Nov. 6, 1997)

Chapter 37

Dieter's Brews Make Tea Time a Dangerous Affair

A cup of hot herbal tea may feel soothing to the soul, but instead of soothing the body, some herbal teas can make you sick.

This is especially true with so-called dieter's teas, herbal teas containing senna, aloe, buckthorn, and other plant-derived laxatives that, when consumed in excessive amounts, can cause diarrhea, vomiting, nausea, stomach cramps, chronic constipation, fainting, and perhaps death.

In recent years, the Food and Drug Administration (FDA) has received "adverse event" reports, including the deaths of four young women, in which dieter's teas may have been a contributing factor.

As a result, FDA is advising consumers to follow package directions carefully when using dieter's teas and other dietary supplements containing senna, aloe, and other stimulant laxatives. Consumers should seek medical attention for persistent diarrhea, abdominal cramps, and other bowel problems to prevent more serious complications.

The agency may consider requiring manufacturers to place a warning about the products' potential side effects on the products' labels. Some manufacturers already are doing so voluntarily.

These products—bought in health food stores and through mail-order catalogs, for example—often are used for weight loss based on some consumers' belief that increased bowel movements will prevent

---

Paula Kurtzweil, *FDA Consumer*, July-August 1997, FDA Pub. No. 97-1286, e-text revised December 1997, http://www.fda.gov/fdac/features/1997/597_tea.html.

193

absorption of calories, thus preventing weight gain. However, a special committee of FDA's Food Advisory Committee concluded in 1995 that studies show that laxative-induced diarrhea does not significantly reduce absorption of calories. This is because the laxatives do not work on the small intestine, where calories are absorbed, but rather on the colon, the lower end of the bowel.

Juice drinks and tablets also may contain stimulant laxatives. FDA usually regulates these products as foods under the Federal Food, Drug, and Cosmetic Act. If the products are represented as dietary supplements, they are regulated under the Dietary Supplement Health and Education Act of 1994.

Stimulant Laxatives

The stimulant laxative teas and dietary supplements FDA is most concerned about contain one or more of the substances senna, aloe, rhubarb root, buckthorn, cascara, and castor oil. These plant-derived products have been used since ancient times for their ability to promote bowel movements and relieve constipation. Several, such as cascara, senna and castor oil, also are available as over-the-counter drug laxatives and are regulated as drugs.

Some of these substances also are used in much smaller quantities as natural flavorings in other foods. As such, they are regulated by FDA as food additives or "generally recognized as safe" substances. FDA has not received any information suggesting that these substances pose a hazard when used in the amounts normally needed to provide flavoring.

Except when used solely as flavorings, the names of these plant substances appear in the ingredient list on the label of these products. Dieter's teas and similar products often list the substances at or near the top because they often are the main ingredients. FDA proposed in December 1995 to require manufacturers to declare dietary ingredients, including proprietary blends, in descending order of predominance by weight on product labels. In the proposed rule, the substance would have to be given by its common or usual name: for example, Tinnevelly senna followed by its Latin name, Cassia angustifolia.

Most consumers who use dieter's teas and similar products know that the products have laxative properties, according to health professionals familiar with the products, even though the product labeling does not specifically state the term "laxative." Instead, the labeling may promote the product as a natural bowel cleanser. Sometimes it may not reflect the laxative qualities at all.

Dieter's Brews Make Tea Time a Dangerous Affair

The product labels may not directly state that the products are for weight loss, although some allude to it. For instance, some products use the terms "dieter's," "diet," "trim," or "slim" in their names. Others may carry information on weight-loss practices, mentioning consumption of the product along with the weight-loss practices. Some of the teas are labeled as "low-calorie." Unless sweetened, they provide essentially no nutrients and no calories.

According to Ara DerMarderosian, Ph.D., professor of pharmacognosy (study of medicinal products in their crude, or unprepared, form) and medicinal chemistry at the Philadelphia College of Pharmacy and Science, users favor the products because they believe that the products may cost less and taste better than over-the-counter laxatives and because they are easy to buy. In addition, he said, people with eating disorders, such as bulimia and anorexia nervosa, may like the products because they act quickly and produce loose, watery stools. Unfortunately, this practice is not only useless for losing weight but can be dangerous for people on severely restricted diets.

Writing in the January 1996 *American Druggist*, DerMarderosian and his colleague Sharon Brudnicki, a registered pharmacist also with the Philadelphia College of Pharmacy and Science, noted that some users like dieter's tea and other stimulant laxatives for their purported "body cleansing" ability.

DerMarderosian was a member of the FDA Food Advisory Committee's 1995 special task group on stimulant laxative substances in food.

Adverse Effects

Reports filed with FDA indicate that users tend to experience adverse effects when they misuse the products by, for example, steeping the tea longer than product labeling recommends or drinking more than the recommended amount. The reports indicate three types of adverse events:

- Short-term: stomach cramps, nausea, vomiting, and diarrhea lasting several days. These symptoms are likely to occur in first-time users who drink more than the recommended amount.

- Chronic: chronic diarrhea, pain, and constipation due to laxative dependency, which causes a sluggish bowel. In one report to FDA, a person who reported using herbal products with stimulant laxatives for decades suffered severe pain and constipation from loss of colon function and required surgery to remove the colon. People who develop chronic problems usually have used these types of products for years.

- Severe: fainting, dehydration and electrolyte disorders (for example, low blood potassium, a condition that can cause paralysis, irregular heartbeat, and possibly death). People who develop severe problems tend to be those who are nutritionally compromised, partly as a result of drastic reductions in food intake—for example, rigorous weight-loss dieters and people with the eating disorders anorexia nervosa and bulimia. Four deaths reported to FDA involved women with a history of such medical problems. According to information presented at a 1995 meeting of FDA's Food Advisory Committee, these herbal stimulant laxatives may have been a contributing factor in their deaths.

Label Warning

At the 1995 meeting, the advisory committee's task group agreed that dietary supplements containing stimulant laxatives can have adverse effects and that a label statement would be helpful in warning consumers about the risks and reducing the incidence of these adverse effects. The group proposed this label warning:

"NOTICE (or WARNING): Contains herbs (insert name of herbs) that can act as stimulant laxatives. Prolonged steeping time can increase the risk of adverse laxative effects, including: nausea, vomiting, abdominal cramps, and diarrhea. Chronic use of laxatives can impair colon function. Use of laxatives may be hazardous in the presence of abdominal pain, nausea, vomiting, or rectal bleeding. Laxative-induced diarrhea does not significantly reduce absorption of food calories. Acute or chronic diarrhea may result in serious injury or death."

The full advisory committee concurred with the recommendations.
California has taken steps to require a similar warning label statement on all food products containing stimulant laxatives sold in that state. Some manufacturers have begun to carry the state's drafted warning statement on their food products. FDA will monitor products sold nationally to be sure that their labels carry information similar to that required in California.

Dieter's Brews Make Tea Time a Dangerous Affair

Consumer Action

The California warning advises all users of these types of dietary supplements to:

- Read and follow package directions carefully.
- Stop using the product if diarrhea, loose stools, or stomach pain develop.
- See a doctor if frequent diarrhea develops.
- See a doctor before using the product if the user is pregnant, nursing, taking medication, or has a medical condition.

Consumers should report adverse effects associated with use of laxative teas or supplements to FDA by calling FDA's MedWatch adverse event and product problem hotline at 1-800-FDA-1088. Additional information about the MedWatch program can be found at www.fda.gov/medwatch/report/consumer/consumer.htm on FDA's website. They also may write to FDA at 5600 Fishers Lane, HFC-160, Rockville, MD 20857.

The report should include:

- name, address and telephone number of the person who became ill
- name and address of the doctor or hospital providing medical treatment
- description of the problem
- name of the product and store where it was bought.

Consumers also should report the problem to the manufacturer or distributor listed on the product's label and to the store where the product was bought.

FDA encourages health professionals to report serious adverse reactions, too, if the reaction appears related to the patient's use of dieter's teas or similar products. Health professionals can call FDA's MedWatch adverse event and product problem hotline at 1-800-FDA-1088. They can get more information about reporting adverse reactions to FDA from www.fda.gov/medwatch/report/hcp.htm on FDA's website.

—by Paula Kurtzweil

Paula Kurtzweil is a member of FDA's public affairs staff.

Chapter 38

A Fat Regulator in the Body

Leptin, a hormone made by the body's fat cells, is thought to play a role in regulating body fat by acting as an appetite suppressor. Leptin was discovered only as recently as 1994. Researchers are trying to understand its underlying mechanisms. Apparently, leptin not only regulates fat, but seems to have additional roles as well.

When leptin functions properly, it signals the body to stop eating by producing a feeling of fullness. High leptin levels in obese individuals may reflect malfunctioning of leptin.

People with high leptin levels in the blood are more likely to have insulin resistance than those with lower levels. Insulin resistance is a condition in which cells do not respond effectively to insulin's message to take up sugar from the bloodstream. People with insulin resistance are at greater risk of developing diabetes, high blood pressure, and low levels of the beneficial high-density lipoprotein (HDL) cholesterol. These conditions can contribute to heart disease development.

Cholesterol is a poor predictor of heart disease. Some people with normal-range blood cholesterol nevertheless have heart attacks. Measuring blood leptin levels might be a better marker for the potential risk of heart disease in people who show none of the traditional signs associated with this condition, including high blood cholesterol.

Leptin may play a role in diseases associated with a fat abdomen, a feature common in aging. A person with an "apple" shaped body, with

---

Beatrice Trum Hunter, *Consumers' Research Magazine*, July 1999, Vol. 82, I. 7, p. 8, copyright 1999 Consumers' Research Inc. Reprinted with permission.

fat deposited mainly around the waist rather than on the thighs or hips, is at greater risk of insulin resistance and heart disease.

In rat studies, leptin enhanced insulin's effects significantly. Moderately obese animals, given an infusion of leptin for eight days, ate less and lost weight. The fat loss from their abdomens was greater than from other body parts.

Leptin may regulate weight in young children. Lactating women have lower concentrations of leptin in their milk than in their blood. The breast may not make or concentrate leptin, but passes leptin to the nursing infant from the mother's blood, indirectly, through the milk. This finding suggests that the leptin delivered in breast milk may lead to some mechanism that regulates the child's weight later in life. If this is confirmed, it adds yet another benefit, among many, offered by breast milk but not available from feeding formulas.

In experiments with mice, injected leptin helped obese animals lose weight. Could this have similar effects in overweight humans? Leptin passed safety tests, and was injected into 70 obese adult volunteers in the Program of Obesity and Metabolism at Tufts University. All participants were on individually tailored weight-reduction diets that provided 500 kilocalories less than each person's basic daily energy needs. By the end of the first month, all participants lost weight. The amounts lost were proportionate to their leptin intake levels. Those injected with the highest leptin amounts lost an average of nearly 16 pounds each over six months. Some participants lost weight at all dose levels, but the amount of weight loss was highly variable.

Leptin may play a role in adult onset type 2 diabetes and in heart disease. A study of 74 healthy men showed that those with the highest leptin concentration in blood were at highest risk of suffering from insulin resistance.

Leptin may play an immunologic role. A group of immune cells, known as helper T cells, have leptin receptors (surface proteins that allow a cell to respond to leptin). Leptin encourages helper T cells to secrete certain chemicals that guide the actions of the immune system. For example, they help ward off viruses, bacteria, and fungi. This finding may explain why malnourished people are so vulnerable to many infectious diseases. Malnourishment leads to extensive metabolic and hormonal changes in the body.

Currently, researchers are investigating leptin to learn whether it can prevent malnourished mice from suffering increased rates of infection. If results are positive, leptin could serve as an immune system booster for low birth weight babies who often experience a wasting syndrome.

A Fat Regulator in the Body

By leptin's signaling malnutrition or starvation, the body knows when to shut down energy-expensive functions. For example, women with little body fat, such as marathon runners or ballet dancers, often stop menstruating. The body may have interpreted a leptin lack as a signal to avoid reproduction. Falling leptin concentrations in the blood may instruct the body to suspend temporarily the actions of the immune system.

Leptin has been found to play another role, in helping to maintain a balance between the blood supply and the fat tissue mass. Leptin may stimulate the growth of new blood vessels needed when fat increases in volume. Also, leptin may spur the growth of endothelial cells that form blood vessels in the maturing egg and early embryo. Also, it may spur wound healing. Leptin may be deployed by some cancer cells to recruit blood vessels. If any tumors are found to make leptin, this finding might serve as a useful tool to control tumor growth.

Commonly used weight-control measures such as diet and exercise, as well as drugs, may produce short-term success but not sustained weight loss. For most people, according to Gerald Bernstein, M.D., president of the American Diabetes Association, "weight loss is an ordeal that requires a truly punitive lifestyle that includes a remarkable reduction in calories." The discovery of leptin as fat regulator, as well as its other roles in the body, contributes fresh insights for long-recognized problems.

Chapter 39

New Drugs, Safer Surgery May Help Overcome Overweight and Obesity

It's official. The fattening of America has reached epidemic proportions. According to the National Institutes of Health, nearly half of American adults are now either overweight or obese—10% and 20% over ideal weight, respectively.

For many people, weight gain is simply a matter of eating too much and exercising too little. But for some, more powerful tools may be needed to manage chronic overweight. With Redux and the now infamous drug combo fen-phen out of the picture, what options are there for those with intractable weight problems?

Meridia

New to the market this year, Meridia (sibutramine), a prescription drug, is the latest weapon in the fight against fat. Much like the now-banned diet drugs Redux and fenfluramine—the "fen" half of fen-phen—Meridia boosts brain levels of serotonin and norepinephrine, natural neurotransmitters thought to help control appetite. Why is Meridia loose on the market, when Redux and fen-phen have been ousted?

While all three drugs raise neurotransmitter levels, each goes about it differently. Redux and fenfluramine work by stimulating the body to churn out more of the brain chemicals, which sometimes results in dangerously high levels. Meridia acts by slowing the body's breakdown of neurotransmitters. Researchers think this results in

Densie Webb, *Environmental Nutrition*, November 1998, p. 1, Copyright 1998 Environmental Nutrition Inc. Reprinted with permission.

only slightly elevated levels, making it theoretically safer. But studies so far have tracked the drug's effects only for one year.

What's the downside? You still have to cut calories and, like most prescription drugs, Meridia comes with a long list of caveats. Most important among them, Meridia can trigger an increase in blood pressure and heart rate in some people, so it is not recommended for those with coronary artery disease, congestive heart failure, arrhythmias or a history of stroke. Less serious side effects include dry mouth, headache and constipation.

To qualify for Meridia you must be healthy, not taking medications that could interact with it, and your Body Mass Index (BMI)—a measure of weight relative to height—must be 30 or more [see the "Practical Dietary Therapy Information" chapter of this sourcebook for information on calculating your BMI]. In other words, this is not a drug for those with only a few pounds to lose.

Xenical

Though not yet approved by the Food and Drug Administration (FDA), Xenical (orlistat) should be available in the U.S. in 1999, according to its maker, Roche Pharmaceuticals [editors note: orlistat was approved by FDA in spring 1999]. Unlike typical diet drugs, which suppress appetite, Xenical is a lipase inhibitor, a true "fat-blocker." It blocks the absorption of up to 30% of fat consumed. Like Meridia and Redux, however, Xenical is intended only for people with serious weight problems (BMI over 30).

And there's a twist. Other diet drugs often come with instructions to follow a low-fat, low-calorie diet, although ignoring that advice only means less weight lost. With Xenical, however, if you don't follow the prescribed low-fat diet, you'll be sorry. Xenical blocks almost one-third of the fat you eat... and it has to go somewhere. The end result of the excess fat can be diarrhea, bloating, and gas. Fat-soluble nutrients are swept away as well, so vitamin supplementation is likely to be a part of the Xenical prescription.

Early concerns about the drug included possible increased risk of breast cancer. But researchers are now convinced that finding was an anomaly. Most studies have found Xenical to be safe and effective for up to two years. One study found an average weight loss of almost 23 pounds in obese people taking the drug for one year, compared to 13 pounds in a control group.

What if Meridia and Xenical are prescribed as a diet-drug duet? Such a combination hasn't been tested, but it's very likely physicians

New Drugs, Safer Surgery May Help

will prescribe both, says Samuel Klein, M.D., of the North American Association for the Study of Obesity. After all, the fen-phen drugs were never tested or approved as a combo either.

Moreover, no study has factored in the new unabsorbable fat-substitute Olean (olestra). One wonders about the potential for literally explosive consequences in someone who is taking Xenical and eating Olean-containing foods.

Leptin

This hormone, produced naturally by fat cells, is believed to dampen appetite and rev up metabolism. Researchers at The Rockefeller University in New York discovered it in 1995, subsequently garnering front-page headlines and generating more excitement than studies warranted.

But a recent study by European researchers found that daily high-dose injections of leptin given to obese people who also followed a reduced-calorie diet resulted in significant weight loss—an average 8% loss over 6 months—with no side effects. Best of all, most of the weight lost was body fat, not lean muscle mass. Though leptin clearly has potential, Klein cautions the findings are preliminary. Expect to hear more about this drug in the future.

Surgery

Obesity surgery, such as stomach banding and gastric bypass, has traditionally been thought of as a last-ditch effort only for the massively obese. That might be changing. Until now, qualifying for surgery required a BMI of at least 40—or about 100 pounds over ideal weight. And surgery was considered risky, at best.

Now, research is showing benefits for a wider group of people and new techniques that are less invasive and less risky. Stomach banding—a method of stomach reduction similar to stomach stapling—can now be performed laparoscopically, resulting in few serious complications. "This may tip the scales in favor of surgery for those with a BMI between 35 and 40," says Klein.

But surgery is still not for everyone. A candidate must be relatively healthy, with medical conditions (e.g. high blood pressure, diabetes) under control and must be prepared to change eating patterns totally. A smaller stomach makes it necessary to eat several small meals, rather than three squares, a day.

Diet vs. Drugs: According to Louis Aronne, M.D., a weight control expert at Cornell University Medical College, those who treat overweight are in the middle of a paradigm shift from looking at obesity as a behavioral problem to viewing it as a medical one. Yet, whether overweight people opt for Meridia, wait for Xenical or leptin, or settle on surgery, a healthful, low-fat, low-calorie diet paired with regular exercise is still an essential part of the weight management equation. One tool without the other just doesn't make sense.

Summary: New and Future Tools to Combat Obesity

Meridia (Sibutramine)

Pros

- elevates serotonin and norepinephrin (natural appetite suppressors) less than now-banned Redux and fenfluramine
- effectively cuts appetite

Cons

- only for those with a BMI over 30
- safety known only for one year of use
- must still follow a low-calorie diet
- some people may experience an increase in blood pressure and heart rate
- side effects include dry mouth, headache, constipation

Xenical (Orlistat)

Pros

- blocks up to 30% of fat consumed
- clinical studies confirm potential for weight loss

Cons

- only for those with a BMI over 30
- safety known only for two-year period of use
- must follow a low-fat diet or will experience diarrhea, bloating and gas
- fat-soluble vitamins lost along with fat

Leptin

Pros

- may curb appetite and rev up metabolism
- weight lost from fat, not muscle
- no side effects noted so far

Cons

- findings too preliminary for marketability yet
- it appears some people may benefit from leptin, but many will not

Laparoscopic Surgery

Pros

- less invasive with fewer complications than traditional stomach reduction surgery

Cons

- only for those with a BMI over 35, who are healthy, with medical conditions under control
- risk associated with any surgery
- requires a change in eating patterns: very small, frequent meals and liquids between meals

—by Densie Webb, Ph.D., R.D.

Chapter 40

Gastric Surgery for Severe Obesity

Introduction

Severe obesity is a chronic condition that is very difficult to treat. Surgery to promote weight loss by restricting food intake or interrupting digestive processes is an option for severely obese people. A body mass index (BMI) above 40—which means about 100 pounds of overweight for men and about 80 pounds for women—indicates that a person is severely obese and therefore a candidate for surgery. Surgery also may be an option for people with a BMI between 35 and 40 who suffer from life-threatening cardiopulmonary problems (for example, severe sleep apnea or obesity-related heart disease) or diabetes. However, as in other treatments for obesity, successful results depend mainly on motivation and behavior.

The Normal Digestive Process

Normally, as food moves along the digestive tract (see Figure 40.1), appropriate digestive juices and enzymes arrive at the right place at the right time to digest and absorb calories and nutrients. After we chew and swallow our food, it moves down the esophagus to the stomach, where a strong acid continues the digestive process. The stomach

---

Weight-Control Information Network (WIN), National Institute of Diabetes, Digestive, and Kidney Diseases (NIDDK), National Institutes of Health (NIH), NIH Pub. No. 96-4006, http://www.niddk.nih.gov/health/nutrit/pubs/gastsurg.htm, April 1996, e-text posted February 20, 1998.

can hold about 3 pints of food at one time. When the stomach contents move to the duodenum, the first segment of the small intestine, bile and pancreatic juice speed up digestion. Most of the iron and calcium in the foods we eat is absorbed in the duodenum. The jejunum and ileum, the remaining two segments of the nearly 20 feet of small intestine, complete the absorption of almost all calories and nutrients. The food particles that cannot be digested in the small intestine are stored in the large intestine until eliminated.

How Does Surgery Promote Weight Loss?

The concept of gastric surgery to control obesity grew out of results of operations for cancer or severe ulcers that removed large portions of the stomach or small intestine.

Because patients undergoing these procedures tended to lose weight after surgery, some physicians began to use such operations to treat severe obesity. The first operation that was widely used for severe obesity was the intestinal bypass. This operation, first used 40 years ago, produces weight loss by causing malabsorption. The idea was that patients could eat large amounts of food, which would be poorly digested or passed along too fast for the body to absorb many calories.

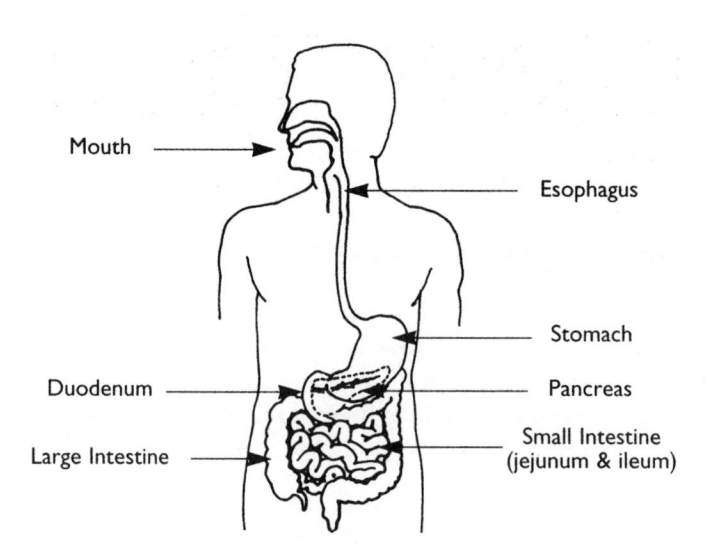

Figure 40.1. The digestive system.

Gastric Surgery for Severe Obesity

The problem with this surgery was that it caused a loss of essential nutrients and its side effects were unpredictable and sometimes fatal. The original form of the intestinal bypass operation is no longer used.

Surgeons now use techniques that produce weight loss primarily by limiting how much the stomach can hold. These restrictive procedures are often combined with modified gastric bypass procedures that somewhat limit calorie and nutrient absorption and may lead to altered food choices.

Two ways that surgical procedures promote weight loss are:

- By decreasing food intake (restriction). Gastric banding, gastric bypass, and vertical-banded gastroplasty are surgeries that limit the amount of food the stomach can hold by closing off or removing parts of the stomach. These operations also delay emptying of the stomach (gastric pouch).

- By causing food to be poorly digested and absorbed (malabsorption). In the gastric bypass procedures, a surgeon makes a direct connection from the stomach to a lower segment of the small intestine, bypassing the duodenum, and some of the jejunum.

Although results of operations using these procedures are more predictable and manageable, side effects persist for some patients.

What Are the Surgical Options?

Restriction Operations

Restriction operations are the surgeries most often used for producing weight loss. Food intake is restricted by creating a small pouch at the top of the stomach where the food enters from the esophagus. The pouch initially holds about 1 ounce of food and expands to 2–3 ounces with time. The pouch's lower outlet usually has a diameter of about 1/4 inch. The small outlet delays the emptying of food from the pouch and causes a feeling of fullness.

After an operation, the person usually can eat only a half to a whole cup of food without discomfort or nausea. Also, food has to be well chewed. For most people, the ability to eat a large amount of food at one time is lost, but some patients do return to eating modest amounts of food without feeling hungry.

Restriction operations for obesity include gastric banding and vertical banded gastroplasty. Both operations serve only to restrict food intake. They do not interfere with the normal digestive process.

Gastric banding. In this procedure, a band made of special material is placed around the stomach near its upper end, creating a small pouch and a narrow passage into the larger remainder of the stomach (see Figure 40.2). In the future, it may be possible to perform gastric banding with smaller incisions through a laparoscope, a flexible fiberoptic tube and light source through which some surgical instruments may be passed. Laparoscopic gastric banding has not yet been approved by the Food and Drug Administration.

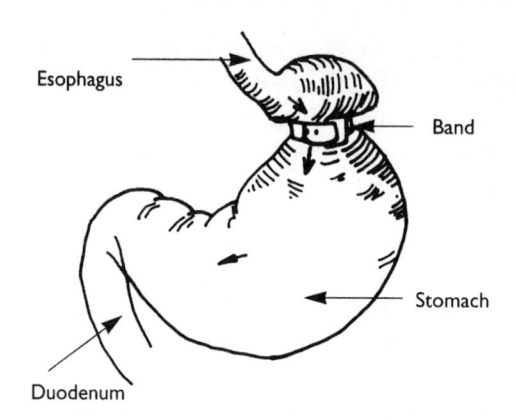

Figure 40.2. Gastric banding.

Vertical banded gastroplasty (VBG). This procedure is the most frequently used restrictive operation for weight control. As the figure illustrates, both a band and staples are used to create a small stomach pouch.

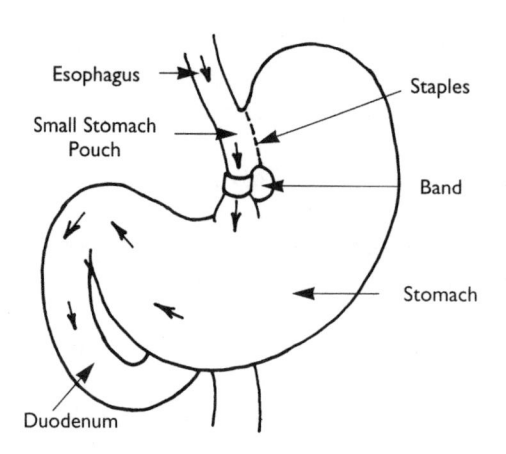

Figure 40.3. Vertical banded gastroplasty (VBG).

Gastric Surgery for Severe Obesity

Restrictive operations lead to weight loss in almost all patients. However, weight regain does occur in some patients. About 30 percent of persons undergoing vertical banded gastroplasty achieve normal weight, and about 80 percent achieve some degree of weight loss. However, some patients are unable to adjust their eating habits and fail to lose the desired weight. In all weight-loss operations, successful results depend on your motivation and behaviors.

A common risk of restrictive operations is vomiting caused by the small stomach being overly stretched by food particles that have not been chewed well. Other risks of VBG include erosion of the band, breakdown of the staple line, and, in a small number of cases, leakage of stomach juices into the abdomen. The latter requires an emergency operation. In a very small number of cases (less than 1 percent) infection or death from complications can occur.

Gastric Bypass Operations

These operations combine creation of small stomach pouches to restrict food intake and construction of bypasses of the duodenum and other segments of the small intestine to cause malabsorption.

Roux-en-Y gastric bypass (RGB). This operation (see Figure 40.4) is the most common gastric bypass procedure. First, a small stomach pouch is created by stapling or by vertical banding. This causes restriction in food intake. Next, a Y-shaped section of the small intestine is attached to the pouch to allow food to bypass the duodenum (the first segment of the small intestine) as well as the first portion of the jejunum (the second segment of the small intestine). This causes reduced calorie and nutrient absorption.

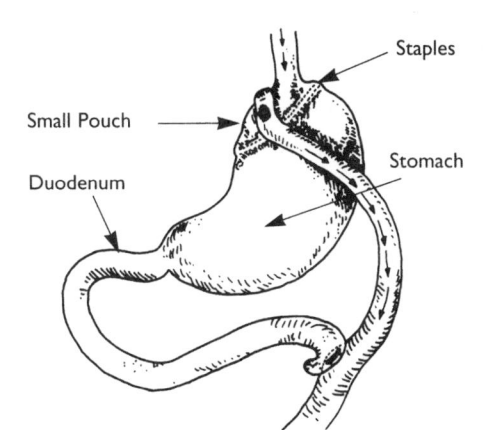

Figure 40.4. Roux-en-Y gastric bypass (RGB)

Obesity Sourcebook, First Edition

Extensive gastric bypass (biliopancreatic diversion). In this more complicated gastric bypass operation, portions of the stomach are removed. The small pouch that remains is connected directly to the final segment of the small intestine, thus completely bypassing both the duodenum and jejunum. Although this procedure successfully promotes weight loss, it is not widely used because of the high risk for nutritional deficiencies.

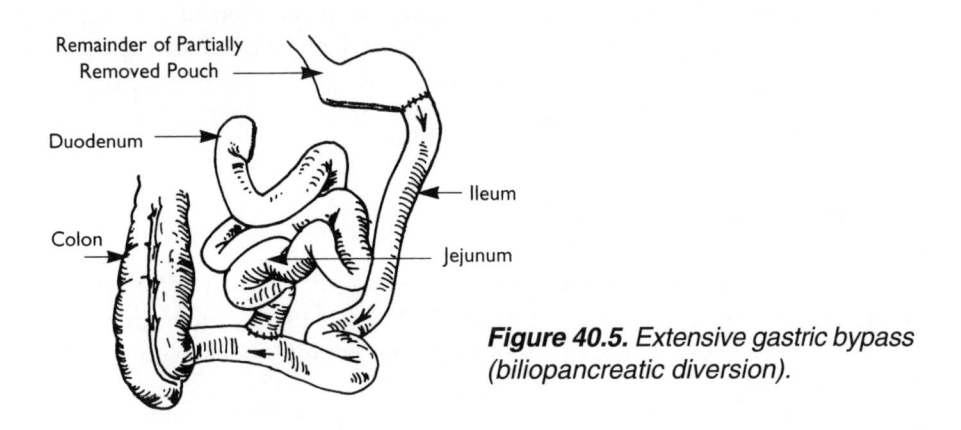

Figure 40.5. Extensive gastric bypass (biliopancreatic diversion).

Gastric bypass operations that cause malabsorption and restrict food intake produce more weight loss than restriction operations that only decrease food intake. Patients who have bypass operations generally lose two-thirds of their excess weight within 2 years.

The risks for pouch stretching, band erosion, breakdown of staple lines, and leakage of stomach contents into the abdomen are about the same for gastric bypass as for vertical banded gastroplasty. However, because gastric bypass operations cause food to skip the duodenum, where most iron and calcium are absorbed, risks for nutritional deficiencies are higher in these procedures. Anemia may result from malabsorption of vitamin B12 and iron in menstruating women, and decreased absorption of calcium may bring on osteoporosis and metabolic bone disease. Patients are required to take nutritional supplements that usually prevent these deficiencies.

Gastric bypass operations also may cause "dumping syndrome," whereby stomach contents move too rapidly through the small intestine. Symptoms include nausea, weakness, sweating, faintness, and, occasionally, diarrhea after eating, as well as the inability to eat

Gastric Surgery for Severe Obesity

sweets without becoming so weak and sweaty that the patient must lie down until the symptoms pass.

The more extensive the bypass operation, the greater is the risk for complications and nutritional deficiencies. Patients with extensive bypasses of the normal digestive process require not only close monitoring, but also life-long use of special foods and medications.

Explore Benefits and Risks

Surgery to produce weight loss is a serious undertaking. Each individual should clearly understand what the proposed operation involves. Patients and physicians should carefully consider the following benefits and risks:

Benefits

Immediately following surgery, most patients lose weight rapidly and continue to do so until 18 to 24 months after the procedure. Although most patients then start to regain some of their lost weight, few regain it all.

Surgery improves most obesity-related conditions. For example, in one study blood sugar levels of most obese patients with diabetes returned to normal after surgery. Nearly all patients whose blood sugar levels did not return to normal were older or had had diabetes for a long time.

Risks

Ten to 20 percent of patients who have weight-loss operations require follow-up operations to correct complications. Abdominal hernias are the most common complications requiring follow-up surgery. Less common complications include breakdown of the staple line and stretched stomach outlets.

More than one-third of obese patients who have gastric surgery develop gallstones. Gallstones are clumps of cholesterol and other matter that form in the gallbladder. During rapid or substantial weight loss a person's risk of developing gallstones is increased. Gallstones can be prevented with supplemental bile salts taken for the first 6 months after surgery.

Nearly 30 percent of patients who have weight-loss surgery develop nutritional deficiencies such as anemia, osteoporosis, and metabolic bone disease. These deficiencies can be avoided if vitamin and mineral intakes are maintained.

Women of childbearing age should avoid pregnancy until their weight becomes stable because rapid weight loss and nutritional deficiencies can harm a developing fetus.

Is the Surgery for You?

For patients who remain severely obese after non-surgical approaches to weight loss have failed, or for patients who have an obesity-related disease, surgery may be the best next step. But for other patients, greater efforts toward weight control, such as changes in eating habits, behavior modification, and increasing physical activity, may be more appropriate. Answers to the following questions may help in your decision to undergo surgery for weight loss.

Are you:

- unlikely to lose weight successfully with (further) non-surgical measures?
- well informed about the surgical procedure and the effects of treatment?
- determined to lose weight and improve your health?
- aware of how your life may change after the operation (adjustment to the side effects of the surgery, including need to chew well and inability to eat large meals)?
- aware of the potential for serious complications, the associated dietary restrictions, and the occasional failures?
- committed to lifelong medical follow-up?

Do you:

- have a BMI of 40 or more?
- have an obesity-related physical problem (such as body size that interferes with employment, walking, or family function)?
- have high-risk obesity-related health problems (such as severe sleep apnea or obesity-related heart disease)?

Remember: There are no guarantees for any method, including surgery, to produce and maintain weight loss. Success is possible only with your fullest cooperation and commitment to behavioral change and medical follow-up—and this cooperation and commitment should be carried out for the rest of your life.

Part Four

Obesity Issues for Special Populations and the Prevention of Obesity

Chapter 41

Obesity in Minority Populations

Overweight and obesity occur at higher rates in racial-ethnic minority populations such as African American and Hispanic Americans, compared with White Americans in the US. Asian-Americans have a relatively low prevalence for obesity. Women and persons of low socioeconomic status within minority populations appear to particularly be affected by overweight and obesity. Cultural factors that influence dietary and exercise behaviors are reported to play a major role in the development of excess weight in minority groups.

Prevalence

Overweight

- Mexican American and black (non-Hispanic) adults in the US, age 20 to 74, are considerably more overweight than whites (non-Hispanic).

- American Indians have very high prevalence rates of overweight. Among the highest rates reported are for American Indians in Arizona at 80% for women and 67% for men.

From the American Obesity Association website, http://www.obesity.org/Obesity_Minority_Populations.htm, September 1999, copyright 1999 American Obesity Association. Reprinted with permission of the American Obesity Association.

Obesity

- Mexican American and black (non-Hispanic) adults in the US also have higher prevalence of obesity than whites (non-Hispanic).

Gender

- For women, the prevalence of overweight is highest among Mexican Americans at 67.6% and the obesity rate is highest among blacks (non-Hispanic) at 37.4 %.
- For men, Mexican Americans have the highest prevalence of overweight at 67.1%, and obesity at 23.1%.

Socioeconomic Status (SES)

- Overweight affects African American women and men across all SES levels.
- Minority women with low income appear to have the greatest likelihood of being overweight.
- Among Mexican American women, age 20 to 74, the rate of overweight is about 13% higher for women living below the poverty line versus above the poverty line.

Health Disparities

- Many obesity-related diseases including diabetes, hypertension, cancer, and heart disease are found in higher rates among various members of racial-ethnic minorities compared with whites.

Diabetes

- Diabetes occurs at a rate of 16% to 26% in Hispanic Americans and black Americans, age 45 to 74, compared with 12% in whites (non-Hispanic) of the same age.
- Higher Body Mass Index (BMI) predicts the risk for type 2 diabetes in Pima Indians. Type 2 diabetes affects about half of the Pima people.
- Among 15 American Indian tribes studied in Oklahoma, 77% of adults screened for diabetes are reported to be obese.

Obesity in Minority Populations

- Among Mexican Americans, obesity and type 2 diabetes are both increasing, unlike other risk factors of cardiovascular disease including smoking and blood pressure, which are declining.

Cancer

- Obesity appears to contribute to the higher risk of pancreatic cancer among black Americans than among whites, particularly for women.

Heart Disease

- Among African Americans, the high prevalence of obesity and obesity-related conditions such as hypertension and type 2 diabetes, are factors reported to contribute to their high death rate from coronary heart disease.
- In a study of older Hispanics, with an average age of 80, obesity was found to be a risk factor for developing coronary artery disease.

Hypertension

- The high prevalence of obesity is reported to be a contributing factor to the high prevalence of hypertension in minority populations, especially among African Americans who have an earlier onset and run a more severe course of hypertension.

Behavioral Risk Factors

Diet and Exercise

- Cultural factors related to dietary choices, physical activity, and acceptance of excess weight among African Americans and other racial-ethnic groups, appear to play a role in interfering with weight loss efforts.
- Sedentary life style, which can contribute to the development of obesity, has been reported by 44% to 60% of Native American men and 40% to 65% of women.
- African Americans and whites report that they exercise less as they get older, however, African American women of all ages report participating in less regular exercise than white women.

- African American men, age 45 and older, report less regular exercise than white men of the same age.

Readers should note that researchers have not always used the same criteria to identify overweight and obesity. In this fact sheet, the American Obesity Association (AOA) has attempted to use the generally accepted definitions for overweight as a Body Mass Index (BMI) of 25–29.9 and obesity as a BMI of 30 or above. We have made an effort to identify studies which have used these specific definitions as well as other scientifically accepted measurements such as waist circumference and waist-to-hip ratio.

Chapter 42

Women and Obesity

Obesity plays a significant role in causing poor health in women, negatively affecting quality of life and shortening quantity of life. More than half of adult U.S. women are overweight, and nearly one quarter are obese. The life expectancy of women in the U.S. is approaching 80 years of age, and more women than ever are expected to turn 65 in the second decade of the new millennium. Prevention and early treatment of obesity are crucial to ensuring a healthy population of women of all ages.

Prevalence

For women, age 20 and above, 50.7% are overweight (Body Mass Index, or BMI greater than 25) and about half of those are obese. The percentage of women in specific categories of excess weight is shown in Table 42.1.

Socioeconomic Status (SES)

- Obesity appears to have a strong inverse relationship with SES (obesity increases as income level decreases) among women in developed societies such as the U.S.

From the American Obesity Association website, http://www.obesity.org/Obesity_Women.htm, September 1999, copyright 1999 American Obesity Association. Reprinted with permission of the American Obesity Association.

- Low-income women in minority populations appear most likely to be overweight.

Age

Women are more likely to become overweight as they become older.

Middle-aged women are at a particularly high risk of becoming obese. The prevalence of obesity among middle-aged women has increased about 1% per year over a 34 year time period from 1960 to 1994. More women between the ages of 30 and 60 are considered obese than nearly 25 years ago.

Race

- More Mexican American and black (non-Hispanic) women are overweight and obese, in all BMI categories, compared to white (non-Hispanic) women.

- The combined prevalence of overweight and obesity for Mexican American women (67.6%) and black (non-Hispanic) women (66.5%) is more than 30% greater in proportion to that of white (non-Hispanic) women (45.5%).

- Over 10% of black (non-Hispanic) women, age 40 to 59, have severe obesity.

Table 42.1. Percentage of women who are overweight (listed according to Body Mass Index, or BMI).

Weight category in Body Mass Index (BMI)	Prevalence (%)
Overweight (BMI: 25 to 29.9)	25.7
Obesity (BMI 30)	24.9
Class I Obesity (BMI: 30 to 34.9)	14.5
Class II Obesity (BMI: 35 to 39.9)	6.6
Class III Severe Obesity (BMI 40)	3.8

Women and Obesity

Mortality

- A direct association has been found between body weight and deaths from all causes in women, age 30 to 55.

- More than 50% of deaths from all causes among adult US women can be attributed to obesity.

Health Effects

- There are many obesity-related conditions, which uniquely or mostly affect women, including those detailed below.

Arthritis

- Women with obesity have almost four times the risk of osteoarthritis as non-obese women.

- A stronger association between osteoarthritis and obesity has been observed in women than in men.

Birth Defects

- Maternal obesity (BMI greater than 29) has been associated with an increased incidence of neural tube defects (NTD) in several studies, although variable results have been found in this area.

- Folate intake, which decreases the risk of NTDs, was found in one study to have a reduced effect with higher pre-pregnancy weight.

Breast Cancer

- After menopause, women with obesity have a higher risk of developing breast cancer. In addition, weight gain after menopause may also increase breast cancer risk.

- Women who gain about 45 pounds or more after age 18 are twice as likely to develop breast cancer after menopause than women with no weight gain.

- Before menopause, high BMI has been associated with a decreased risk of breast cancer. However, a recent study found an increased risk of the most lethal form of breast cancer, called inflammatory breast cancer (IBC), in women with BMI as low as 26.7 regardless of menopausal status.

- Before menopause, women who are overweight and have breast cancer appear to have a shorter life span than women with lower BMI.

Endometrial Cancer (EC)

- Women with obesity have three to four times the risk of EC than women with lower BMI.
- An estimated 34% to 56% of EC risk can be attributed to overweight.
- Body size is a risk factor for EC regardless of where fat is distributed in the body. Women with obesity and diabetes have a 3-fold increase in risk for EC above the risk of obesity alone. Cardiovascular Disease (CVD)
- In middle and old age groups, heavier weight is associated with CVD and its risk factors, particularly for women.

Gallbladder Disease

- Obesity is the best-established predictor of gallbladder disease in women.
- Women with obesity have at least twice the risk of gallstone disease than women of normal weight.

Infertility

- Obesity has been found to affect ovulation, response to fertility treatment, pregnancy rates and pregnancy outcome.
- Infertile women with obesity who lose weight have shown improvement in becoming pregnant and reaching full term.

Obstetric and Gynecological Complications

- In addition to infertility, excess body fat can lead to complications such as menstrual abnormality, miscarriage, and difficulties in performing assisted reproduction.
- The frequency of menstrual disturbance in women with severe obesity is three times greater than for women of normal weight.

Women and Obesity

- High pre-pregnancy weight is associated with an increased risk of pregnancy hypertension, gestational diabetes, urinary infection, Cesarean section delivery, and toxemia.

- Women with obesity are 13 times more likely to have overdue births, longer labors, induced labor, and blood loss.

- Complications after childbirth related to obesity include an increased risk of wound and endometrial infection, endometritis, and urinary tract infection.

Urinary Stress Incontinence

- Obesity is a well-documented risk factor for the involuntary loss of urine as well as urgency.

- Obesity has been found to be a strong risk factor for women of several urinary symptoms after childbirth.

Stigma and Discrimination

- Women with obesity appear to have much more prejudice and discrimination directed against them than men with obesity.

- Obesity contributes to unemployment for women. After undergoing surgery to reduce obesity, a drop in unemployment rate from 84% to 64% was reported for women.

- Women with obesity face significant barriers in establishing and maintaining social relationships in a society that emphasizes thinness as physical attractiveness.

- Women with obesity have reported attending fewer years of college and receiving less financial support for higher education than women who are non-obese.

Readers should note that researchers have not always used the same criteria to identify overweight and obesity. In this fact sheet, the American Obesity Association (AOA) has attempted to use the generally accepted definitions for overweight as a Body Mass Index (BMI) of 25–29.9 and obesity as a BMI of 30 or above. We have made an effort to identify studies which have used these specific definitions as well as other scientifically accepted measurements such as waist circumference and waist to hip ratio.

Chapter 43

Native Americans: Helping Researchers Understand Obesity

History paints a colorful portrait of the American Indians who live today in the Gila River Indian Community. Their ancestors were among the first people to set foot in the Americas 30,000 years ago. They have lived in the Sonoron Desert near the Gila River in what is now southern Arizona for at least 2,000 years.

Called the Pima Indians by exploring Spaniards who first encountered them in the 1600s, these early Americans called themselves "O'Odham," the river people, and those with whom they intermarried, "Tohono O'Odham," the desert people.

Archaeological finds suggest that the Pima Indians descended from the Hohokam, "those who have gone," a prehistoric people who originated in Mexico. Strong runners, the Pima Indians were also master weavers and farmers who could make the desert bloom. Once trusted scouts for the U.S. Cavalry, the Pima Indians are pathfinders for health, helping scientists from the National Institute of Diabetes and Digestive and Kidney Diseases (NIDDK), a part of the National Institutes of Health (NIH), learn the secrets of diabetes, obesity, and their complications.

Migrating from Mexico, the people settled the land up to where the Gila River and the Salt River meet, in what is now Arizona. They established a sophisticated system of irrigation that made the desert fruitful

---

This chapter contains text from *The Pima Indians, Pathfinders for Health*, on the National Institute of Diabetes and Digestive and Kidney Diseases (NIDDK) website, National Institutes of Health (NIH), http://www.niddk.nih.gov/health/diabetes/pima/pathfind/pathfind.htm, 1995.

with wheat, beans, squash and cotton. The women of the community made exquisite baskets so intricately woven that they were watertight.

They were also a generous people. They sheltered the Pee Posh (or Maricopa Indians) who fled attack by hostile tribes, and who also became part of the Gila River community. Anyone who followed the Gila river, the main southern route to the Pacific, encountered these peaceful and productive traders who gave hospitality to travellers for hundreds of years. "Bread is to eat, not to sell. Take what you want," they told Kit Carson in 1846.

Today, the Pima Indians of the Gila River Indian Community are still an agricultural people, nurturing orchards of orange trees, pistachios and olives. They are still giving, too. Eleven thousand strong, the members of the Gila River Indian Reservation have participated in 30 years of research that will help people avoid diabetes, have healthier eyes, hearts, and kidneys, and to understand how and why people gain weight and what can be done to prevent it.

"The Pima Indians are giving a great gift to the world by continuing to volunteer for research studies. Their generosity contributes to better health for all people, and we are all in their debt," says Dr. Peter Bennett, Chief of the Phoenix Epidemiology and Clinical Research Branch of the NIDDK.

The Pima Indians' help is so important to the ability of doctors to understand and treat diabetes, obesity, and kidney disease because of the uniqueness of the community. There are few like it in the world.

Young Pima Indians often marry other Pimas. Many Pima families have lived in the Gila River Indian Community for generations. Because of this, scientists can search for root causes of disease through several generations of many families. The length of NIDDK's study and the number of families involved allows scientists an invaluable perspective on how the disease progresses. The more generations studied, the deeper and better the understanding of how diabetes affects people, and the greater the opportunity to develop drug or genetic therapy, or lifestyle changes that will slow or prevent the coming of disease.

The research takes so long, says NIH scientist Dr. Bill Knowler, because diseases like obesity and diabetes are so hard to understand. There seem to be several different causes, and the complex interaction between the genes a person inherits and the lifestyle a person chooses can make it hard to find treatments and cure. Scientists are trying to find a path through this maze.

Thirty years of research show that exercising and eating lower fat, fiber-rich foods can at least delay diabetes. "If you delay it long enough," adds Dr. Knowler, "It's almost as good as preventing it."

Native Americans: Helping Researchers Understand Obesity

This cooperative search between the Pima Indians and the NIH began in 1963 when the NIDDK (then called the National Institute of Arthritis, Diabetes and Digestive and Kidney Diseases), made a survey of rheumatoid arthritis among the Pimas and the Blackfeet of Montana. They discovered an extremely high rate of diabetes among the Pima Indians. Two years later, the Institute, the Indian Health Service, and the Pima community set out to find some answers to this mystery. They hoped to shed light on an even broader question: Why do Native Americans, Hispanics and other non-white peoples have up to ten times the rate of diabetes as Caucasians?

Three decades' collective efforts by scientists and volunteers have laid the foundation for eventually curing or preventing diabetes and its complications. The work begun in 1965 has yielded a definition of diabetes that is now used worldwide, and set out diagnostic criteria used by doctors from Sacaton, Arizona to Sicily to identify and treat diabetes and to anticipate how it is likely to develop.

Doctors can best treat a disease when they understand what causes it and how it progresses. By studying Pima volunteers for many years, NIH doctors learned that unhealthy weight is a strong predictor of diabetes. Eighty percent of people with diabetes are overweight. They also discovered that high levels of insulin in the blood, or hyperinsulinemia, is another strong risk factor.

Studying this clue, researchers working with patients found that high levels of insulin were linked to insulin resistance. Normally, the pancreas releases insulin to regulate the amount of sugar or glucose in the blood. People who have non-insulin-dependent or Type II diabetes (hereafter referred to simply as "diabetes") produce insulin, but their bodies don't respond to it effectively. NIH researchers have made it clear that people with insulin resistance are those most likely to get diabetes.

By studying Pima Indian volunteers, Dr. Clifton Bogardus and his colleagues established that glucose not needed for immediate energy is converted to glycogen and stored in skeletal muscle. However, several enzymes that drive this natural process appear different in insulin resistant people, according to the researchers, and they continue to study the biochemistry of insulin resistance to understand this breakdown and how it might be repaired.

By studying Pima Indian volunteers, researchers have determined that diabetes runs in families, as does insulin resistance, and obesity. Scientists believe that some people also have a gene that makes them more likely to have the kidney disease that occurs in people who have had diabetes a long time. Looking for these genes is a key part of the search now being conducted by NIH and the Pima Indians.

Researchers are working on this complex genetic puzzle by studying blood drawn from every member of the Pima community who comes into the NIH clinic at Hu Hu Kam Memorial Hospital for an examination. Blood is checked for healthy levels of blood sugar, cholesterol, and other nutrients. Then, each person's blood and serum are typed and some is reduced to a very small pellet of DNA, the genetic material that instructs a person's cells to function one way or another. When NIH researchers find a family with one parent who is diabetic and one who is not, they are able to study the genes of both parents and their children in an effort to find the gene or genes shared by those who have diabetes.

After finding these genes, scientists hope to break the codes that cause insulin resistance, obesity, diabetes and kidney disease of diabetes. "If we can locate the genes contributing to disease—some enzyme being made or not being made," explains Dr. Knowler, "we can identify which people are at high risk for the disease and figure out ways to intervene." Finding these genes will help doctors identify youngsters at risk and begin prevention before disease sets in.

Another important finding has already made a difference in how diabetes patients are treated. The complications that come with long-term diabetes—kidney disease, eye disease, and amputations caused by nerve damage—are the major reasons for illness and death among the Pima Indians. When Dr. Knowler began his research in Phoenix, few understood what he and his colleagues would discover by working with Pima volunteers: that high blood pressure predicts complications of diabetes such as eye and kidney disease, and that lowering blood pressure may slow the onset of diabetes and the progress of already existing kidney disease. Because of this work, doctors today are not only aware of the need to treat high blood pressure in people with diabetes, but they begin treating it sooner than in the past.

"Our greatest pride," says Dr. Knowler, "is in conducting research that affects clinical practice."

Other research with important implications for future generations is Dr. David Pettitt's study of high blood sugar and diabetes in pregnant women. By working with Pima volunteers, Dr. Pettitt found that children born to diabetic women are more likely to be overweight and more likely to develop diabetes than children of women who have not developed diabetes.

Dr. Eric Ravussin conducts studies that measure food intake, metabolism, and energy expenditure to evaluate their interaction and contribution to a genetic predisposition to obesity.

Native Americans: Helping Researchers Understand Obesity

Now NIH and the Pima Indians are building on these accomplishments. "The search goes forward on two fronts," says Dr. Knowler. "We're working hard on the genetics of the disease. We're optimistic we will find one or more genes. It's still hard to predict how we might prevent diabetes, but we might, for example, be able eventually to correct the genetic difference that causes disease. More immediately, identifying the diabetes genes would allow us to identify the people most likely to get the disease."

The second strategy is to encourage those who are at high risk to change behaviors that can lead to diabetes, such as eating a high fat diet, being physically inactive, and being overweight.

The NIH has begun a major nation-wide program to prevent diabetes in people who increase exercise and eat lower fat foods. Fifty percent of the volunteers will be American Indians and other minorities, and once again, the Pima Indians will be prominent among them. Health for this and future generations: that's the NIH-Pima goal.

—by Jane DeMouy

Chapter 44

Helping Your Overweight Child

Introduction

In the United States at least one child in five is overweight and the number of overweight children continues to grow. Over the last 2 decades, this number has increased by more than 50 percent, and the number of "extremely" overweight children has nearly doubled (*Arch Pediatr Adolesc Med*. 1995: 149: 1085-91). A doctor determines if children are overweight by measuring their height and weight. Although children have fewer weight-related health problems than adults, overweight children are at high risk of becoming overweight adolescents and adults. Overweight adults are at risk for a number of health problems including heart disease, diabetes, high blood pressure, stroke, and some forms of cancer.

What Causes Children to Become Overweight?

Children become overweight for a variety of reasons. The most common causes are genetic factors, lack of physical activity, unhealthy eating patterns, or a combination of these factors. In rare cases, a medical problem, such as an endocrine disorder, may cause a child to become overweight. Your physician can perform a careful physical exam and some blood tests, if necessary, to rule out this type of problem.

Weight-Control Information Network (WIN), National Institute of Diabetes, Digestive, and Kidney Diseases (NIDDK), National Institutes of Health (NIH), NIH Pub. No. 97-4096, http://www.niddk.nih.gov/health/nutrit/pubs/helpchld.htm, January 1997, e-text updated February 10, 1998.

Genetic Factors

Children whose parents or brothers or sisters are overweight may be at an increased risk of becoming overweight themselves. Although weight problems run in families, not all children with a family history of obesity will be overweight. Genetic factors play a role in increasing the likelihood that a child will be overweight, but shared family behaviors such as eating and activity habits also influence body weight.

Lifestyle

A child's total diet and his or her activity level both play an important role in determining a child's weight. The increasing popularity of television and computer and video games contributes to children's inactive lifestyles. The average American child spends approximately 24 hours each week watching television—time that could be spent in some sort of physical activity.

Is My Child Overweight?

If you think that your child is overweight, it is important to talk with your child's doctor. A doctor is the best person to determine whether your child has a weight problem. Physicians will measure your child's weight and height to determine if your child's weight is within a healthy range. A physician will also consider your child's age and growth patterns to determine whether your child is overweight. Assessing overweight in children is difficult because children grow in unpredictable spurts.

For example, it is normal for boys to have a growth spurt in weight and catch up in height later. It is best to let your child's doctor determine whether your child will "grow into" a normal weight. If your doctor finds that your child is overweight, he or she may ask you to make some changes in your family's eating and activity habits.

How Can I Help My Overweight Child?

Be Supportive

One of the most important things you can do to help overweight children is to let them know that they are okay whatever their weight. Children's feelings about themselves often are based on their parents' feelings about them. If you accept your children at any weight, they

Helping Your Overweight Child

will be more likely to accept and feel good about themselves. It is also important to talk to your children about weight, allowing them to share their concerns with you. Your child probably knows better than anyone else that he or she has a weight problem. For this reason, overweight children need support, acceptance, and encouragement from their parents.

Focus on the Family

Parents should try not to set children apart because of their weight, but focus on gradually changing their family's physical activity and eating habits. Family involvement helps to teach everyone healthful habits and does not single out the overweight child.

Increase Your Family's Physical Activity

Regular physical activity, combined with healthy eating habits, is the most efficient and healthful way to control your weight. It is also an important part of a healthy lifestyle. Some simple ways to increase your family's physical activity include the following:

- Be a role model for your children. If your children see that you are physically active and have fun, they are more likely to be active and stay active for the rest of their lives.

- Plan family activities that provide everyone with exercise and enjoyment, like walking, dancing, biking, or swimming. For example, schedule a walk with your family after dinner instead of watching TV. Make sure that you plan activities that can be done in a safe environment.

- Be sensitive to your child's needs. Overweight children may feel uncomfortable about participating in certain activities. It is important to help your child find physical activities that they enjoy and that aren't embarrassing or too difficult.

- Reduce the amount of time you and your family spend in sedentary activities, such as watching TV or playing video games.

- Become more active throughout your day and encourage your family to do so as well. For example, walk up the stairs instead of taking the elevator, or do some activity during a work or school break-get up and stretch or walk around.

The point is not to make physical activity an unwelcome chore, but to make the most of the opportunities you and your family have to be active.

Teach Your Family Healthy Eating Habits

Teaching healthy eating practices early will help children approach eating with the right attitude—that food should be enjoyed and is necessary for growth, development, and for energy to keep the body running. The best way to begin is to learn more about children's nutritional needs by reading or talking with a health professional and then to offer them some healthy options, allowing your children to choose what and how much they eat.

Here Are Some Ways to Help Your Child Develop Good Attitudes about Eating

Don't Place Your Child on a Restrictive Diet

Children should never be placed on a restrictive diet to lose weight, unless a doctor supervises one for medical reasons. Limiting what children eat may be harmful to their health and interfere with their growth and development.

To promote proper growth and development and prevent overweight, parents should offer the whole family a wide variety of foods from each of the food groups displayed in the Food Guide Pyramid. The Food Guide Pyramid applies to healthy people ages 2 years and older.

The Food Guide Pyramid illustrates the importance of balance among food groups in a daily eating pattern. Select most of your daily servings of food from the food groups that are the largest in the picture and closest to the bottom of the Pyramid [see the "Weight Loss for Life" chapter of this Sourcebook for a diagram of the Food Guide Pyramid].

- Most of the foods in your diet should come from the grain products group (6-11 servings), the vegetable group (3-5 servings), and the fruit group (2-4 servings). (See below for suggested serving sizes.)

- Your diet should include moderate amounts of foods from the milk group (2-3 servings) and the meat and beans group (2-3 servings).

Helping Your Overweight Child

- Foods that provide few nutrients and are high in fat and sugars should be used sparingly. Fat should not be restricted in the diets of children younger than 2 years of age.

Note: Serving sizes are for children and adults ages 2 years and older. A range of servings is given for each food group. The smaller number is for children who consume about 1,300 calories a day, such as 2–4 years of age. The larger number is for those who consume about 3,000 calories a day, such as boys 15–18 years of age.

One Serving Equals...

Bread, cereal, rice, and pasta group.

- 1 slice of bread
- 1 ounce of ready to eat cereal
- 1/2 cup of cooked cereal, rice, or pasta

Milk, yogurt, and cheese group.

- 1 cup of milk or yogurt
- 1 1/2 ounces of natural cheese
- 2 ounces of processed cheese

Vegetable group.

- 1 cup of raw vegetables or 1/2 cup of frozen leafy vegetables (cooked)
- 1/2 cup of other vegetables—cooked or chopped raw
- 3/4 cup of vegetable juice

Meat, poultry, fish, dry beans, and nuts group.

- 2–3 ounces of cooked lean meat, poultry, or fish
- 1/2 cup of cooked dry beans or 1 egg counts as 1 ounce of lean meat
- 2 tablespoons of peanut butter or 1/3 cup of nuts count as 1 ounce of meat

Fruit group.

- 1 medium apple, banana, or orange
- 1/2 cup of chopped, cooked, or canned fruit
- 3/4 cup of fruit juice

If you are unsure about how to select and prepare a variety of foods for your family, consult a physician or registered dietitian for nutrition counseling. You may also want to refer to the readings and organizations listed at the end of this fact sheet for more information on healthy eating.

Carefully Cut Down on the Amount of Fat in Your Family's Diet

Reducing fat is a good way to cut calories without depriving your child of nutrients. Simple ways to cut the fat in your family's diet include eating lowfat or nonfat dairy products, poultry without skin and lean meats, and lowfat or fat-free breads and cereals. Making small changes to the amount of fat in your family's diet is a good way to prevent excess weight gain in children: however, major efforts to change your child's diet should be supervised by a health professional. In addition, fat should not be restricted in the diets of children younger than 2 years of age. After that age, children should gradually adopt a diet that contains no more than 30 percent of calories from fat by the time the child is about 5 years old.

Don't Overly Restrict Sweets or Treats

While it is important to be aware of the fat, salt, and sugar content of the foods you serve, all foods—even those that are high in fat or sugar-have a place in the diet, in moderation.

Guide Your Family's Choices Rather Than Dictate Foods

Make a wide variety of healthful foods available in the house. This practice will help your children learn how to make healthy food choices.

Encourage Your Child to Eat Slowly

A child can detect hunger and fullness better when eating slowly.

Eat Meals Together as a Family as Often as Possible

Try to make mealtimes pleasant with conversation and sharing, not a time for scolding or arguing. If mealtimes are unpleasant, children may try to eat faster to leave the table as soon as possible. They then may learn to associate eating with stress.

Helping Your Overweight Child

Involve Children in Food Shopping and Preparing Meals

These activities offer parents hints about children's food preferences, teach children about nutrition, and provide children with a feeling of accomplishment. In addition, children may be more willing to eat or try foods that they help prepare.

Plan for Snacks

Continuous snacking may lead to overeating, but snacks that are planned at specific times during the day can be part of a nutritious diet, without spoiling a child's appetite at mealtimes. You should make snacks as nutritious as possible, without depriving your child of occasional chips or cookies, especially at parties or other social events. Below are some ideas for healthy snacks.

Healthy Snacks

- fresh, frozen, or canned vegetables and fruit served either plain or with lowfat or fat-free cheese or yogurt
- dried fruit, served with nuts or sunflower or pumpkin seeds
- breads and crackers made with enriched flour and whole grains, served with fruit spread or fat-free cheese
- frozen desserts, such as nonfat or lowfat ice cream, frozen yogurt, fruit sorbet, popsicles, water ice, and fruit juice bars

Note: Children of preschool age can easily choke on foods that are hard to chew, small and round, or sticky, such as hard vegetables, whole grapes, hard chunks of cheese, raisins, nuts, and seeds, and popcorn. Its important to carefully select snacks for children in this age group.

Discourage Eating Meals or Snacks While Watching TV

Try to eat only in designated areas of your home, such as the dining room or kitchen. Eating in front of the TV may make it difficult to pay attention to feelings of fullness, and may lead to overeating.

Try Not to Use Food to Punish or Reward Your Child

Withholding food as a punishment may lead children to worry that they will not get enough food. For example, sending children to bed without any dinner may cause them to worry that they will go hungry. As a result, children may try to eat whenever they get a chance. Similarly, when foods, such as sweets, are used as a reward, children may assume that these foods are better or more valuable than other foods. For example, telling children that they will get dessert if they eat all of their vegetables sends the wrong message about vegetables.

Make Sure Your Child's Meals Outside the Home Are Balanced

Find out more about your school lunch program, or pack your child's lunch to include a variety of foods. Also, select healthier items when dining at restaurants.

Set a Good Example

Children are good learners, and they learn best by example. Setting a good example for your kids by eating a variety of foods and being physically active will teach your children healthy lifestyle habits that they can follow for the rest of their lives.

Is Additional Help Available?

If you need to make changes to your family's eating and exercise habits, but are finding it difficult, a registered dietitian (RD) may be able to help. Your physician may be able to refer you to an RD, or you can call the National Center for Nutrition and Dietetics of The American Dietetic Association at 800-366-1655 and ask for the name of an RD in your area.

If your efforts at home are unsuccessful in helping your child reach a healthy weight and your physician determines that your child's health is at risk unless he or she loses weight steadily, you may want to consider a formal treatment program. To locate a weight-control program for your child, you may want to contact a local university-based medical center.

Look for the following characteristics when choosing a weight-control program for your child. The program should:

- be staffed with a variety of health professionals. The best programs may include RDs, exercise physiologists, pediatricians or family physicians, and psychiatrists or psychologists.

Helping Your Overweight Child

- perform a medical evaluation of the child. Before being enrolled in a program, your child's weight, growth, and health should be reviewed by a physician. During enrollment, your child's weight, growth, and health should be monitored by a health professional at regular intervals.
- focus on the whole family, not just the overweight child.
- be adapted to the specific age and capabilities of the child. Programs for 4-year-olds are different from those developed for children 8 or 12 years of age in terms of degree of responsibility of the child and parents.
- focus on behavioral changes.
- teach the child how to select a variety of foods in appropriate portions.
- encourage daily activity and limit sedentary activity, such as watching TV.
- include a maintenance program and other support and referral resources to reinforce the new behaviors and to deal with underlying issues that contributed to overweight.

The overall goal of a successful treatment program should be to help the whole family focus on making healthy changes to their eating and activity habits that they will be able to maintain throughout life.

Chapter 45

Promoting Healthier Lifestyles and Active Living for Childhood Obesity

Childhood Obesity: Healthier Lifestyles Are Needed to Treat This Growing Problem

Count your blessings if your child's weight is in the normal range. Unfortunately, the number of overweight or obese children and teens in the United States is increasing dramatically—a trend that many health officials are now calling a public health crisis.

The third National Health and Nutrition Examination Survey (NHANES III), conducted from 1988 to 1994 by the National Center for Health Statistics, a division of the Centers for Disease Control and Prevention (CDC), shows that approximately one in five children in the United States between the ages of 6 and 17 is overweight. In the 30 years since NHANES I was conducted, the number of overweight children in the U.S. has more than doubled. And, it seems, children are just keeping up with their parents. The NHANES III study found that over one-third of adults are overweight.

This chapter contains text from "Childhood Obesity: Healthier Lifestyles Are Needed to Treat This Growing Problem," http://www.mayohealth.org/mayo/9705/htm/overweig.htm, May 15, 1997, copyright 1997 Mayo Foundation for Medical Education and Research, reprinted from Mayo Clinic Health Oasis (www.mayohealth.org), with permission of Mayo Foundation for Medical Education and Research, Rochester, MN 55905, and "Promoting Lifelong Physical Activity—at a Glance," Centers for Disease Control and Prevention (CDC), National Center for Chronic Disease Prevention and Health Promotion, http://www.cdc.gov/nccdphp/dash/00binaries/phactaag.pdf, March 1997.

For the NHANES III study, children and adolescents were defined as "overweight" if their body mass index (BMI) exceeded the 95th percentile of BMI for those of their same age and sex. Pediatricians often use a growth chart to determine if a child is overweight. Because there is no universally accepted definition for "overweight," it's difficult to estimate exactly how many children fit the description.

Obese Children Often Become Obese Adults

Overweight children do face some health risks. Being overweight can mean higher blood pressure and blood cholesterol levels, particularly in children genetically prone to these conditions. Overweight children are likely to suffer social and psychological stresses because they appear "different" from their peers.

The greatest risk, however, comes if children remain overweight into adulthood, which studies show is a strong possibility. Obese children who become obese adults are at greater risk—at a younger age—for developing heart disease, diabetes, high blood pressure, high cholesterol, gallbladder disease, arthritis and certain cancers.

Early Intervention

"If you can intervene with overweight children before they are fully grown, you can often help them grow into their weight and prevent them from becoming overweight adults," explains Dr. David J. Driscoll, a pediatric cardiologist and head of Mayo Clinic's Cardiovascular Health Clinic for the Young. "Some overweight children don't need to lose weight as much as they need to gain weight at a slower rate," he adds.

During infancy and early adolescence, fat normally increases faster than muscle. Overeating and underactivity during these times make children particularly vulnerable to excessive weight gain.

Some research supports the fat cell theory of obesity. According to this concept, fat cells that are formed in childhood stay with you throughout life. Developing abnormally high numbers of fat cells also may increase your appetite, which makes it harder to lose weight.

What Causes Obesity?

Weight gain among children is likely due to a combination of factors including: poor dietary habits, genetic makeup, family lifestyle, socioeconomic status, and a child's ethnicity. Obesity is more prevalent

Promoting Healthier Lifestyles and Active Living

among Hispanic, African-American and American Indian children, particularly girls.

Overweight children are not necessarily overeaters. Unfortunately, much of the food they enjoy contains high amounts of calories. A child doesn't have to eat huge quantities of food to put on excess weight. An extra 200 calories a day (the amount in four home-made chocolate chip cookies) can cause your child to gain almost one-half pound a week.

Studies show that children's excessive consumption of high-calorie soft drinks and fruit beverages may be adding to the problem. The average teen drinks almost 65 gallons of soft drinks annually; school-age children have more than doubled their consumption of these beverages in the past two decades. Children also eat a lot of fast-food, which tends to be high in fat and calories.

Inactivity Most Likely to Blame

Weight control involves balancing food intake with the energy burned in everyday activities. Although diet is a factor, low levels of physical activity may play a greater role in childhood obesity than eating lots of high-calorie food.

Why are children today less active? Many blame increased television viewing. Watching TV doesn't require much energy and often is accompanied by snacking on high-calorie foods. The American Heart Association reports that, on average, children watch 17 hours of television a week. And that's not counting the time spent playing video and computer games. One study found the odds of being overweight were nearly five times greater for youth watching more than five hours of television per day compared with those who watched from zero to two hours per day.

According to a 1996 U.S. Surgeon General's report on fitness, nearly half of young people ages 12 to 21 are not vigorously active. The American College of Sports Medicine reports that, due to financial constraints, only one-third of schools now offer physical education classes and many children today find team sports too competitive or costly to join.

Heredity Has Strong Influence

The risk of becoming obese is greatest among children who have two obese parents. Danish adoption records provide a unique perspective on the issue of heredity versus environment when studying obesity in children. Researchers studied 540 adopted Danish children, who are now adults. The scientists wanted to know if weights of the children were closer to their biological or adoptive parents. They found no relationship between the weight of the adoptive parents and adopted children. But there was a strong link between the weight of the adopted children and their biological parents, even though 90 percent of the children had been adopted before the age of 1.

The researchers concluded that genetic factors are important in determining obesity in adults. And when a genetic tendency is combined with habits that promote weight gain, it's more likely that a child will be overweight. Important: if obesity is common in your family, pay extra attention to diet and exercise.

Treatment Is a Family Affair

Weight control is not easy at any age, but it can be nearly impossible for overweight children and teenagers if loved ones make fun of them. The whole family needs to promote healthy living in a way that is fun and inviting to the child. Parents need to practice what they preach, setting good dietary and exercise examples.

Sometimes the encouragement of family members may not be enough. A physician and registered dietitian can assess the severity of the weight problem and suggest specific foods and amounts for your child, taking into account nutrient needs for normal growth. Support groups whose members are the same age as your child may provide an opportunity for discussing mutual problems and solutions. Special clinics designed to meet the needs of overweight children may be an option, but insurance companies usually don't cover the cost of obesity programs.

With careful, loving attention, your child can develop healthy patterns of eating and activity. Managing childhood obesity will help you and your child get started. Diet and exercise guidelines for overweight children will keep you going with practical advice.

Promoting Lifelong Physical Activity—at a Glance

Young people can build healthy bodies and establish healthy lifestyles by including physical activity in their daily lives. However, many young people are not physically active on a regular basis, and physical activity declines dramatically during adolescence. School and community programs can help young people get active and stay active.

Promoting Healthier Lifestyles and Active Living

Benefits of Physical Activity

Regular physical activity in childhood and adolescence

- improves strength and endurance
- helps build healthy bones and muscles
- helps control weight
- reduces anxiety and stress and increases self-esteem
- may improve blood pressure and cholesterol levels

In addition, young people say they like physical activity because it is fun; they do it with friends; and it helps them learn skills, stay in shape, and look better.

Consequences of Physical Inactivity

- The percentage of young people who are overweight has more than doubled in the past 30 years.
- Inactivity and poor diet cause at least 300,000 deaths a year in the United States. Only tobacco use causes more preventable deaths.
- Adults who are less active are at greater risk of dying of heart disease and developing diabetes, colon cancer, and high blood pressure.

Physical Inactivity among Young People

- Almost half of young people aged 12–21, and more than a third of high school students do not participate in vigorous physical activity on a regular basis.
- Seventy-two percent of 9th graders participate in vigorous physical activity on a regular basis, compared with only 55% of 12th graders.
- Daily participation in physical education classes by high school students dropped from 42% in 1991 to 25% in 1995.
- The time students spend being active in physical education classes is decreasing; among high school students enrolled in a physical education class, the percentage who were active for at

least 20 minutes during an average class dropped from 81% in 1991 to 70% in 1995.

How Much Physical Activity Do Young People Need?

Everyone can benefit from a moderate amount of physical activity on most, if not all, days of the week. Young people should select activities they enjoy, that fit into their daily lives. Examples of moderate activity include

- walking 2 miles in 30 minutes or running 1 1/2 miles in 15 minutes
- bicycling 5 miles in 30 minutes or 4 miles in 15 minutes
- dancing fast for 30 minutes or jumping rope for 15 minutes
- playing basketball for 15–20 minutes or volleyball for 45 minutes

Increasing the frequency, time, or intensity of physical activity can bring even more health benefits—up to a point. Too much physical activity can lead to injuries and other health problems.

Chapter 46

Diet and Exercise Guidelines for Overweight Children

Childhood obesity presents the special challenge of managing weight while maintaining growth. Children must receive adequate vitamins, minerals, protein, and calories to build strong, healthy bodies. Severely restricted diets, while generally unhealthy, are a special risk for children.

Overweight children shouldn't be put on the same diets as some adults. Instead, many nutrition experts now advocate dietary guidelines specific to children. Unlike adults, where low fat is the name of the game, the average child needs a certain amount of fat for normal growth. If they get too little, they risk nutrient deficiencies and impaired growth. "However, a diet too high in fat can lead to excess calories and weight gain," notes Susan K. Eckert, registered dietitian at Mayo Clinic, Rochester, Minn.

Government dietary guidelines currently recommend that after the age of 2 years, children gradually adopt a diet that, by about age 5, contains no more than 30 percent of calories from fat. A diet low in fat, saturated fat and cholesterol (less than 300 mg per day) is encouraged for most school-age children and adolescents.

Mayo dietitians support a common-sense approach to dietary guidelines for children. "Parents of overweight children need to emphasize the

---

"Diet and Exercise Guidelines for Overweight Children," http://www.mayohealth.org/mayo/9705/htm/over_2sb.htm, May 15, 1997, copyright 1997 Mayo Foundation for Medical Education and Research, reprinted from Mayo Clinic Health Oasis (www.mayohealth.org), with permission of Mayo Foundation for Medical Education and Research, Rochester, MN 55905.

good foods from the Food Guide Pyramid, and teach children to go easy on fats, sweets and oils," explains Mayo registered dietitian Jennifer K. Nelson [see the "Weight Loss for Life" chapter of this sourcebook for a diagram of the Food Guide Pyramid].

Proper diet is half the battle; the other is getting inactive children off the couch and exercising. The U.S. Surgeon General's Report on Physical Activity and Health recommends 30 minutes of moderate to vigorous physical activity per day for children and adults. Different health agencies and medical groups suggest more or less activity, but the theme is the same: get children moving.

Overweight children may be more prone to injuries of the joints, so it's recommended they start exercising slowly. Lower impact exercise, such as swimming, biking, and the use of some fitness machines, is recommended over high-impact sports, such as running or high-intensity aerobics. Proper warm-up and cool-down exercises are especially important for overweight children.

Before beginning any weight-loss regimen, overweight children should visit a physician for a thorough physical examination. Physicians may recommend consultation with a physical therapist to plan an exercise program specific to the child's needs and goals. The idea is for children to learn fitness for life.

"It's extremely important for the whole family to adopt a healthier lifestyle along with the overweight child," says Timothy J. McLean, a physical therapist at Mayo's Sports Medicine Center, who has worked with slightly overweight as well as extremely obese children. "Overweight children who have families that exercise together—and have fun in the process—fare better in maintaining a healthy weight than children whose families never exercise," he notes.

Dr. David Driscoll, a pediatric cardiologist and head of Mayo Clinic's Cardiovascular Health Clinic for the Young, agrees that family involvement is key to managing a child's weight. "Mom and Dad can't be eating high-fat foods while telling their children to be on a low-fat diet. The whole family has to learn to prepare and choose nutritionally balanced, healthy meals together." He recommends families of overweight children see a dietitian for guidance.

Chapter 47

Television-Watching Is Associated with Obesity

Intervention strategies to promote lifelong physical activity among U.S. children are needed to stem the adverse health consequences of inactivity, such as obesity, according to the findings of a recent study.

Researchers conducted a study to assess participation in vigorous activity and television-watching habits and their relationship to body weight in U.S. children. The study was a nationally representative cross-sectional survey that included an in-person interview and medical examination.

Between 1988 and 1994, 4,063 children ages eight to 16 were studied. Mexican Americans and non-Hispanic blacks were oversampled to produce reliable estimates in those groups.

The children were measured for episodes of weekly vigorous activity and daily hours of television watched, and their relationship to body mass index and body fatness.

Eighty percent of the children reported three or more bouts of vigorous activity each week, although the rates were lower in non-Hispanic black and Mexican American girls (69 percent and 73 percent, respectively). Twenty percent of children participated in vigorous activity twice or fewer times each week, and this rate was higher in girls (26 percent) than in boys (17 percent).

Overall, 26 percent of U.S. watched four or more hours of television per day and 67 percent watched at least two hours of television

The Brown University Child and Adolescent Behavior Letter, July 1998, Vol. 14, N. 7, p. 4, copyright 1998 Manisses Communications Group Inc. Reprinted with permission.

per day. The highest rates of television-watching occurred among non-Hispanic black children (42 percent), who watched four or more hours of television per day.

Not surprisingly, boys and girls who watched four or more hours of television each day had greater body fat and greater body mass index levels than did children who watched less than two hours of television a day.

"Many U.S. children watch a great deal of television and are inadequately vigorously active," the authors conclude. "Vigorous activity levels are lowest among girls, non-Hispanic blacks and Mexican Americans."

References

Andersen RE, Crespo CJ, Bartlett SJ, et al.: "Relationship of physical activity and television watching with body weight and level of fatness among children." *Journal of the American Medical Association* 1998; 279:938–942. For reprints, contact Ross E. Andersen, Ph.D., Johns Hopkins School of Medicine, 333 Cassell Drive, Suite 1640, Baltimore, MD 21124.

Chapter 48

Growing Older, Eating Better

When Bernadette Harkins, 89, of Rockville, Md., could no longer feed herself properly, she moved to an assisted-living residence. Today, she can enjoy three meals a day served to her and about 30 other people in their home-like communal dining room.

When Harry, 85, of Moscow, Pa., could no longer feed himself properly, he moved in with his daughter and her family. With her guidance, he ate six times a day, snacking on high-calorie, high-protein foods, and maintaining a near-normal weight.

Harry, who asked that his last name not be used, and Harkins typify many of today's older generation. Living alone in most cases, they often are unable to meet their dietary needs and are forced to make compromises.

Harry didn't know how to cook. He developed cancer, which made it even more important that he eat a well-balanced diet. Harkins knew how to cook but didn't take time to prepare adequate meals for herself.

"I would snack is what I'd do," she said. "I would think about getting a meal and then just have a cup of tea and toast. I knew I wasn't doing the right thing as far as nutrition was concerned."

Their eating problems stemmed from loneliness and lack of desire or skill to cook. Other older people may eat poorly for other reasons, ranging from financial difficulties to physical problems.

Paula Kurtzweil, *FDA Consumer*, March 1996, e-text revised December 1996, FDA Pub. No. 97-2301, http://www.fda.gov/fdac/features/296_old.html.

The solutions can be just as varied, from finding alternative living arrangements to accepting home-delivered meals to using the food label recently revised by the Food and Drug Administration and the U.S. Department of Agriculture. Physical activity also is important in maintaining a healthy lifestyle.

Why the Concern?

Nutrition remains important throughout life. Many chronic diseases that develop late in life, such as osteoporosis, can be influenced by earlier poor habits. Insufficient exercise and calcium intake, especially during adolescence and early adulthood, can significantly increase the risk of osteoporosis, a disease that causes bones to become brittle and crack or break.

But good nutrition in the later years still can help lessen the effects of diseases prevalent among older Americans or improve the quality of life in people who have such diseases. They include osteoporosis, obesity, high blood pressure, heart disease, certain cancers, gastrointestinal problems, and chronic undernutrition.

Studies show that a good diet in later years helps both in reducing the risk of these diseases and in managing the diseases' signs and symptoms. This contributes to a higher quality of life, enabling older people to maintain their independence by continuing to perform basic daily activities, such as bathing, dressing and eating.

Poor nutrition, on the other hand, can prolong recovery from illnesses, increase the costs and incidence of institutionalization, and lead to a poorer quality of life.

The Single Life

Whether it happens at age 65 or 85, older people eventually face one or more problems that interfere with their ability to eat well.

Social isolation is a common one. Older people who find themselves single after many years of living with another person may find it difficult to be alone, especially at mealtimes. They may become depressed and lose interest in preparing or eating regular meals, or they may eat only sparingly.

In a study published in the July 1993 *Journals of Gerontology*, researchers found that newly widowed people, most of whom were women, were less likely to say they enjoy mealtimes, less likely to report good appetites, and less likely to report good eating behaviors than their married counterparts. Nearly 85 percent of widowed subjects reported a weight change during the two years following their spouse's death, as compared with 30 percent of married subjects. The widowed group was more likely to report an average weight loss of 7.6 pounds (17 kilograms).

According to the study, most of the women said they had enjoyed cooking and eating when they were married, but, as widows, they found those activities "a chore," especially since there was no one to appreciate their cooking efforts.

For many widowed men who may have left the cooking to their wives, the problem may extend even further: They may not know how to cook and prepare foods. Instead, they may snack or eat out a lot, both of which may lead people to eat too much fat and cholesterol and not get enough vitamins and minerals.

Special Diets

At the same time, many older people, because of chronic medical problems, may require special diets: for example, a low-fat, low-cholesterol diet for heart disease, a low-sodium diet for high blood pressure, or a low-calorie diet for weight reduction. Special diets often require extra effort, but older people may instead settle for foods that are quick and easy to prepare, such as frozen dinners, canned foods, lunch meats, and others that may provide too many calories, or contain too much fat and sodium for their needs.

On the other hand, Mona Sutnick, Ed.D., a registered dietitian in private practice in Philadelphia, pointed out that some people may go overboard on their special diets, overly restricting foods that may be more beneficial than detrimental to their health.

"My advice for a 60-year-old person might be 'watch your fat' but for an 80-year-old who's underweight, I'd say, 'eat the fat, get the calories,'" Sutnick said.

Physical Problems

Some older people may overly restrict foods important to good health because of chewing difficulties and gastrointestinal disturbances, such as constipation, diarrhea, and heartburn. Because missing teeth and poorly fitting dentures make it hard to chew, older people may forego fresh fruits and vegetables, which are important sources of vitamins, minerals and fiber. Or they may avoid dairy products, believing they cause gas or constipation. By doing so, they miss out on important sources of calcium, protein and some vitamins.

Adverse reactions from medications can cause older people to avoid certain foods. Some medications alter the sense of taste, which can adversely affect appetite. This adds to the problem of naturally diminishing senses of taste and smell, common as people age.

Other medical problems, such as arthritis, stroke or Alzheimer's disease, can interfere with good nutrition. It may be difficult, if not impossible, for example, for people with arthritis or who have had a stroke to cook, shop, or even lift a fork to eat. Dementia associated with Alzheimer's and other diseases may cause them to eat poorly or forget to eat altogether.

Money Matters

Lack of money is a particular problem among older Americans who may have no income other than Social Security. According to 1994 U.S. Census Bureau data, nearly 12 percent of people 65 and over are below the average poverty level for their age group. In 1994, the poverty level for a person 65 and over was $7,108 a year.

According to the 1994 data, the mean annual income for people 65 and over was $16,709, almost $10,000 less than what they earned on average between ages 55 and 64.

Lack of money may lead older people to scrimp on important food purchases—for example, perishable items like fresh fruits, vegetables and meat—because of higher costs and fear of waste. They may avoid cooking or baking foods like meats, stews and casseroles because recipes for these foods usually yield large quantities.

Financial problems also may cause older people to delay medical and dental treatments that could correct problems that interfere with good nutrition.

Food Programs

Many older people may find help under the Older Americans Act, which provides nutrition and other services that target older people who are in greatest social and economic need, with particular attention on low-income minorities. According to the U.S. Administration on Aging, which administers the Older Americans Act, the nutrition programs were set up to address the dietary inadequacy and social isolation among older people.

Home-delivered meals and congregate nutrition services are the primary nutrition programs. The congregate meal program allows seniors to gather at a local site, often the local senior citizen center,

Growing Older, Eating Better

school or other public building or a restaurant, for a meal and other activities, such as games and lectures on nutrition and other topics of interest to older people.

Available since 1972, these programs, funded by the federal, state and local governments, ensure that senior citizens get at least one nutritious meal five to seven days a week. Under current standards, that meal must comply with the Dietary Guidelines for Americans and provide at least one-third of the Recommended Dietary Allowances for an older person. Often, people receive foods that correspond with their special dietary needs, such as no-added-salt foods for those who need to restrict their sodium intake or ground meat for those who have trouble chewing.

Other nutrition services provided under the Older Americans Act are nutrition education, screening and counseling.

While these nutrition programs target poor people, they are available to other older people regardless of income, according to Jean Lloyd, a registered dietitian and nutrition officer with the Administration on Aging. Although no one is charged for the meals, older people can voluntarily and confidentially donate money, she said.

The meals provide not only good nutrition, but they also give older people a chance to socialize—a key factor in preventing the adverse nutritional effects of social isolation.

For those who qualify, food stamps are another aid for improving nutrition. Under this program, a one-person household can receive up to $115 a month in food stamps to buy most grocery items.

For the homebound, grocery-shopping assistance is available in many areas. Usually provided by non-government organizations, this service shops for and delivers groceries to people at their request. The recipient pays for the groceries and sometimes a service fee.

In some communities, private organizations also sell home-delivered meals.

Other Assistance

Family members and friends can help ensure that older people take advantage of food programs by putting them in touch with the appropriate agencies or organizations and helping them fill out the necessary forms. Some other steps they can take include:

- looking in occasionally to ensure that the older person is eating adequately

- preparing foods for and making them available to the older person
- joining the older person for meals

In some cases, they may help see that the older person is moved to an environment, such as their home, an assisted-living facility, or a nursing home, that can help ensure that the older person gets proper nutrition.

Whatever an older person's living situation, proper medical and dental treatment is important for treating medical problems, such as gastrointestinal distress and chewing difficulties, that interfere with good nutrition. If a medication seems to ruin an older person's taste and appetite, a switch to another drug may help.

A review of basic diet principles may help improve nutrition. Explaining to older people the importance of good nutrition in the later years may motivate them to make a greater effort to select nutritious foods.

Look to the Label

The food label can help older people select a good diet. Revamped in 1992, the label gives the nutritional content of most foods and enables consumers to see how a food fits in with daily dietary recommendations.

Some of the information appears as claims describing the food's nutritional benefits: for example, "low in cholesterol" or "high in vitamin C." Under strict government rules, these claims can be used only if the food meets certain criteria. This means that claims can be trusted. For example, a "low-cholesterol" food can provide no more than 20 milligrams (mg) of cholesterol and no more than 2 grams of saturated fat per serving. A high-potassium food must provide at least 700 mg of potassium per serving.

Less common but also helpful are label claims linking a nutrient or food to the risk of a disease or health-related condition. So far, Food and Drug Administration (FDA) allows only eight of these claims because they are the only ones supported by scientific evidence. One claim links sodium, a nutrient found in salt and used in many processed foods, to high blood pressure. On the food label, this claim would read something like this:

"Diets low in sodium may reduce the risk of high blood pressure, a disease associated with many factors."

More in-depth information is found on the "Nutrition Facts" panel on the side or back of the food label. This information is required on almost all food packages. Unlike before, this nutrition information is easier to read because it appears in bigger type and is usually on a white or other neutral contrasting background, when practical.

Some nutrition information also may be available for many raw meats, poultry and fish and fresh fruits and vegetables at the point of purchase. The information may appear in brochures or on posters or placards.

Physical Activity

Besides diet, physical activity is part of a healthy lifestyle at any age. It can help reduce and control weight by burning calories. Moderate exercise that places weight on bones, such as walking, helps maintain and possibly even increases bone strength in older people. A study published in the Dec. 28, 1994, *Journal of the American Medical Association* found that intensive strength training can help preserve bone density and improve muscle mass, strength and balance in postmenopausal women. In the study, subjects used weight machines for strength training.

Also, scientists looking into the benefits of exercise for older people agree that regular exercise can improve the functioning of the heart and lungs, increase strength and flexibility, and contribute to a feeling of well-being.

Any regular physical activity is good, from brisk walking to light gardening. Common sense is the key. But, before a vigorous exercise program is started or started after a long period of rest, a doctor should be consulted.

Taking time out for exercise, using the food label to help pick nutritious foods, taking advantage of the several assistance programs available, and getting needed medical attention can go a long way in helping older people avoid the nutritional pitfalls of aging and more fully enjoy their senior years.

—by Paula Kurtzweil

Paula Kurtzweil is a member of FDA's public affairs staff.

Chapter 49

Obesity in Older Persons

Introduction

Obesity among older persons is a growing concern. Not only are greater numbers of persons living beyond 65 years, but higher percentages of this population are considered overweight. The prevalence of obesity in this population has continued to increase in national surveys despite the objectives of Healthy People 2000 to decrease the prevalence of obesity to 20% by the year 2000.[1] This trend has adverse medical, functional, psychosocial, and health-care resource consequences. Possible causes for this trend and treatment recommendations will be suggested in this chapter.

The Problem

Body mass index (BMI, measured as kg/m^2) is a useful tool to estimate body size and fatness and has been applied widely in population studies. Studies that have controlled for smoking have clarified that excess body weight increases risk of death from any cause and that the desirable BMI range for optimal health may be somewhat lower than previously thought.[2-4] An increased mortality rate from all causes extends into the seventh decade for overweight persons, although the relative risk is higher for younger subjects.[2] A healthy range for BMI has been suggested as 19 to 24.9.[5] The new federal

---

Copyright The American Dietetic Association. Reprinted by permission from Journal of the American Dietetic Association, Vol. 98, I. 11, p. 1308.

obesity guidelines define overweight as a BMI of 25 to 29.9 and obesity as a BMI of 30 and above.[6]

These guidelines have elicited much consternation, because approximately 1 in 2 adult Americans are now classified as overweight, and 1 in 5 are obese.[6] The growing prevalence of obesity (BMI greater than or equal to 30) is noteworthy, climbing from 14.1% reported in the first National Health and Nutrition Examination Survey (NHANES I) to 14.5% in NHANES II to 22.5% in NHANES III.[7] Trends were similar for all sex, age, and race/ethnic groups.[7] A remarkable 33% of a rural Pennsylvania sample of Medicare risk participants (mean age = 71 years) met this obesity threshold.[8] Obesity guidelines are not yet available that specifically apply to older persons, but we can conclude that obesity is growing in prevalence in this age group too, and that many older Americans would benefit from achieving a healthier weight.

Causes

Obesity is common into the sixth and seventh decades of life and then declines. Many obese older persons were obese middle-aged adults. Reduced energy expenditure plays a major role in this pattern. A retrospective review of physically active vs. sedentary older women (mean age = 71 years) in the Netherlands found that the sedentary group had greater body weight from age 25 years forward.[9] Their current body weight was 12 kg greater than that of their active counterparts. Their excess body weight had persisted throughout adult life.

Sedentary lifestyles may be the dominant factor and contribute to obesity across the generations. However, older persons face an even greater challenge: many view weight gain and sedentary living as an inevitable part of the aging process. However, a 1994 study of resistance exercise intervention among older persons suggests that the decline in lean body mass and increase in fat mass typically seen in older persons need not occur.[10]

Although obesity remains a subject in need of clinical research, limited data are available about characteristics of obesity in older persons. Obesity tends to be somewhat more prevalent among older women than men.[7,8] The middle-age increase in body mass and proportion of body fat typically occurs in men after 40 years of age and in women at menopause; peak body fatness tends to occur somewhat later in women than men, and may extend into the fifth and sixth decades of life. At the same time, a linear decline in food intake with aging has been noted in men and women.[11] It is also likely, however, that energy intake of older persons is greater today than previously. Mean energy intakes for adults are 100 to 300 kcal higher in NHANES III (1988–1991) compared with NHANES II (1976–1980).[12] These observations suggest that the obesity in older persons is predominately caused by a decrease in physical activity, an alteration in metabolic rate, or an increase in the efficiency by which fat is stored.[11]

Consequences

Excess body weight and modest weight gain (greater than or equal to 5 kg) during middle age may be associated with comorbidities in old age. These include hypertension, diabetes mellitus, cardiovascular disease, and osteoarthritis.[2,13–27]

Although obesity (BMI greater than or equal to 30) has no known medical benefit, the incidence of osteoporosis appears to be somewhat lower in moderately overweight women (BMI 25 to 28) than in those of lower weight.[28] Early population studies also suggested that risk of death might be somewhat reduced for moderately overweight older persons. This finding was attributed to increased metabolic reserve against chronic disease or illness.[29] It is worth reemphasizing that studies that have controlled for smoking have found that excess body weight increases the risk of death from any cause.[2,3] It must also be emphasized that these studies do not suggest any benefit from severe obesity.

Obesity in older persons may also have profound functional and psychosocial consequences. Although middle-aged adults with obesity may be fairly functional, the same is often not true for older persons. Observations from multiple studies show that high BMI (past or current) is associated with greater risk for self-reported functional limitation (especially mobility) among older persons.[30–34] A 1996 study[35] has also suggested a relationship between measured physical performance limitation and obesity among older persons. Functional impairment in older persons may result in their withdrawal from social activities and their dependence on others for the activities of daily living. As older adults suffer functional limitation, activity levels and consequent energy expenditure are further reduced. This decrease in function and increase in dependence may be considered failure to thrive as a result of obesity.[36] Physiologic and performance capabilities have been improved through progressive resistance training in frail older persons,[10] and may have benefit for the obese older person.

Depression is common in obese and older persons. Evaluation and appropriate treatment of depression should not be overlooked. Self-reported quality of life has been found to worsen as a patient's weight increases. The subject's perception of mobility and health was most notably affected with increasing age.[37] Obesity treatment in the older population needs to focus on interventions that address psychosocial concerns.

Because obesity is associated with increased risk of chronic disease, health-care resource use is increased in younger and older obese persons. The estimated cost associated with treatment of the health outcomes of the current overweight population of middle-aged American women during the next 25 years is a staggering $16 billion.[38] The annual direct cost of type 2 diabetes, coronary heart disease, hypertension, and gallstones in the general population for persons with a BMI greater than 30 was estimated at $22.62 billion health-care dollars, compared with $5.89 billion for lean persons with a BMI of 23 to 24.9.[39] Screening of rural older persons identified a BMI of greater than 27 as a variable significantly associated with increased monthly health-care costs.[8]

Interventions

Dietitians are crucial participants in the multidisciplinary effort necessary for successful weight reduction in the obese older person. Although dietitians have well-defined roles in dietary assessment, dietary instruction, and behavior modification, there are clearly opportunities for expanded roles in medical assessment and follow-up, exercise prescription, and surveillance for complications. The precise roles for a dietitian in a particular setting will depend on available personnel and resources. Appropriate mentorship and training are prerequisites to an assumption of expanded roles.

Medical evaluation of older adults should occur before they begin a weight reduction program. Patients often respond favorably to physician reinforcement of the need for weight reduction, and continued medical intervention is often necessary to manage changes in dosages of medications, such as antihypertensives, insulin, and hypoglycemics as weight loss occurs. A thorough history and physical will allow the physician to identify medical concerns before appropriate recommendations for exercise, diet, and weight reduction goals are established. This is often prerequisite to obtaining reimbursement for any weight reduction effort.

Changing the lifestyle of obese older persons presents some unique challenges. An increasing burden of disease and poor quality of life may motivate patients to change, or older persons may feel no need to change at this point in their life. Societal expectations reinforce sedentary living and other adverse health behaviors; for example, older persons are often discouraged from active sports participation. Educational programs to effect lifestyle improvement in older persons must include participation by family members or caregivers and take into consideration that older adult learners may also face obstacles such as impaired hearing and eyesight, limited resources, and multiple medical problems. After an initial educational session, regular visits with a health-care team, which may include a dietitian, physician, nurse, exercise specialist, and mental health professional, can provide incentive to patients to maintain their improved behaviors. The dietitian may review food and exercise records, weight change, and problems encountered. Together, the dietitian and the patient develop behavioral goals and strategies for the future.

Modest goals are a key component of a weight management program for older adults. For persons with a BMI greater than 27, weight loss goals should focus first on a 10% to 20% reduction of the starting body weight, and then on maintaining this loss. Inappropriate or unrealistic weight loss goals are likely to result in failure. There is no need to make the obese older person into a "small" person—only into a "smaller" person. Moderate weight loss goals are consistent with the healthier weight approach[5] and are in contrast with ideal body weight goals, which require substantial weight losses that are rarely maintained.

The use of very-low-energy diets or protein-sparing modified fasts is not recommended in older persons unless the patient can be monitored closely by skilled practitioners. These interventions require drastic dietary changes and can result in dramatic fluid, electrolyte, and weight shifts that may not be tolerated in older patients. Although very-low-energy diets and protein-sparing modified fasts may appear attractive to consumers because they result in a precipitous weight loss, recidivism is common with the transition back to a conventional diet.

Dietary guidelines for obese older persons should focus on adopting a healthful diet that provides moderate reduction in energy, is low in fat (less than 30% of energy), and is high in fiber. Maintaining adequate intakes of protein (1 g/kg per day), fluids, and other nutrients is essential. A multivitamin with minerals may be recommended. Modest reductions in energy intake (e.g., 1,200 to 1,500 total kcal for women and 1,500 to 1,800 total kcal for men) are recommended. Self-monitoring through the use of a food log may be helpful in modifying energy intake. Simply reducing serving sizes and eliminating high-fat snacks may be sufficient if patients are able to increase their physical activity.

Exercise strategies for older adults must be individually determined with consideration of age, diseases, and disability. A 15-item tool is available to screen patients to determine who should be evaluated by a physician for clearance before beginning an exercise program.[40] Thirty minutes a day of moderate-intensity physical activity is recommended for every US adult.[41] These activities may be divided into several daily periods that total 30 minutes. Routine activities like mall walking, water aerobics, dancing, playing with grandchildren, and gardening should be encouraged. It should be emphasized that all activities count in daily energy expenditure, including walking to the mailbox and housecleaning chores.

Because low fitness levels may prevent many sedentary older men and women from expending much energy, resistance training may be of benefit.[42] Strength conditioning or progressive resistance training can improve muscle strength and enhance the ability of obese persons to lose weight and improve function. Resistance exercises can be done using resistance machines, elastic bands, or simple weight-lifting devices. Velcro-strapped wrist and ankle bags or moderately heavy household objects such as plastic milk jugs or food cans can be used. Performing these exercises 2 to 3 times a week is recommended. Even very old or disabled patients can participate in these types of activities.

The use of appetite suppressant medications in the older population is not recommended for weight reduction. The serious side effects of valvular heart disease and pulmonary hypertension,[43] along with the increased risk of drug interactions due to the use of multiple medications, make the use of these medications undesirable in older adults. Many older persons may already be taking antidepressants, which are serotonergic reuptake inhibitors and have an appetite suppressant effect. They should not receive multiple pharmacologic agents of this type.

Older persons are particularly susceptible to unsubstantiated health or weight loss claims for herbal or natural remedies. These products may not be reported during a routine review of medications and health-care professionals should ask specific questions about their use. They are often costly, have little evidence of efficacy, and may even be toxic. Resources of the patient should be directed toward the purchase of healthful foods, not gimmicks.

Outcomes of Weight Management

What outcomes would determine success in a weight management program designed for older persons? Small changes in lifestyle can have enormous benefit in terms of function, health, and quality of life even without large weight losses. Studies indicate that overweight women who achieve a weight loss of 5 kg may reduce their subsequent risk for developing hypertension, diabetes, or osteoarthritis by 50% or more.[14,16,23,25] The Nonpharmacologic Intervention in the Elderly (TONE) trial[44] randomly assigned 585 obese, older (aged 60 to 80 years) persons to groups for reduced sodium intake, weight loss, both, or usual care. Hypertension was less prevalent at the 15- to 36-month follow up in those who received either intervention, but risk reduction was greatest in those who received both. Weight loss of 3.5 to 4.5 kg was described as a safe and effective therapy for hypertension in older persons.

Conclusion

The growing prevalence of obesity in the older population constitutes a national public health crisis. Dietitians must take the lead in promoting awareness of obesity as a serious health concern for older persons. Programs that target prevention of obesity in all age groups are the key to addressing this problem. Treatment of obese older adults may be plagued by the recidivism seen in other populations. The focus must be on achieving a more healthful weight to promote improved health, function, and quality of life.

References

1. US Dept of Health and Human Services. "Healthy People 2000: National Health Promotion and Disease Prevention Objectives." Boston, Mass: Jones and Bantbett; 1992.

2. Stevens J, Cai J, Pamuk ER, Williamson DF, Thun MJ, Wood JL. "The effect of age on the association between body mass index and mortality." *N Engl J Med*. 1998;338:1–7.

3. Kushner RF. "Body weight and mortality." *Nutr Rev*. 1993;51:127–136.

4. Kuczmarski RJ, Carroll MD, Flegal KM, Troiano RP. "Varying body mass index cutoff points to describe overweight prevalence among U.S. adults: NHANES III (1988 to 1994)." *Obes Res*. 1997;5:542–546.

5. Meisler J, St Jeor SJ. "Summary and recommendations from the American Health Foundation's Expert Panel on Healthy Weight." *Am J Clin Nutr*. 1996;63(suppl):474S–477S.

6. "Clinical Guidelines on the Identification, Evaluation, and Treatment of Overweight and Obesity in Adults." Bethesda, Md: National Institutes of Health, National Heart, Lung, and Blood Institute; Preprint June 1998.

7. Flegal KM, Carroll MD, Kuczmarski RJ, Johnson CL. "Overweight and obesity in the United States: prevalence and trends, 1960–1994." *Int J Obes.* 1998;22:39–47.

8. Jensen G, Kita K, Fish J, Heydt D, Frey C. "Nutrition risk screening characteristics of rural older persons: relation to functional limitations and health-care charges." *Am J Clin Nutr.* 1997;66:819–828.

9. Voorrips LE, Meijers JH, Sol P, Seidell JC, van Staveren WA. "History of body weight and physical activity of elderly women differing in current physical activity." *Int J Obes Relat Metab Disord.* 1992;16:199–205.

10. Fiatarone MA, O'Neill EF, Ryan ND, Clements KM, Solares GR, Nelson ME, Roberts SB, Kehayias JJ, Lipsitz LA, Evans WJ. "Exercise training and nutritional supplementation for physical frailty in very elderly people." *N Engl J Med.* 1994;330:1769–1775.

11. Morley J. "Anorexia of aging: physiologic and pathologic." *Am J Clin Nutr.* 1997;66:760.773.

12. McDowell MA, Briefel RR, Alaimo K, Bischof AM, Caughman CR, Carroll MD, Loria CM, Johnson CL. "Energy and macronutrient intakes of persons age 2 months and over in the United States: Third National Health and Nutrition Examination Survey, phase 1, 1998–91." *Advance Data.* 1994;255:1–3.

13. McCarron A, Reusser M. "Body weight and blood pressure regulation." *Am J Clin Nutr.* 1996;63(suppl):4238–4258.

14. Huang Z, Willst WC, Manson JE, Rosner B, Stampfer MJ, Speizer FE, Colditz GA. "Body change, weight change, and risk for hypertension in women." *Ann Intern Med.* 1998;128:81–88.

15. Pi-Sunyer F. "Weight and non-insulin-dependent diabetes mellitus." *Am J Clin Nutr.* 1996;63 (suppl):428.498.

16. Colditz GA, Willet WC, Rotnitzky A, Manson JE. "Weight gain as a risk factor for clinical diabetes in women." *Ann Intern Med.* 1995;122:481.486.

17. Kannel W, D'Agostino R, Cabb J. "Effect of weight and cardiovascular disease." *Am J Clin Nutr.* 1996;63(suppl):4198–422S.

18. Harris TB, Launer LJ, Madans J, Feldman JJ. "Cohort study of effect of being overweight and change in weight on risk of coronary heart disease in old age." *BMJ.* 1997;314:1791–1794.

19. Anderson J, Felson DT. "Factors associated with osteoarthritis of the knee in the first National Health and Nutrition Examination Survey (NHANES I)." *Am J Epidemiol.* 1988;128:179–189.

20. Davis MA, Ettinger WH, Neuhaus JM. "The role of metabolic factors and blood pressure in the association of obesity with osteoarthritis of the knee." *J Rheumatol.* 1988;15;1827–1832.

21. Davis MA, Ettinger WH, Neuhaus JM. "Obesity and osteoarthritis of the knee: evidence from the National Health and Nutrition Examination Survey (NHANES I)." *Semin Arthritis Rheum.* 1990;20:34.41.

22. Felson DT. "The epidemiology of knee osteoarthritis: results from the Framingham Osteoarthritis Study." *Semin Arthritis Rheum.* 1990; 20:42–50.

23. Felson DT, Zhang Y, Anthony JM, Naimark A, Anderson JJ. "Weight loss reduces risk for symptomatic knee osteoarthritis in women." *Ann Intern Med.* 1992;116:535–539.

24. Hochberg MC, Lethbridge-Cejku M, Scott WW, Reichle R, Plato CC, Tobin JD. "The association of body weight, body fatness and body fat distribution with osteoarthritis of the knee: data from the Baltimore Longitudinal study of Aging." *J Rheumatol.* 1995;22:488–493.

25. Felson D. "Weight and osteoarthritis." *Am J Clin Nutr.* 1996;63 (suppl):430S–432S.

26. Martin K, Lethbridge-Cejku M, Muller DC, Elahi D, Andres R, Tobin JD, Hochberg MC. "Metabolic correlates of obesity and radiographic features of knee osteoarthritis: data from

the Baltimore Longitudinal Study of Aging." *J Rheumatol.* 1997;24;702–707.

27. Manninen P, Rilhimaki H, Heliovaara M, Makela P. "Overweight, gender and knee osteoarthritis." *Int J Obes Relat Metab Disord.* 1996;20:595–597.

28. Wardlaw G. "Putting bodyweight and osteoporosis into perspective." *Am J Clin Nutr.* 1996;63(suppl):433S–436S.

29. Build Study 1979. "Chicago, Ill: Society of Actuaries and Association of Life Insurance Medical Directors; 1980."

30. Hubert HB, Bloch DA, Fries JF. "Risk factors for physical disability in an aging cohort: the NHANES I Epidemiologic Follow-up Study." *J Rheumatol.* 1293;20:480–488.

31. Galanos A, Dieper C, Corcni-Huntly J, Bales C, Fillenbaum G. "Nutrition and function: is there a relationship between body mass index and functional capabilities of community-dwelling elderly?" *J Am Geriatr Soc.* 1994;42:368–374.

32. Launer LJ, Harris T, Rumpel C, Madana J. "Body mass index, weight change, and risk of mobility disability in middle-aged and older women." *JAMA.* 1994;271:1093–1098.

33. Ensrud KE, Nevitt MC, Yunis C, Cauley JA, Seeley DG, Fox KM, Cushings SR. "Correlates of impaired function in older women." *J Am Geriatr Soc.* 1994;42:481–489.

34. Jordan JM, Luta G, Renner JB, Linder GF, Dragomir A, Hochberg MC, Fryer JG. "Self-reported functional status in osteoarthritis of the knee in a rural southern community: the role of sociodemographic factors, obesity, and knee pain." *Arthritis Care Res.* 1998;9:272–278.

35. Apovian C, Frey C, Rogers J, McDermott B, Jensen G. "Body mass index and physical function in obese older women." *J Am Geriatr Soc.* 1996;44:1487–1488.

36. Still C, Apovian C, Jensen G. "Failure to thrive in older adults [letter]." *Ann Intern Med.* 1997;126:668.

37. Kolotkin R, Head S, Hamilton M, Tse C. "Assessing impact of weight on quality of life." *Obes Res.* 1995;3:49–56.

38. Gorsky RD, Pamuk E, Williamson DF, Shaffer PA, Kaplan JP. "The 25-year health costs of women who remain overweight after 40 years of age." *Am J Prev Med.* 1996;12:388–394.

9. Wolf A, Colditz G, "Social and economic effects of body weight in the United States." *Am J Clin Nutr.* 1996;63(suppl):4668–4698.

40. Thomas S, Reading J, Shepard RJ. "Revision of the physical activity readiness questionnaire (PAR-Q)." *Can J Sports Sci.* 1992;17:338–345.

41. Pate R, Pratt M, Blair S, Haskel W, Macera C, Haskell WL, Bouchard C, Buchner D, Ettinger W, Heath GW, King AC, Kriska A, Leon AS, Marcus BH, Morris J. "Physical activity and public health." *JAMA.* 1995; 273:402–407.

42. Evans WJ, Cyr-Campbell D. "Nutrition, exercise, and healthy aging." *J Am Diet Assoc.* 1997;97:632–638.

43. Connolly HM, Crary JL, McGoon MD, Hensrud DD, Edwards BS, Edwards WD, Schaff HV. "Valvular heart disease associated with fenfluramine-phentermine." *N Engl J Med.* 1997;337:581–588.

44. Whelton PK, Appel LL, Espeland MA, Applegate WB, Ettinger WH Jr, Kostis JB, Kumanyika S, Lacy CR, Johnson KC, Folmar S, Cutler J A. "Sodium reduction and weight loss in the treatment of hypertension in older persons: a randomized controlled trial of nonpharmacologic interventions in the elderly (TONE). TONE Collaborative Research Group." *JAMA.* 1998;279:839–846.

—by Gordon L. Jensen

G. L. Jensen is an associate professor of medicine with the Division of Gastroenterology at Vanderbilt University Medical Center, Nashville, Tenn. J. Rogers is a clinical nurse specialist at the Penn State Geisinger Medical Center, Danville, Pa.

Part Five

Additional Help and Information

Chapter 50

Glossary of Terms Related to Obesity and Its Management

A

abdominal fat: Fat (adipose tissue) that is centrally distributed between the thorax and pelvis and that induces greater health risk.

absolute risk: The observed or calculated probability of an event in a population under study, as contrasted with the relative risk.

aerobic exercise: A type of physical activity that includes walking, jogging, running, and dancing. Aerobic training improves the efficiency of the aerobic energy-producing systems that can improve cardio-respiratory endurance.

age-adjusted: Summary measures of rates of morbidity or mortality in a population using statistical procedures to remove the effect of age differences in populations that are being compared. Age is probably the most important and the most common variable in determining the risk of morbidity and mortality.

anorexiant: A drug, process, or event that leads to anorexia.

anthropometric measurements: Measurements of human body height, weight, and size of component parts, including skinfold measurement. Used to study and compare the relative proportions under normal and abnormal conditions.

"Clinical Guidelines on the Identification, Evaluation, and Treatment of Overweight and Obesity in Adults: Glossary of Terms," pp. 167-177, http://www.nhlbi.nih.gov/guidelines/obesity/ob_gdlns.pdf, 1998.

atherogenic: Causing the formation of plaque in the lining of the arteries.

behavior therapy: Behavior therapy constitutes those strategies, based on learning principles such as reinforcement, that provide tools for overcoming barriers to compliance with dietary therapy and/or increased physical activity.

biliopancreatic diversion: A surgical procedure for weight loss that combines a modest amount of gastric restriction with intestinal malabsorption.

B

BMI: Body mass index; the body weight in kilograms divided by the height in meters squared (wt/ht2) used as a practical marker to assess obesity; often referred to as the Quetelet Index. An indicator of optimal weight for health and different from lean mass or percent body fat calculations because it only considers height and weight.

body composition: The ratio of lean body mass (structural and functional elements in cells, body water, muscle, bone, heart, liver, kidneys, etc.) to body fat (essential and storage) mass. Essential fat is necessary for normal physiological functioning (e.g., nerve conduction). Storage fat constitutes the body's fat reserves, the part that people try to lose.

C

carbohydrates: A nutrient that supplies 4 calories/gram. They may be simple or complex. Simple carbohydrates are called sugars, and complex carbohydrates are called starch and fiber (cellulose). An organic compound-containing carbon, hydrogen, and oxygen-that is formed by photosynthesis in plants. Carbohydrates are heat producing and are classified as monosaccharides, disaccharides, or polysaccharides.

cardiovascular disease (CVD): Any abnormal condition characterized by dysfunction of the heart and blood vessels. CVD includes atherosclerosis (especially coronary heart disease, which can lead to heart attacks), cerebrovascular disease (e.g., stroke), and hypertension (high blood pressure).

central fat distribution: The waist circumference is an index of body fat distribution. Increasing waist circumference is accompanied by

Glossary of Terms Related to Obesity and Its Management

increasing frequencies of overt noninsulin-dependent diabetes mellitus, dyslipidemia, hypertension, coronary heart disease, stroke, and early mortality. In the body fat patterns called android type (apple shaped) fat is deposited around the waist and upper abdominal area and appears most often in men. Abdominal body fat is thought to be associated with a rapid mobilization of fatty acids rather than resulting from other fat depots, although it remains a point of contention. If abdominal fat is indeed more active than other fat depots, it would then provide a mechanism by which we could explain (in part) the increase in blood lipid and glucose levels. The latter have been clearly associated with an increased risk for cardiovascular disease hypertension and type 2 diabetes mellitus. The gynoid type (pear-shaped) of body fat is usually seen in women. The fat is deposited around the hips, thighs, and buttocks, and presumably is used as energy reserve during pregnancy and lactation.

cholecystectomy: Surgical removal of the gallbladder and gallstones, if present.

cholecystitis: Inflammation of the gallbladder, caused primarily by gallstones. Gallbladder disease occurs most often in obese women older than 40 years of age.

cholesterol: A soft, waxy substance manufactured by the body and used in the production of hormones, bile acid, and vitamin D and present in all parts of the body, including the nervous system, muscle, skin, liver, intestines, and heart. Blood cholesterol circulates in the bloodstream. Dietary cholesterol is found in foods of animal origin.

cimetidine: A weight loss drug that is thought to work by suppression of gastric acid or suppression of hunger by blocking histamine H2 receptors. It is not approved by the Food and Drug Administration (FDA).

cognitive behavior therapy: A system of psychotherapy based on the premise that distorted or dysfunctional thinking, which influences a person's mood or behavior, is common to all psychosocial problems. The focus of therapy is to identify the distorted thinking and to replace it with more rational, adaptive thoughts and beliefs.

comorbidity: Two or more diseases or conditions existing together in an individual.

computed tomography (CT) scans: A radiographic technique for direct visualization and quantification of fat that offers high image contrast and clear separation of fat from other soft tissues. CT can estimate total body adipose tissue volume and identify regional, subcutaneous, visceral, and other adipose tissue depots. Radiation exposure, expense, and unavailability restrict the epidemiologic use of CT.

confounding: Extraneous variables resulting in outcome effects that obscure or exaggerate the "true" effect of an intervention.

coronary heart disease (CHD): A type of heart disease caused by narrowing of the coronary arteries that feed the heart, which needs a constant supply of oxygen and nutrients carried by the blood in the coronary arteries. When the coronary arteries become narrowed or clogged by fat and cholesterol deposits and cannot supply enough blood to the heart, CHD results.

cue avoidance: A stimulus control technique often used in weight loss programs in which individuals are asked to reduce their exposure to certain food cues by making a variety of changes in their habits. The rationale is to make it easier on oneself and reduce temptation by reducing contact with food cues. For example, coming home from work and feeling tired is a time when many people reach for the high fat foods if they are available. By not having the high fat foods within reach, one can avoid eating them.

D

dexfenfluramine: A serotonin agonist drug used to treat obesity. FDA approval has been withdrawn.

diabetes: A complex disorder of carbohydrate, fat, and protein metabolism that is primarily a result of relative or complete lack of insulin secretion by the beta cells of the pancreas or a result of defects of the insulin receptors.

diastolic blood pressure: The minimum pressure that remains within the artery when the heart is at rest.

diethylproprion: An appetite suppressant prescribed in the treatment of obesity.

dopamine: A catecholamine neurotransmitter that is found primarily in the basal ganglia of the central nervous system. Major functions include the peripheral inhibition and excitation of certain muscles; cardiac excitation; and metabolic, endocrine and central nervous system actions.

Glossary of Terms Related to Obesity and Its Management

dual energy X-ray absortiometry (DEXA): A method used to estimate total body fat and percent of body fat. Potential disadvantages include whole body radiation and the long time required for scanning while the subject lies on a hard table.

dyslipidemia: Disorders in the lipoprotein metabolism; classified as hypercholesterolemia, hypertriglyceridemia, combined hyperlipidemia, and low levels of high-density lipoprotein (HDL) cholesterol. All of the dyslipidemias can be primary or secondary. Both elevated levels of low-density lipoprotein (LDL) cholesterol and low levels of HDL cholesterol predispose to premature atherosclerosis.

E

efficacy: The extent to which a specific intervention, procedure, regimen, or service produces a beneficial result under ideal conditions. Ideally, the determination of efficacy is based on the results of a randomized control trial.

energy balance: Energy is the capacity of a body or a physical system for doing work. Energy balance is the state in which the total energy intake equals total energy needs.

energy deficit: A state in which total energy intake is less than total energy need.

ephedrine: A sympathomimetic drug that stimulates thermogenesis in laboratory animals and humans. Animal studies show that it may reduce fat content and, therefore, body weight by mechanisms that probably involve increased expenditure and reduced food intake.

extreme obesity: A body mass index greater than 40.

F

femoxetine: A selective serotonin reuptake inhibitor drug used in obese patients for weight loss.

fenfluramine: A serotonin agonist drug used in the treatment of obesity. FDA approval has been withdrawn.

fibrinogen: A plasma protein that is converted into fibrin by thrombin in the presence of calcium ions. Fibrin is responsible for the semisolid character of a blood clot.

fluoxetine: An antidepressant drug used to promote weight loss whose action is mediated by highly specific inhibition of serotonin reuptake into presynaptic neurons. Serotonin acts in the brain to alter feeding and satiety by decreasing carbohydrate intake, resulting in weight reduction.

G

gallstones: Constituents in the gallbladder that are not reabsorbed, including bile salts and lipid substances such as cholesterol that become highly concentrated. They can cause severe pain (obstruction and cramps) as they move into the common bile duct. Risk factors for cholesterol gallstone formation include female gender, weight gain, overweight, high energy intake, ethnic factors (Pima Indians and Scandinavians), use of certain drugs (clofibrate, estrogens, and bile acid sequestrants), and presence of gastrointestinal disease. Gallstones sometimes develop during dieting for weight reduction. There is an increased risk for gallstones and acute gallbladder disease during severe caloric restriction.

gastric banding: Surgery to limit the amount of food the stomach can hold by closing part of it off. A band made of special material is placed around the stomach near its upper end, creating a small pouch and a narrow passage into the larger remainder of the stomach. The small outlet delays the emptying of food from the pouch and causes a feeling of fullness.

gastric bubble/balloon: A free-floating intragastric balloon used in the treatment of obesity.

gastric bypass: A surgical procedure that combines the creation of small stomach pouches to restrict food intake and the construction of bypasses of the duodenum and other segments of the small intestine to cause food malabsorption. Patients generally lose two-thirds of their excess weight after 2 years.

gastric exclusion: Same as gastric partitioning and Rouxen Y bypass. A small stomach pouch is created by stapling or by vertical banding to restrict food intake. A Y-shaped section of the small intestine is attached to the pouch to allow food to bypass the duodenum as well as the first portion of the jejunum.

gastric partitioning: See gastric exclusion.

Glossary of Terms Related to Obesity and Its Management

gastroplasty: See also jejuno-ileostomy. A surgical procedure that limits the amount of food the stomach can hold by closing off part of the stomach. Food intake is restricted by creating a small pouch at the top of the stomach where the food enters from the esophagus. The pouch initially holds about 1 ounce of food and expands to 2-3 ounces with time. The pouch's lower outlet usually has a diameter of about 1/4 inch. The small outlet delays the emptying of food from the pouch and causes a feeling of fullness.

genotype: The entire genetic makeup of an individual. The fundamental constitution of an organism in terms of its hereditary factors. A group of organisms in which each has the same hereditary characteristics.

glucose tolerance: The power of the normal liver to absorb and store large quantities of glucose and the effectiveness of intestinal absorption of glucose. The glucose tolerance test is a metabolic test of carbohydrate tolerance that measures active insulin, a hepatic function based on the ability of the liver to absorb glucose. The test consists of ingesting 100 grams of glucose into a fasting stomach; blood sugar should return to normal approximately 2 hours after ingestion.

H

hemoglobin A1c: Microvascular diseases in patients with insulin-dependent diabetes mellitus (IDDM, or type I) are clearly related to the level of hemoglobin (Hb)A1c (i.e., glycemia). HbA1c levels are used by clinicians as a measure of long-term control of plasma glucose (normal, 4 to 6 percent). Generally, complications are substantially lower among patients with HbA1c levels of 7 percent or less than in patients with HbA1c levels of 9 percent or more.

hemorrhagic stroke: A disorder involving bleeding within ischemic brain tissue. Hemorrhagic stroke occurs when blood vessels that are damaged or dead from lack of blood supply (infarcted), located within an area of infarcted brain tissue, rupture and transform an "ischemic" stroke into a hemorrhagic stroke. Ischemia is inadequate tissue oxygenation caused by reduced blood flow; infarction is tissue death resulting from ischemia. Bleeding irritates the brain tissues, causing swelling (cerebral edema). Blood collects into a mass (hematoma). Both swelling and hematoma will compress and displace brain tissue.

heritability: The proportion of observed variation in a particular trait that can be attributed to inherited genetic factors in contrast to environmental ones.

high-density lipoproteins (HDL): Lipoproteins that contain a small amount of cholesterol and carry cholesterol away from body cells and tissues to the liver for excretion from the body. Low-level HDL increases the risk of heart disease, so the higher the HDL level, the better. The HDL component normally contains 20 to 30 percent of total cholesterol, and HDL levels are inversely correlated with coronary heart disease risk.

hypercholesterolemia (high blood cholesterol): Cholesterol is the most abundant steroid in animal tissues, especially in bile and gallstones. The relationship between the intake of cholesterol and its manufacture by the body to its utilization, sequestration, or excretion from the body is called the cholesterol balance. When cholesterol accumulates, the balance is positive; when it declines, the balance is negative. In 1993 NHLBI National Cholesterol Education Program (NCEP) Expert Panel on Detection, Evaluation, and Treatment of High Blood Cholesterol in Adults issued an updated set of recommendations for monitoring and treatment of blood cholesterol levels. The NCEP guidelines recommended that total cholesterol levels and subfractions of high-density lipoprotein (HDL) cholesterol be measured beginning at age 20 in all adults, with subsequent periodic screenings as needed. Even in the group of patients at lowest risk for coronary heart disease (total cholesterol less than 200 mg/dL and HDL greater than 35 mg/dL), the NCEP recommended that rescreening take place at least once every 5 years or upon physical examination.

hypertension: High blood pressure (i.e., abnormally high blood pressure tension involving systolic and/or diastolic levels). The Sixth Report of the Joint National Committee on Prevention, Detection, Evaluation, and Treatment of High Blood Pressure defines hypertension as a systolic blood pressure of 140 mm Hg or greater, a diastolic blood pressure of 90 mm Hg or greater, or taking hypertensive medication. The cause may be adrenal, benign, essential, Goldblatt's, idiopathic, malignant pate, portal, postpartum, primary, pulmonary, renal or renovascular.

hypertriglyceridemia: An excess of triglycerides in the blood that is an autosomal dominant disorder with the phenotype of hyperlipoproteinemia, type IV. The National Cholesterol Education

Program defines a high level of triglycerides as being between 400 and 1,000 mg/dL.

I

incidence: The rate at which a certain event occurs (i.e., the number of new cases of a specific disease occurring during a certain period).

insulin-dependent diabetes mellitus (type I diabetes): A disease characterized by high levels of blood glucose resulting from defects in insulin secretion, insulin action, or both. Autoimmune, genetic, and environmental factors are involved in the development of type I diabetes. Insulin-dependent diabetes mellitus (type I diabetes): A disease characterized by high levels of blood glucose resulting from defects in insulin secretion, insulin action, or both. Autoimmune, genetic, and environmental factors are involved in the development of type I diabetes.

ischemic stroke: A condition in which the blood supply to part of the brain is cut off. Also called "plug-type" stokes. Blocked arteries starve areas of the brain controlling sight, speech, sensation, and movement so that these functions are partially or completely lost. Ischemic stroke is the most common type of stroke, accounting for 80 percent of all strokes. Most ischemic strokes are caused by a blood clot called a thrombus, which blocks blood flow in the arteries feeding the brain, usually the carotid artery in the neck, the major vessel bringing blood to the brain. When it becomes blocked, the risk of stoke is very high.

J

jejuno-ileostomy: See gastroplasty.

j-shaped relationship: The relationship between body weight and mortality.

L

lipoprotein: Protein-coated packages that carry fat and cholesterol throughout the bloodstream. There are four general classes: high-density, low-density, very low-density, and chylomicrons.

locus/loci: A general anatomical term for a site in the body or the position of a gene on a chromosome.

longitudinal study: Also referred to as a "cohort study" or "prospective study"; the analytic method of epidemiologic study in which subsets of a defined population can be identified who are, have been, or in the future may be exposed or not exposed, or exposed in different degrees, to a factor or factors hypothesized to influence the probability of occurrence of a given disease or other outcome. The main feature of this type of study is to observe large numbers of subjects over an extended time, with comparisons of incidence rates in groups that differ in exposure levels.

low-calorie diet (LCD): Caloric restriction of about 800 to 1,500 calories (approximately 12 to 15 kcal/kg of body weight) per day.

low-density lipoprotein (LDL): Lipoprotein that contains most of the cholesterol in the blood. LDL carries cholesterol to the tissues of the body, including the arteries. A high level of LDL increases the risk of heart disease. LDL typically contains 60 to 70 percent of the total serum cholesterol and both are directly correlated with CHD risk.

lower-fat diet: An entire plan in which 30 percent or less of the day's total calories are from fat.

M

macronutrients: Nutrients in the diet that are the key sources of energy, namely protein, fat, and carbohydrates.

magnetic resonance imaging (MRI): Magnetic resonance imaging uses radio frequency waves to provide direct visualization and quantification of fat. The sharp image contrast of MRI allows clear separation of adipose tissue from surrounding nonlipid structures. Essentially the same information provided by CT is available from MRI, including total body and regional adipose tissue, subcutaneous adipose, and estimates of various visceral adipose tissue components. The advantage of MRI is its lack of ionizing radiation and hence its presumed safety in children, younger adults, and pregnant women. The minimal present use of MRI can be attributed to the expense, limited access to instrumentation, and long scanning time.

menopause: The cessation of menstruation in the human female, which begins at about the age of 50.

monounsaturated fat: An unsaturated fat that is found primarily in plant foods, including olive and canola oils.

Glossary of Terms Related to Obesity and Its Management

myocardial infarction (MI): Gross necrosis of the myocardium as a result of interruption of the blood supply to the area; it is almost always caused by atherosclerosis of the coronary arteries, upon which coronary thrombosis is usually superimposed.

N

NHANES: National Health and Nutrition Examination Survey; conducted every 10 years by the National Center for Health Statistics to survey the dietary habits and health of U.S. residents.

O

obesity: The condition of having an abnormally high proportion of body fat. Most overweight persons are obese. Defined as a body mass index (BMI) of greater than or equal to 30. Subjects are generally classified as obese when body fat content exceeds 30 percent in women and 25 percent in men.

observational study: An epidemiologic study that does not involve any intervention, experimental or otherwise. Such a study may be one in which nature is allowed to take its course, with changes in one characteristic being studied in relation to changes in other characteristics. Analytical epidemiologic methods, such as case-control and cohort study designs, are properly called observational epidemiology because the investigator is observing without intervention other than to record, classify, count, and statistically analyze results.

Orlistat: A lipase inhibitor used for weight loss. Lipase is an enzyme found in the bowel that assists in lipid absorption by the body. Orlistat blocks this enzyme, reducing the amount of fat the body absorbs by about 30 percent. It is known colloquially as a "fat blocker." Because more oily fat is left in the bowel to be excreted, Orlistat can cause an oily anal leakage and fecal incontinence. Orlistat may not be suitable for people with bowel conditions such as irritable bowel syndrome or Crohn's disease.

osteoarthritis: Noninflammatory degenerative joint disease occurring chiefly in older persons, characterized by degeneration of the articular cartilage, hypertrophy of bone at the margins, and changes in the synovial membrane. It is accompanied by pain and stiffness.

overweight: An excess of body weight but not necessarily body fat; a body mass index of 25 to 29.9 kg/m2.

P

peripheral regions: Other regions of the body besides the abdominal region (i.e., the gluteal-femoral area).

pharmacotherapy: A regimen of using appetite suppressant medications to manage obesity by decreasing appetite or increasing the feeling of satiety. These medications decrease appetite by increasing serotonin or catecholamine-two brain chemicals that affect mood and appetite.

phenotype: The entire physical, biochemical, and physiological makeup of an individual as determined by his or her genes and by the environment in the broad sense.

phentermine: An adrenergic isomeric with amphetamine, used as an anorexic; administered orally as a complex with an ion-exchange resin to produce a sustained action.

polyunsaturated fat: An unsaturated fat found in greatest amounts in foods derived from plants, including safflower, sunflower, corn, and soybean oils.

postprandial plasma blood glucose: Glucose tolerance test performed after ingesting food.

prevalence: The number of events, e.g., instances of a given disease or other condition, in a given population at a designated time. When used without qualification, the term usually refers to the situation at specific point in time (point prevalence). Prevalence is a number not a rate.

prospective study: An epidemiologic study in which a group of individuals (a cohort), all free of a particular disease and varying in their exposure to a possible risk factor, is followed over a specific amount of time to determine the incidence rates of the disease in the exposed and unexposed groups.

protein: A class of compounds composed of linked amino acids that contain carbon, hydrogen, nitrogen, oxygen, and sometimes other atoms in specific configurations.

R

randomization: Also called random allocation. Is allocation of individuals to groups, e.g., for experimental and control regimens, by

Glossary of Terms Related to Obesity and Its Management

chance. Within the limits of chance variation, random allocation should make the control and experimental groups similar at the start of an investigation and ensure that personal judgment and prejudices of the investigator do not influence allocation.

randomized clinical trial (RCT): An epidemiologic experiment in which subjects in a population are randomly allocated into groups, usually called study and control groups, to receive or not to receive an experimental prevention or therapeutic product, maneuver, or intervention. The results are assessed by rigorous comparison of rates of disease, death, recovery, or other appropriate outcome in the study and control groups, respectively. RCTs are generally regarded as the most scientifically rigorous method of hypothesis testing available in epidemiology.

recessive gene: A gene that is phenotypically expressed only when homozygous.

refractory obesity: Obesity that is resistant to treatment.

resting metabolic rate (RMR): RMR accounts for 65 to 75 percent of daily energy expenditure and represents the minimum energy needed to maintain all physiological cell functions in the resting state. The principal determinant of RMR is lean body mass (LBM). Obese subjects have a higher RMR in absolute terms than lean individuals, an equivalent RMR when corrected for LBM and per unit surface area, and a lower RMR when expressed per kilogram of body weight. Obese persons require more energy for any given activity because of a larger mass, but they tend to be more sedentary than lean subjects.

risk: The probability that an event will occur. Also, a nontechnical term encompassing a variety of measures of the probability of a generally unfavorable outcome.

Roux-en Y bypass: See gastric exclusion; the most common gastric bypass procedure.

S

saturated fat: A type of fat found in greatest amounts in foods from animals, such as fatty cuts of meat, poultry with the skin, whole-milk dairy products, lard, and in some vegetable oils, including coconut, palm kernel, and palm oils. Saturated fat raises blood cholesterol more than anything else eaten. On a Step I Diet, no more than 8 to 10 percent of total calories should come from saturated fat, and in the Step II Diet, less than 7 percent of the day's total calories should come from saturated fat.

secular trends: A relatively long-term trend in a community or country.

serotonin: A monoamine vasoconstrictor, found in various animals from coelenterates to vertebrates, in bacteria, and in many plants. In humans, it is synthesized in the intestinal chromaffin cells or in the central or peripheral neurons and is found in high concentrations in many body tissues, including the intestinal mucosa, pineal body, and central nervous system. Produced enzymatically from tryptophan by hydroxylation and decarboxylation, serotonin has many physiologic properties (e.g., inhibits gastric secretion, stimulates smooth muscle, serves as central neurotransmitter, and is a precursor of melatonin).

sibutramine: A drug used for the management of obesity that helps reduce food intake and is indicated for weight loss and maintenance of weight loss when used in conjunction with a reduced-calorie diet. It works to suppress the appetite primarily by inhibiting the reuptake of the neurotransmitters norepinephrine and serotonin. Side effects include dry mouth, headache, constipation, insomnia, and a slight increase in average blood pressure. In some patients it causes a higher blood pressure increase.

sleep apnea: A serious, potentially life-threatening breathing disorder characterized by repeated cessation of breathing due to either collapse of the upper airway during sleep or absence of respiratory effort.

social pressure: A strategy used in behavior therapy in which individuals are told that they possess the basic self-control ability to lose weight, but that coming to group meetings will strengthen their abilities. The group is asked to listen and give advice, similar to the way many self-help groups, based on social support, operate.

stoma size: The size of a new opening created surgically between two body structures.

stress incontinence: An involuntary loss of urine that occurs at the same time that internal abdominal pressure is increased, such as with laughing, sneezing, coughing, or physical activity.

Glossary of Terms Related to Obesity and Its Management

stress management: A set of techniques used to help an individual cope more effectively with difficult situations in order to feel better emotionally, improve behavioral skills, and often to enhance feelings of control. Stress management may include relaxation exercises, assertiveness training, cognitive restructuring, time management, and social support. It can be delivered either on a one-to-one basis or in a group format.

stroke: Sudden loss of function of part of the brain because of loss of blood flow. Stroke may be caused by a clot (thrombosis) or rupture (hemorrhage) of a blood vessel to the brain.

submaximal heart rate test: Used to determine the systematic use of physical activity. The submaximal work levels allow work to be increased in small increments until cardiac manifestations such as angina pain appear. This provides a more precise manipulation of workload and gives a reliable and quantitative index of a person's functional impairment if heart disease is detected.

surgical procedures: See jejuno-ileostomy, gastroplasty, gastric bypass, gastric partitioning, gastric exclusion, Roux-en Y bypass, and gastric bubble.

systolic blood pressure: The maximum pressure in the artery produced as the heart contracts and blood begins to flow.

T

triglyceride: A lipid carried through the bloodstream to tissues. Most of the body's fat tissue is in the form of triglycerides, stored for use as energy. Triglycerides are obtained primarily from fat in foods.

type 2 diabetes mellitus: Usually characterized by a gradual onset with minimal or no symptoms of metabolic disturbance and no requirement for exogenous insulin. The peak age of onset is 50 to 60 years. Obesity and possibly a genetic factor are usually present.

V

validity: The degree to which the inferences drawn from study results, especially generalization extending beyond the study sample, are warranted when account is taken of the study methods, the representativeness of the study sample, and the nature of the population from which it is drawn.

vertical banded gastroplasty: A surgical treatment for extreme obesity; an operation on the stomach that involves constructing a small pouch in the stomach that empties through a narrow opening into the distal stomach and duodenum.

very low-calorie diet (VLCD): The VLCD of 800 (approximately 6-10 kcal/kg body weight) or fewer calories per day is conducted under physician supervision and monitoring and is restricted 177 to severely obese persons.

very low-density lipoprotein (VLDL): The lipoprotein particles that initially leave the liver, carrying cholesterol and lipid. VLDLs contain 10 to 15 percent of the total serum cholesterol along with most of the triglycerides in the fasting serum; VLDLs are precursors of LDL, and some forms of VLDL, particularly VLDL remnants, appear to be atherogenic (from ATP II).

visceral fat: One of the three compartments of abdominal fat. Retroperitoneal and subcutaneous are the other two compartments.

VO 2 max: Maximal oxygen uptake is known as VO2 max and is the maximal capacity for oxygen consumption by the body during maximal exertion. It is used as an indicator of cardio-respiratory fitness.

W

waist circumference: To define the level at which the waist circumference is measured, a bony landmark is first located and marked. The subject stands, and the technician, positioned to the right of the subject, palpates the upper hip bone to locate the right ileum. Just above the uppermost lateral border of the right ileum, a horizontal mark is drawn and then crossed with a vertical mark on the midaxillary line. The measuring tape is then placed around the trunk, at the level of the mark on the right side, making sure that it is on a level horizontal plane on all sides. The tape is then tightened slightly without compressing the skin and underlying subcutaneous tissues. The measure is recorded in centimeters to the nearest millimeter.

waist-hip ratio (WHR): The ratio of a person's waist circumference to hip circumference. WHR looks at the relationship between the differences in the measurements of waist and hips. Most people store body fat in two distinct ways, often called the "apple" and "pear" shapes, either the middle (apple) or the hips (pear). For most people,

Glossary of Terms Related to Obesity and Its Management

carrying extra weight around their middle increases health risks more than carrying extra weight around their hips or thighs. Overall obesity, however, is still of greater risk than body fat storage locations or WHR. A WHR greater than or equal to 1.0 is in the danger zone, with risks of heart disease and other ailments connected with being overweight. For men, a ratio of .90 or less is considered safe, and for women .80 or less.

List of Abbreviations

AAFP: American Academy of Family Physicians

ADA: American Diabetes Association

AHCPR: Agency for Health-Care Policy and Research

AHI: Apnea and Hypopnea Index

ATP II: Second Report of the Expert Panel on the Detection, Evaluation, and Treatment of High Blood Cholesterol in Adults (Adult Treatment Panel II)

BED: Binge Eating Disorder

BMI: Body Mass Index

BN: Bulimia Nervosa

CAD: Coronary Artery Disease

CARDIA: Coronary Artery Risk Development in Young Adults

CDC: Centers for Disease Control and Prevention

CHD: Coronary Heart Disease

CHF: Congestive Heart Failure

CPAP: Continuous Positive Airway Pressure

CRSS: Critical Review Status Sheet

CT: Computed Tomography

CVD: Cardiovascular Disease

DEXA: Dual-Energy X-ray Absorpiometry

DNA: Deoxyribonucleic Acid

FDA: Food and Drug Administration

HDL: High-Density Lipoprotein

HHANES: Hispanic Health and Nutrition Examination Survey

HMO: Health Maintenance Organization

IGT: Impaired Glucose Tolerance

IOM: Institute of Medicine

LCD: Low-Calorie Diets

LDL: Low-Density Lipoprotein

MEDLINE MEDLARS: (Medical Literature Analysis and Retrieval System) On-Line

MeSH: Medical Subject Headings

MMPI: Minnesota Multiphasic Personality Inventory

MRI: Magnetic Resonance Imaging

NAASO: North American Association of the Study of Obesity

NCEP: National Cholesterol Education Program

NHANES: National Health and Nutrition Examination Survey

NHBPEP: National High Blood Pressure Education Program

NHCS: National Center for Health Statistics (CDC)

NHES: National Health Examination Survey

NHIS: National Health Interview Survey

NHLBI: National Heart, Lung, and Blood Institute

NIDDK: National Institute of Diabetes and Digestive and Kidney iseases

NIH: National Institutes of Health

NLM: National Library of Medicine

RCTs: Randomized Controlled Trials

RDI: Respiratory Disturbance Index

SOS: Swedish Obesity Study

SSRIs: Selective Serotonin Reuptake Inhibitors

TAIM: Trial of Antihypertensive Interventions and Management

Glossary of Terms Related to Obesity and Its Management

TONE: Trial of Nonpharmacologic Interventions in the Elderly

VLCD: Very Low-Calorie Diets

VLDL: Very Low-Density Lipoprotein

VO 2 max: Oxygen Consumption

WHR: Waist-to-Hip Ratio

Chapter 51

Practical Dietary Therapy Information

This chapter contains helpful charts, shopping lists, nutrition information, calorie charts, and low-fat menus. The chapter also includes tips for healthy eating out. The Body Mass Index (BMI) table [shown in Table 51.1] is referred to extensively in other chapters in this sourcebook and is an increasingly accepted standard for determining obesity.

Shopping—What to Look for

Low-Calorie Shopping List

Make a shopping list. Include the items you need for your menus and any low-calorie basics you need to restock in your kitchen.

Dairy Case

- low-fat (1%) or fat free (skim) milk
- low-fat or reduced-fat cottage cheese
- fat-free cottage cheese
- low-fat cheeses
- low-fat or nonfat yogurt
- light or diet margarine (tub, squeeze or spray)
- reduced-fat or fat-free sour cream
- fat-free cream cheese
- eggs/Egg substitutes

Excerpted from "Clinical Guidelines on the Identification, Evaluation, and Treatment of Overweight and Obesity in Adults: Appendix VI Practical Dietary Therapy Information," pp. 138–163, http://www.nhlbi.nih.gov/guidelines/obesity/ob_gdlns.pdf, 1998.

Breads, Muffins, Rolls

- bread, bagels, pita bread
- English muffins
- yeast breads (whole wheat, rye, pumpernickel, multi-grain, raisin)
- corn tortillas (not fried)
- low-fat flour tortillas
- fat-free biscuit mix
- foccacia
- rice crackers
- challah

Cereals, Crackers, Rice, Noodles, and Pasta

- plain cereal, dry or cooked
- saltines, soda crackers (low sodium or unsalted tops)
- graham crackers
- other low-fat crackers
- rice (brown, white, etc.)
- pasta (noodles, spaghetti)
- bulgur, couscous, kasha
- potato mixes (made without fat)
- rice mixes (made without fat)
- wheat mixes
- tabouli grain salad
- hominy
- polenta
- polvillo
- hominy grits
- quinoa
- millet
- aramanth

Meat Case

- white meat chicken and turkey (without skin)
- fish (not battered)
- beef, round or sirloin
- extra lean ground beef such as ground round
- pork tenderloin
- 95% fat-free lunch meats or low-fat deli meats
- meat equivalents:
- tofu (or bean curd)
- beans (see bean list)
- eggs/egg substitutes (see dairy list)

Practical Dietary Therapy Information

Fresh Fruit

- apples
- oranges
- pears
- grapefruit
- apricot
- dried fruits
- cherries
- raisins
- plums
- melons
- lemons
- limes
- plantains
- mango
- papaya
- kiwi
- olives
- figs
- quinces
- currants
- persimmons
- pomegranates
- anon
- caimito
- chirimoya
- guanabana
- mamey
- papayas
- zapote
- guava
- starfruit
- ugli fruit
- dried pickled plums
- litchee nuts
- winter melons

Canned Fruit
(in Juice or Water)

- canned pineapple
- applesauce
- other canned fruits (mixed or plain)

Frozen Fruits
(without Added Sugar)

- frozen blueberries
- frozen raspberries
- frozen 100% fruit juice

Dried Fruit

- raisins/dried fruit (these tend to be higher in calories than fresh fruit)

Fresh Vegetables

- broccoli
- peas
- cauliflower
- squash
- green Beans
- spinach
- cabbage
- artichokes
- cucumber
- asparagus
- mushrooms
- carrots or celery
- onions
- potatoes
- tomatoes
- green peppers
- chilies
- tomatillos

Canned Vegetables
(Low Sodium or No Salt Added)

- canned tomatoes
- tomato sauce or pasta
- other canned vegetables
- canned vegetable soup, reduced sodium

Frozen Vegetables
(without Added Fats)

- frozen broccoli
- frozen spinach
- frozen mixed medley, etc.
- frozen yucca

Exotic Fresh Vegetables

- okra
- dandelions
- eggplant
- grape leaves
- mustard greens
- kale
- leeks
- boniato
- chayote

- borenjena
- plantain
- cassava
- prickly pear cactus
- bamboo shoots
- Chinese celery
- water chestnuts
- bok choy
- burdock root

- napa cabbage
- taro
- seaweed
- bean sprouts
- amaranth
- choy sum
- calabacita
- sea vegetables
- rhubarb

Beans and Legumes (If Canned, No Salt Added)

- lentils
- black beans
- red beans (kidney beans)
- navy beans
- black beans
- pinto beans
- black-eyed peas
- fava beans

- mung beans
- Italian white beans
- great white northern beans
- chickpeas (garbanzo beans)
- dried beans, peas, and lentils (without flavoring packets)
- canned bean soup

Practical Dietary Therapy Information

Baking Items

- flour
- sugar
- imitation butter (flakes or buds)
- non-stick cooking spray
- canned evaporated milk—fat free (skim) or reduced-fat (2%)
- nonfat dry milk powder
- cocoa powder, unsweetened
- baking powder
- baking soda
- cornstarch
- unflavored gelatin
- gelatin, any flavor (reduced calorie)
- pudding mixes (reduced calorie)
- angel food cake mix
- other low-fat mixes
- other

Frozen Foods

- frozen fish fillets—unbreaded
- egg substitute
- frozen 100 percent fruit juices (no sugar added)
- frozen fruits (no sugar added)
- frozen vegetables (plain)
- other frozen foods

Condiments, Sauces, Seasonings, and Spreads

- low-fat or nonfat salad dressings
- mustard (Dijon, etc.)
- catsup
- barbecue sauce
- other low-fat sauces
- jam, jelly, or honey
- spices
- flavored vinegars
- hoisin sauce, plum sauce
- salsa or picante sauce
- canned green chilies
- soy sauce (low sodium)
- bouillon cubes/granules (low sodium)

Miscellaneous / Other Foods

- peas/whole legumes
- baked beans
- millet
- mushrooms
- oatmeal

Beverages

- no-calorie drink mixes
- diet soda
- reduced-calorie juices
- unsweetened iced tea
- carbonated water
- water

We live in a fast-moving world. To reduce the time you spend in the kitchen you can improve your organization by using a shopping list and keeping a well-stocked kitchen. Shop for quick low-fat food items, and fill your kitchen cupboards with a supply of low-calorie basics.

Read labels as you shop. Pay attention to the serving size and the servings per container. All labels list total calories in a serving size of the product. Compare the total calories in the product you choose with others like it; choose the one that is lowest in calories. Figure 51.1 shows a label that identifies important information.

Practical Dietary Therapy Information

Product:

Nutrition Facts
Serving Size 1 cup (228g)
Servings Per Container 2

Amount Per Serving	
Calories 250 Calories from Fat 110	
	% Daily Value*
Total Fat 12g	18%
Saturated Fat 3g	15%
Cholesterol 30mg	10%
Sodium 470mg	20%
Total Carbohydrate 31g	10%
Dietary Fiber 0g	0%
Sugars 5g	
Protein 5g	

Vitamin A 4% • Vitamin C 2%
Calcium 20% • Iron 4%

* Percent Daily Values are based on a 2,000 calorie diet. Your daily values may be higher or lower depending on your calorie needs:

	Calories:	2,000	2,500
Total Fat	Less than	65g	80g
Sat Fat	Less than	20g	25g
Cholesterol	Less than	300mg	300mg
Sodium	Less than	2,400mg	2,400mg
Total Carbohydrate		300g	375g
Dietary Fiber		25g	30g

Calories per gram:
Fat 9 • Carbohydrates 4 • Protein 4

Check for:

- Serving size
- Number of servings

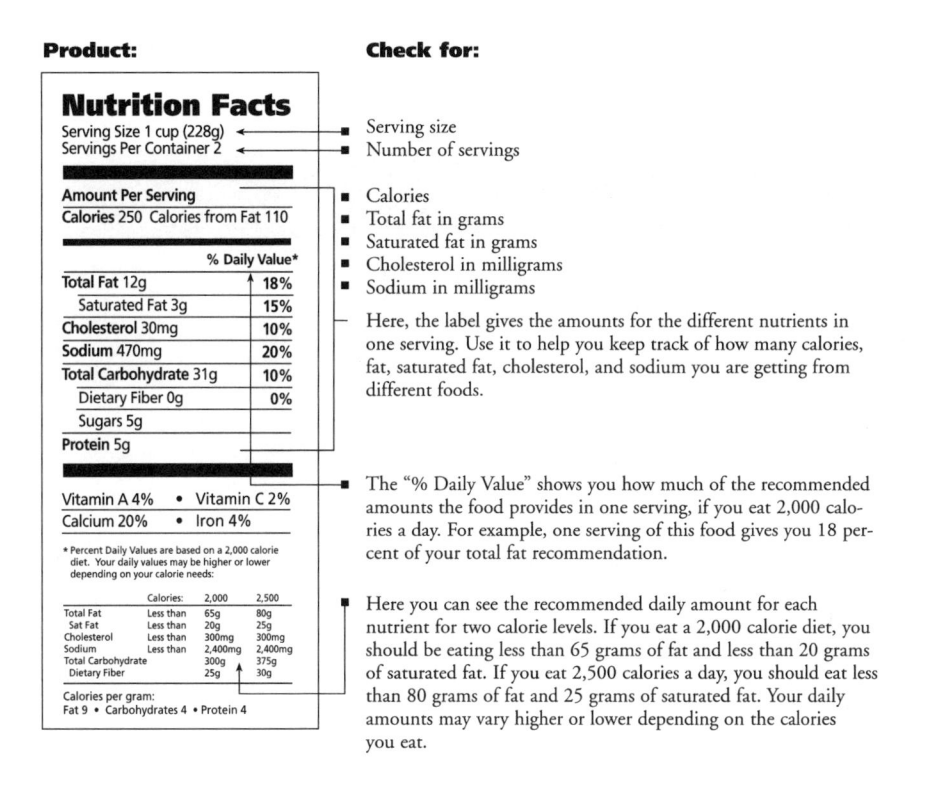

- Calories
- Total fat in grams
- Saturated fat in grams
- Cholesterol in milligrams
- Sodium in milligrams

Here, the label gives the amounts for the different nutrients in one serving. Use it to help you keep track of how many calories, fat, saturated fat, cholesterol, and sodium you are getting from different foods.

The "% Daily Value" shows you how much of the recommended amounts the food provides in one serving, if you eat 2,000 calories a day. For example, one serving of this food gives you 18 percent of your total fat recommendation.

Here you can see the recommended daily amount for each nutrient for two calorie levels. If you eat a 2,000 calorie diet, you should be eating less than 65 grams of fat and less than 20 grams of saturated fat. If you eat 2,500 calories a day, you should eat less than 80 grams of fat and 25 grams of saturated fat. Your daily amounts may vary higher or lower depending on the calories you eat.

Figure 51.1. The "Nutrition Facts" label.

Obesity Sourcebook, First Edition

Table 51.1a. The Body Mass Index (BMI) table (continued on next page).

To use the table, find the appropriate height in the left-hand column. Move across to a given weight. The number at the top of the column is the BMI at that height and weight. Pounds have been rounded off.

Body Mass Index	19	20	21	22	23	24	25	26	27	28	29	30	31	32	33	34	35
Height (inches)								Body Weight (pounds)									
58	91	96	100	105	110	115	119	124	129	134	138	143	148	153	158	162	167
59	94	99	104	109	114	119	124	128	133	138	143	148	153	158	163	168	173
60	97	102	107	112	118	123	128	133	138	143	148	153	158	163	168	174	179
61	100	106	111	116	122	127	132	137	143	148	153	158	164	169	174	180	185
62	104	109	115	120	126	131	136	142	147	153	158	164	169	175	180	186	191
63	107	113	118	124	130	135	141	146	152	158	163	169	175	180	186	191	197
64	110	116	122	128	134	140	145	151	157	163	169	174	180	186	192	197	204
65	114	120	126	132	138	144	150	156	162	168	174	180	186	192	198	204	210
66	118	124	130	136	142	148	155	161	167	173	179	186	192	198	204	210	216
67	121	127	134	140	146	153	159	166	172	178	185	191	198	204	211	217	223
68	125	131	138	144	151	158	164	171	177	184	190	197	203	210	216	223	230
69	128	135	142	149	155	162	169	176	182	189	196	203	209	216	223	230	236
70	132	139	146	153	160	167	174	181	188	195	202	209	216	222	229	236	243
71	136	143	150	157	165	172	179	186	193	200	208	215	222	229	236	243	250
72	140	147	154	162	169	177	184	191	199	206	213	221	228	235	242	250	258
73	144	151	159	166	174	182	189	197	204	212	219	227	235	242	250	257	265
74	148	155	163	171	179	186	194	202	210	218	225	233	241	249	256	264	272
75	152	160	168	176	184	192	200	208	216	224	232	240	248	256	264	272	279
76	156	164	172	180	189	197	205	213	221	230	238	246	254	263	271	279	287

Practical Dietary Therapy Information

Table 51.1b. The Body Mass Index (BMI) table (continued from previous page).

BODY MASS INDEX

Height (inches)	36	37	38	39	40	41	42	43	44	45	46	47	48	49	50	51	52	53	54
58	172	177	181	186	191	196	201	205	210	215	220	224	229	234	239	244	248	253	258
59	178	183	188	193	198	203	208	212	217	222	227	232	237	242	247	252	257	262	267
60	184	189	194	199	204	209	215	220	225	230	235	240	245	250	255	261	266	271	276
61	190	195	201	206	211	217	222	227	232	238	243	248	254	259	264	269	275	280	285
62	196	202	207	213	218	224	229	235	240	246	251	256	262	267	273	278	284	289	295
63	203	208	214	220	225	231	237	242	248	254	259	265	270	278	282	287	293	299	304
64	209	215	221	227	232	238	244	250	256	262	267	273	279	285	291	296	302	308	314
65	216	222	228	234	240	246	252	258	264	270	276	282	288	294	300	306	312	318	324
66	223	229	235	241	247	253	260	266	272	278	284	291	297	303	309	315	322	328	334
67	230	236	242	249	255	261	268	274	280	287	293	299	306	312	319	325	331	338	344
68	236	243	249	256	262	269	276	282	289	295	302	308	315	322	328	335	341	348	354
69	243	250	257	263	270	277	284	291	297	304	311	318	324	331	338	345	351	358	365
70	250	257	264	271	278	285	292	299	306	313	320	327	334	341	348	355	362	369	376
71	257	265	272	279	286	293	301	308	315	322	329	338	343	351	358	365	372	379	386
72	265	272	279	287	294	302	309	316	324	331	338	346	353	361	368	375	383	390	397
73	272	280	288	295	302	310	318	325	333	340	348	355	363	371	378	386	393	401	408
74	280	287	295	303	311	319	326	334	342	350	358	365	373	381	389	396	404	412	420
75	287	295	303	311	319	327	335	343	351	359	367	375	383	391	399	407	415	423	431
76	295	304	312	320	328	336	344	353	361	369	377	385	394	402	410	418	426	435	443

Table 51.2. Low-calorie, lower-fat alternatives. These low-calorie alternatives provide new ideas for old favorites. When making a food choice, remember to consider vitamins and minerals. Some foods provide most of their calories from sugar and fat but give you few if any vitamins and minerals.

This guide is not meant to be an exhaustive list. We stress reading labels to find out just how many calories are in the specific products you decide to buy.

Higher-Fat Foods	Lower-Fat Foods
	Dairy Products
Evaporated whole milk	Evaporated fat-free (skim) or reduced-fat (2%) milk
Whole milk	Low-fat (1%), reduced-fat (2%), or fat-free skim milk
Ice cream	Sherbet, low fat or fat-free frozen yogurt, or ice milk (check label for calorie content)
Whipping cream	Imitation whipped cream (made with fat free (skim) milk) or low-fat vanilla yogurt
Sour cream	Plain low-fat yogurt
Cream cheese	Neufchatel or "light" cream cheese or fat-free cream cheese
Cheese (cheddar, Swiss, jack)	Reduced-calorie cheese, low-calorie processed cheeses, etc.
American cheese	Fat-free cheese
Regular (4%) cottage cheese	Fat-free American cheese or other types of fat-free cheeses
Whole milk mozzarella cheese	Part-skim milk, low-moisture mozzarella cheese
Whole milk ricotta cheese	Part-skim milk ricotta cheese
Coffee cream (half and half) or nondairy creamer (liquid, powder)	Low-fat (1%) or reduced-fat (2%) milk or non-fat dry milk powder or non-dairy creamer
	Cereals, Grains, and Pasta
Ramen noodles	Rice or noodles (spaghetti, macaroni, etc.)
Pasta with white sauce (alfredo)	Pasta with red sauce (marinara)
Pasta with cheese sauce	Pasta with vegetables (primavera)
Granola	Bran flakes, crispy rice, etc.
	Cooked grits or oatmeal
	Reduced-fat granola

Practical Dietary Therapy Information

Table 51.2. Low-calorie, lower-fat alternatives (continued from previous page)

Higher-Fat Foods	Lower-Fat Foods
	Meat, Fish, and Poultry
Coldcuts or lunch meats (bologna, salami, liverwurst)	Low-fat coldcuts (95 to 97% fat-free lunch meats, low-fat pressed meats)
Hot dogs (regular)	Lower-fat hot dogs
Bacon or sausage	Canadian bacon or lean ham
Regular ground beef	Extra lean ground beef such as ground round or ground turkey (read labels)
Chicken or turkey with skin, duck, or goose	Chicken or turkey without skin (white meat)
Oil-packed tuna	Water-packed tuna (rinse to reduce sodium content)
Beef (chuck, rib, brisket)	Beef (round, loin) (trimmed of external fat) (choose select grades)
Pork (spareribs, untrimmed loin)	Pork tenderloin or trimmed, lean smoked ham
Frozen breaded fish or fried fish (homemade or commercial)	Fish or shellfish, unbreaded (fresh, frozen, canned in water)
Whole eggs	Egg whites or egg substitutes
Frozen TV dinners (containing more than 13 grams of fat per serving)	Frozen TV dinners (containing less than 13 grams of fat per serving and lower in sodium)
Chorizo sausage	Turkey sausage, drained well (read label) Vegetarian sausage (made with tofu)
	Baked Goods
Croissants, brioches, etc.	Hard French rolls or soft brown 'n serve rolls
Donuts, sweet rolls, muffins, scones, or pastries	English muffins, bagels, reduced-fat, or fat-free muffins or scones
Party crackers	Low-fat crackers (choose lower in sodium) Saltine or soda crackers (choose lower in sodium)
Cake (pound, chocolate, yellow)	Cake (angel food, white, gingerbread)
Cookies	Reduced-fat or fat-free cookies (graham crackers, ginger snaps, fig bars) (compare calorie level)

Table 51.2. Low-calorie, lower-fat alternatives (continued from previous pages)

Higher-Fat Foods	Lower-Fat Foods
	Snacks and Sweets
Nuts	Popcorn (air-popped or light microwave), fruits, vegetables
Ice cream, e.g., cones or bars	Frozen fruit or chocolate pudding bars, or frozen yogurt
Custards or puddings (made with whole milk)	Puddings (made with skim milk)
	Fats, Oils, and Salad Dressings
Regular margarine or butter	Light spread margarines, diet margarine, or whipped butter, tub or squeeze bottle
Regular mayonnaise	Light or diet mayonnaise or mustard
Regular salad dressings	Reduced-calorie or fat-free salad dressings, lemon juice, or plain or herb flavored or wine vinegar
Butter or margarine on toast or bread	Jelly, jam, or honey on bread or toast
Oils, shortening, or lard	Non-stick cooking spray for stir-frying or sautéing
	As a substitute for oil or butter, use applesauce or prune puree in baked goods
	Miscellaneous
Canned cream soups	Canned broth-based soups
Canned beans and franks	Canned baked beans in tomato sauce
Gravy (homemade with fat and/or milk)	Gravy mixes made with water or homemade with the fat skimmed off and fat-free milk
Fudge sauce	Chocolate sauce
Avocado on sandwiches	Cucumber slices or lettuce leaves
Guacamole dip or refried beans with lard	Salsa

Practical Dietary Therapy Information

Fat-Free Versus Regular—Calorie Comparison

A calorie is a calorie is a calorie...whether it comes from fat or carbohydrate. Anything eaten in excess can lead to weight gain. You can lose weight by eating less calories and by increasing your physical activity. Reducing the amount of fat and saturated fat that you eat is one easy way to limit your overall calorie intake. However, eating fat-free or reduced-fat foods isn't always the answer to weight loss. For example, if you eat twice as many fat-free cookies as regular cookies you may not have reduced your overall calorie intake. The following list of foods and their fat-free varieties will show you that just because a product is fat-free, it doesn't mean that it is "calorie-free." And, calories do count!

Table 51.3. Fat-free versus regular calorie comparison.

Fat-Free or Reduced Fat	Calories	Regular	Calories
Reduced-Fat Peanut Butter, 2 tablespoons	190	Regular Peanut Butter, 2 tablespoons	190
Cookies: Reduced-Fat Chocolate Chip Cookie, 1 cookie	128	Cookies: Regular Chocolate Chip Cookie, 1 cookie	136
Fat-Free Fig Cookie, 1 cookie	70	Fig Cookie, 1 cookie	50
Ice Cream: Premium Nonfat Frozen Yogurt, ½ cup	190	Ice Cream: Regular Ice Cream, ½ cup	180
Premium Reduced-Fat Ice Cream, ½ cup	190	Regular Ice Cream, ½ cup	180
Fat-Free Caramel Topping, 2 tablespoons	130	Butterscotch Caramel Topping, 2 tablespoons	130
Reduced-Fat Granola Cereal, ¼ cup	110	Granola Cereal, ¼ cup	130
Reduced-Fat Croissant Roll, 1 roll	110	Regular Croissant Roll, 1 roll	130
Baked Tortilla Chips, 1 ounce	110	Regular Tortilla Chips, 1 ounce	130
Reduced-Fat Breakfast Bar, 1 bar	140	Breakfast Bar, 1 bar	130

Good Sources of Calcium

Calcium is not just for growing children. It is an important mineral that adults also need to keep their bones and teeth strong and their muscles functioning. Many people do not eat enough calcium everyday. The following is a list of good sources of calcium and tips on how to include more calcium in your diet everyday.

Table 51.4. Good sources of calcium.

Source	Calcium (milligrams)
Milk (1 cup)	
Whole	300
2% reduced-fat	300
1%* low-fat	300
Fat free*	300
Yogurt* (1 cup)	
Plain, low-fat	415
Flavored, low-fat	315
Plain, fat free	315
Cheese (1 ounce)	
Reduced-fat Cheddar*	120
American	175
Swiss Cheese	270
Mozzarella, part-skim	185
Cottage Cheese (½ cup)	
2% reduced-fat	75
Calcium fortified cottage cheese	300
Ice Cream	
Regular, ½ cup	90
Low-fat, ½ cup	100
Frozen Yogurt	
Low-fat, ½ cup	100
Beans, dried cooked, 1 cup	90
Salmon, with bones, 3 ounces	205
Tofu, processed with calcium sulfate, ½ cup	435
Spinach, fresh cooked	244
Turnip Greens, fresh cooked, 1 cup	100
Kale, fresh cooked	94
Broccoli, fresh cooked	75
Waffle, 7" diameter	180
Pancakes, (2) 4" diameter	115
Pizza, with vegetables, ¼ 12" pie	180

* Low-fat and nonfat varieties of foods are still good sources of calcium.

Practical Dietary Therapy Information

Calcium Requirements

- women ages 19–24: 1,200 mg
- women ages 25–50: 1,000 mg
- men ages 19–24: 1,200 mg
- men ages 25–50: 800 mg

Tips for Fitting in Calcium

- Eat cereal with fat-free milk. Try adding fresh fruit.
- Drink an extra glass of milk every day, try calcium-fortified milk.
- Spread calcium-fortified cottage cheese on crackers or bagel. Add fresh fruit.
- Drink calcium-fortified orange juice.
- Blend a yogurt smoothie with low-fat or fat-free yogurt and milk, and fresh or frozen fruit.
- Make instant pudding with low-fat or fat-free milk.
- Choose frozen yogurt for dessert instead of cake or cookies.
- Add a slice of low-fat or fat-free cheese to sandwiches.
- Substitute calcium fortified tofu in stir-fries for chicken, shrimp, or beef.
- Sauté greens (kale, bok choy, collard greens) in cooking spray and lemon juice and herbs.
- Read food labels for products with added calcium.

Food Preparation—What to Do

Low-Calorie, Low-Fat Cooking/Serving Methods

Cooking low-calorie, low-fat dishes may not take a long time, but best intentions can be lost with the addition of butter or other added fats at the table. It is important to learn how certain ingredients can add unwanted calories and fat to low fat dishes—making them no longer lower in calories and lower in fat! The following list provides examples of lower fat-cooking methods and tips on how to serve your low-fat dishes.

These cooking methods tend to be lower in fat:

- bake
- broil
- microwave
- roast—for vegetables and/or chicken without skin
- steam
- lightly stir-fry or sauté in cooking spray, small amounts of vegetable oil, or reduced sodium broth
- grill seafood, chicken or vegetables

Look at the following examples for how to save calories and fat when preparing and serving foods. You might be surprised at how easy it is!

- Two tablespoons of butter on a baked potato can add an extra 200 calories and 22 grams of fat! However, 1/2 cup salsa only adds 18 calories and no fat!
- Two tablespoons of regular clear Italian salad dressing will add an extra 136 calories and 14 grams of fat. Reduced fat Italian dressing only adds 30 calories and 2 grams of fat!

Try these low-fat flavorings—added during preparation or at the table.

- herbs—oregano, basil, cilantro, thyme, parsley, sage, or rosemary
- spices—cinnamon, nutmeg, pepper, or paprika
- reduced-fat or fat-free salad dressing
- mustard
- catsup
- fat-free or reduced-fat mayonnaise
- fat-free or reduced-fat sour cream
- fat-free or reduced-fat yogurt
- reduced sodium soy sauce

Practical Dietary Therapy Information

- salsa
- lemon or lime juice
- vinegar
- horseradish
- fresh ginger
- sprinkle of buttered flavor (not made with real butter)
- red pepper flakes
- sprinkle of parmesan cheese (stronger flavor than most cheese)
- sodium-free salt substitute
- jelly or fruit preserves on toast or bagels

Dining out—How to Choose

Whether or not you're trying to lose weight, you can eat healthy when dining out or bringing in food, if you know how. The following tips will help you move toward healthier eating as you limit your calories, as well as fat, saturated fat, cholesterol, and sodium when eating out.

- Ask for what you want! Most restaurants will honor your requests.
- Ask questions! Don't be intimidated by the menu—your server will be able to tell you how foods are prepared or suggest substitutions on the menu.
- If you wish to reduce portion sizes—try ordering appetizers as your main meal.

General tips. Limiting your calories and fat can be easy as long as you know what to order. Try asking these questions when you call ahead or before you order. Ask the restaurant, do you or would you on request:

- serve margarine (rather than butter) with the meal?
- serve fat-free (skim) milk rather than whole milk or cream?
- use less oil when cooking?
- trim visible fat off poultry or meat?
- leave all butter, gravy, or sauces off a side dish or entree?

- serve salad dressing on the side?
- accommodate special requests if made in advance by telephone or in person?
- above all else, don't get discouraged. There are usually several healthy choices to choose from at most restaurants.

Reading the Menu

- Choose lower-calorie, low-fat cooking methods. Look for terms like steamed, in its own juice (au jus), garden fresh, broiled, baked, roasted, poached, tomato juice, dry boiled (in wine or lemon juice), and lightly sautéed or stir-fried.
- Be aware of foods high in calories, fat, and saturated fat. Watch out for terms like butter sauce, fried, crispy, creamed, in cream or cheese sauce, au gratin, au fromage, escalloped, parmesan, hollandaise, bernaise, marinated (in oil), stewed, basted, sautéed, stir-fried, casserole, hash, prime, pot pie and pastry crust.

Specific Tips for Healthy Choices

Breakfast

- fresh fruit or small glass of citrus juice
- whole grain bread, bagel or English muffin with jelly or honey
- whole grain cereal with low-fat (1%) or fat-free milk
- oatmeal with fat-free milk topped with fruit
- omelet made with egg whites or egg substitute
- multigrain pancakes without butter on top
- nonfat yogurt (try adding cereal or fresh fruit)

Beverages

- water with lemon
- flavored sparkling water (non-caloric)
- juice spritzer (half fruit juice and half sparkling water)
- iced tea
- tomato juice (reduced sodium)

Practical Dietary Therapy Information

Bread

Most bread and breadsticks are low in calories and low in fat. The calories add up when you add butter, margarine, or olive oil to the bread. Also, eating a lot of bread in addition to your meal will fill you up with extra unwanted calories and not leave enough room for fruits and vegetables.

Appetizers

- steamed seafood
- shrimp cocktail (limit cocktail sauce—it's high in sodium)
- melons or fresh fruit
- bean soups
- salad with reduced fat dressing (or add lemon juice or vinegar)
- If you are on a cholesterol-lowering diet, eat shrimp and other shellfish in moderation.

Entree

- poultry, fish, shellfish, and vegetable dishes are healthy choices
- pasta with red sauce or with vegetables (primavera)
- look for terms like baked, broiled, steamed, poached, lightly sautéed, or stir-fried
- ask for sauces and dressings on the side
- limit the amount of butter, margarine, and salt you use at the table

Salads/Salad Bars

- fresh greens, lettuce and spinach
- fresh vegetables—tomato, mushroom, carrots, cucumber, peppers, onion, radishes, and broccoli
- beans, chick peas, and kidney beans
- skip the non-vegetable choices: deli meats, bacon, egg, cheese, croutons
- choose lower-calorie, reduced-fat or fat-free dressing, lemon juice, or vinegar

Side Dish

- Plain vegetables and starches (rice, potato, noodles) make good additions to meals and can also be combined for a lower-calorie alternative to higher-calorie entrees.
- Ask for side dishes without butter or margarine.
- Ask for mustard, salsa or low-fat yogurt instead of sour cream or butter.

Dessert / Coffee

- fresh fruit
- nonfat frozen yogurt
- sherbet or fruit sorbed (these are usually fat free, but check the calorie content)
- try sharing a dessert
- ask for low-fat milk for your coffee (instead of cream or half-'n-half)

Tips for Healthy Multicultural Dining out

If you're dining out or bringing in, it is easy to find healthy foods. Knowing about American food terms, as well as other ethnic cuisines can help make your dining experience healthy and enjoyable! The following list includes healthy food choices (lower in calories and fat) and terms to look for when making your selection.

Chinese

Choose more often...

- steamed
- jum (poached)
- chu (boiled)
- kow (roasted)
- shu (barbecued)
- hoison sauce with assorted Chinese vegetables: broccoli, mushroom, onion, cabbage, snow peas, scallions, bamboo shoots, water chestnuts, asparagus

Practical Dietary Therapy Information

- oyster sauce (made from seafood)
- lightly stir-fried in mild sauce
- cooked in light wine sauce
- hot and spicy tomato sauce
- sweet and sour sauce
- hot mustard sauce
- reduced sodium soy sauce
- dishes without MSG added
- garnished with spinach or broccoli
- fresh fish filets, shrimp, scallops
- chicken, without skin
- lean beef
- bean curd (tofu)
- moo Shu vegetable, chicken or shrimp
- steamed rice
- lychee fruit

French

    Choose more often...

- dinner salad with vinegar or lemon juice dressing (or other reduced fat dressing)
- crusty bread without butter
- fresh fish, shrimp, scallops, steamed mussels (without sauces)
- chicken breast, without skin
- rice and noodles without cream or added butter or other fat
- fresh fruit for dessert

Italian

    Choose more often...

- lightly sautéed with onions
- shallots
- peppers and mushrooms

- artichoke hearts
- sun-dried tomatoes
- red sauces—spicy marinara sauce (arrabiata), marinara sauce or cacciatore
- light red sauce or light red or white wine sauce
- light mushroom sauce
- red clam sauce
- primavera (no cream sauce)
- lemon sauce
- capers
- herbs and spices—garlic and oregano
- crushed tomatoes and spices
- florentine (spinach)
- grilled (often fish or vegetables)
- piccata (lemon)
- manzanne (eggplant)

Middle Eastern

Choose more often ...

- lemon dressing, lemon juice
- blended or seasoned with Middle Eastern spices
- herbs and spices
- mashed chickpeas
- fava beans
- smoked eggplant
- with tomatoes, onions, green peppers, and cucumbers
- spiced ground meat
- special garlic sauce
- basted with tomato sauce
- garlic
- chopped parsley and/or onion
- couscous (grain)
- rice or bulgur (cracked wheat)

Practical Dietary Therapy Information

- stuffed with rice and imported spices
- grilled on a skewer
- marinated and barbecued
- baked
- charbroiled or charcoal broiled
- fresh fruit

Japanese

Choose more often...

- house salad with fresh ginger and cellophane (clear rice) noodles
- rice
- nabemono
- chicken, fish or shrimp teriyaki, broiled in sauce
- menrui or soba noodles, often used in soups
- yakimono (broiled)
- tofu or bean curd
- grilled vegetables

Indian

Choose more often...

- tikka (pan roasted)
- cooked with or marinated in yogurt
- cooked with green vegetables, onions, tomatoes, peppers, and mushrooms
- with spinach (saag)
- baked leavened bread
- masala
- tandoori
- paneer
- cooked with curry, marinated in spices
- lentils, chick beans, garbanzo beans, beans

- garnished with dried fruits
- chickpeas (garbanzo) and potatoes
- basmati rice (pullao)
- matta (peas)
- chicken or shrimp kebab

Mexican

   Choose more often...

- shredded spicy chicken
- rice and black beans
- rice
- ceviche (fish marinated in lime juice and mixed with spices)
- served with salsa (hot red tomato sauce)
- served with salsa verde (green chili sauce)
- covered with enchilada sauce
- topped with shredded lettuce, diced tomatoes and onions
- served with or wrapped in a corn or wheat flour (soft) tortilla
- grilled
- marinated
- picante sauce
- simmered with chili vegetarian tomato sauce

Thai

   Choose more often...

- barbecued, sautéed, broiled, boiled, or steamed, braised, marinated
- charbroiled
- basil sauce, basil or sweet basil leaves
- lime sauce or lime juice
- chili sauce or crushed dried chili flakes
- thai spices
- served in hollowed-out pineapple
- fish sauce

Practical Dietary Therapy Information

- hot sauce
- napa, bamboo shoots, black mushrooms, ginger, garlic
- bed of mixed vegetables
- scallions, onions

Steakhouses

Choose more often...

- lean broiled beef (no more than 6 ounces) London broil, filet mignon, round, and flank steaks
- baked potato without added butter, margarine, or sour cream. Try low-fat yogurt or mustard.
- green salad with reduced fat dressing
- steamed vegetables without added butter or margarine. Try lemon juice and herbs.
- seafood dishes (usually indicated as "surf" on menus)

Fast Food

Choose more often...

- grilled chicken breast sandwich without mayonnaise
- single hamburger without cheese
- grilled chicken salad with reduced-fat dressing
- garden salad with reduced-fat dressing
- low-fat or nonfat yogurt
- fat-free muffin
- cereal with low-fat milk

Deli/Sandwich Shop

Choose more often...

- fresh sliced vegetables in pita bread with low-fat dressing, yogurt, or mustard
- cup of bean soup (lentil, minestrone)
- turkey breast sandwich with mustard, lettuce, tomato
- fresh fruit

Table 51.5. Sample reduced-calorie menus. This is a summary chart for the reduced calorie menus on the following pages.

SAMPLE REDUCED-CALORIE MENUS

	Calories	Total CHO % kcal	Total Fat % kcal	Sodium (mg)	SFA % kcal	Cholesterol (mg)	Protein % kcal
Traditional Cuisine							
1,600	1,613	55	29	1,341	8	142	19
1,200	1,247	58	26	1,043	7	96	19
Asian-American Cuisine							
1,600	1,609	56	27	1,296	8	148	20
1,200	1,220	55	27	1,043	8	117	21
Southern Cuisine							
1,600	1,653	53	28	1,231	8	172	20
1,200	1,225	50	31	867	9	142	21
Mexican-American Cuisine							
1,600	1,638	56	27	1,616	9	143	20
1,200	1,239	58	26	1,364	8	91	19
Lacta-Ovo Vegetarian Cuisine							
1,600	1,650	56	27	1,829	8	82	19
1,200	1,205	60	25	1,335	7	44	18

Practical Dietary Therapy Information

Table 51.6.

SAMPLE MENU: TRADITIONAL AMERICAN CUISINE, REDUCED CALORIE

	1,600 Calories	1,200 Calories
Breakfast		
Whole Wheat Bread	1 slice	1 slice
Jelly, regular	2 tsp	2 tsp
Cereal, Shredded Wheat	1 cup	½ cup
Milk, 1% low-fat	1 cup	1 cup
Orange Juice	¾ cup	¾ cup
Coffee, Regular	1 cup	1 cup
Milk, 1% low-fat	1 oz	—
Lunch		
Roast Beef Sandwich		
Whole Wheat Bread	2 slices	2 slices
Lean Roast Beef, unseasoned	2 oz	2 oz
American Cheese, low-fat, low-sodium	1 slice (¾ oz)	—
Lettuce	1 leaf	1 leaf
Tomato	3 slices	3 slices
Mayonnaise, low-calorie	2 tsp	1 tsp
Apple	1 medium	1 medium
Water	1 cup	1 cup
Dinner		
Salmon	3 oz	2 oz
Vegetable Oil	1½ tsp	1½ tsp
Baked Potato	¾ medium	¾ medium
Margarine	1 tsp	1 tsp
Carrots seasoned with	½ cup	½ cup
margarine	½ tsp	—
Green Beans seasoned with	½ cup	½ cup
margarine	½ tsp	½ tsp
White Dinner Roll	1 medium	1 small
Ice Milk	½ cup	—
Iced Tea, unsweetened	1 cup	1 cup
Water	2 cups	2 cups
Snack		
Popcorn, air popped	2½ cups	2½ cups
Margarine	1½ tsp	¾ tsp

Calories:	1,613	Calories:	1,247
Total Carb, % kcals:	55	Total Carb, % kcals:	58
Total Fat, % kcals:	29	Total Fat, % kcals:	26
*Sodium, mg:	1,341	*Sodium, mg:	1,043
SFA, % kcals:	8	SFA, % kcals:	7
Cholesterol, mg:	142	Cholesterol, mg:	96
Protein, % kcals:	19	Protein, % kcals:	19

1,600: 100% RDA met for all nutrients except: Vit E 99%, Iron 73%, Zinc 91%
1,200: 100% RDA met for all nutrients except: Vit E 80%, Vit B$_2$ 96%, Vit B$_6$ 94%, Calcium 68%, Iron 63%, Zinc 73%
* No salt added in recipe preparation or as seasoning. Consume at least 32 oz. water.

Table 51.7.

SAMPLE MENU: ASIAN-AMERICAN CUISINE, REDUCED CALORIE

	1,600 Calories	1,200 Calories
Breakfast		
Banana	1 small	1 small
Whole Wheat Bread	2 slices	1 slice
Margarine	1 tsp	1 tsp
Orange Juice	¾ cup	¾ cup
Milk, 1% low-fat	¾ cup	¾ cup
Lunch		
Beef Noodle Soup, canned, low-sodium	½ cup	½ cup
Chinese Noodle and Beef Salad		
Beef Roast	3 oz	2 oz
Peanut Oil	1½ tsp	1 tsp
Soy Sauce, low-sodium	1 tsp	1 tsp
Carrots	½ cup	½ cup
Zucchini	½ cup	½ cup
Onion	¼ cup	¼ cup
Chinese Noodles, soft-type	¼ cup	¼ cup
Apple	1 medium	1 medium
Tea, unsweetened	1 cup	1 cup
Dinner		
Pork Stir-fry with Vegetables		
Pork Cutlet	2 oz	2 oz
Peanut Oil	1 tsp	1 tsp
Soy Sauce, low-sodium	1 tsp	1 tsp
Broccoli	½ cup	½ cup
Carrots	1 cup	½ cup
Mushrooms	¼ cup	½ cup
Steamed White Rice	1 cup	½ cup
Tea, unsweetened	1 cup	1 cup
Snack		
Almond Cookies	2 cookies	—
Milk, 1% low-fat	¾ cup	¾ cup

Calories:	1,609	Calories:	1,220
Total Carb, % kcals:	56	Total Carb, % kcals:	55
Total Fat, % kcals:	27	Total Fat, % kcals:	27
*Sodium, mg:	1,296	*Sodium, mg:	1,043
SFA, % kcals:	8	SFA, % kcals:	8
Cholesterol, mg:	148	Cholesterol, mg:	117
Protein, % kcals:	20	Protein, % kcals:	21

1,600: 100% RDA met for all nutrients except: Zinc 95%, Iron 87%, Calcium 93%
1,200: 100% RDA met for all nutrients except: Vit E 75%, Calcium 84%, Magnesium 98%, Iron 66%, Zinc 77%
* No salt added in recipe preparation or as seasoning. Consume at least 32 oz. water.

Practical Dietary Therapy Information

Table 51.8.

Sample Menu: Southern Cuisine, Reduced Calorie		
	1,600 Calories	**1,200 Calories**
Breakfast		
Oatmeal, prepared with 1% low-fat milk	½ cup	½ cup
Milk, 1% low-fat	½ cup	½ cup
English Muffin	1 medium	—
Cream Cheese, light, 18% fat	1 T	—
Orange Juice	¾ cup	½ cup
Coffee	1 cup	1 cup
Milk, 1% low-fat	1 oz	1 oz
Lunch		
Baked Chicken, without skin	2 oz	2 oz
Vegetable Oil	1 tsp	½ tsp
Salad		
Lettuce	½ cup	½ cup
Tomato	½ cup	½ cup
Cucumber	½ cup	½ cup
Oil and Vinegar Dressing	2 tsp	1 tsp
White Rice, seasoned with	½ cup	¼ cup
margarine, diet	½ tsp	½ tsp
Baking Powder Biscuit, prepared with vegetable oil	1 small	½ small
Margarine	1 tsp	1 tsp
Water	1 cup	1 cup
Dinner		
Lean Roast Beef	3 oz	2 oz
Onion	¼ cup	¼ cup
Beef Gravy, water-based	1 T	1 T
Turnip Greens, seasoned with	½ cup	½ cup
margarine, diet	½ tsp	½ tsp
Sweet Potato, baked	1 small	1 small
Margarine, diet	½ tsp	¼ tsp
Ground Cinnamon	1 tsp	1 tsp
Brown Sugar	1 tsp	1 tsp
Cornbread prepared with margarine, diet	½ medium slice	½ medium slice
Honeydew Melon	¼ medium	⅛ medium
Iced Tea, sweetened with sugar	1 cup	1 cup
Snack		
Saltine Crackers, unsalted tops	4 crackers	4 crackers
Mozzarella Cheese, part-skim, low-sodium	1 oz	1 oz

Calories:	1,653	Calories:	1,225
Total Carb, % kcals:	53	Total Carb, % kcals:	50
Total Fat, % kcals:	28	Total Fat, % kcals:	31
*Sodium, mg:	1,231	*Sodium, mg:	867
SFA, % kcals:	8	SFA, % kcals:	9
Cholesterol, mg:	172	Cholesterol, mg:	142
Protein, % kcals:	20	Protein, % kcals:	21

1,600: 100% RDA met for all nutrients except: Vit E 97%, Magnesium 98%, Iron 78%, Zinc 90%
1,200: 100% RDA met for all nutrients except: Vit E 82%, Vit B_1 & B_2 95%, Vit B_3 99%, Vit B_6 88%, Magnesium 83%, Iron 56%, Zinc 70%
* No salt added in recipe preparation or as seasoning. Consume at least 32 oz. water.

Table 51.9.

SAMPLE MENU: MEXICAN-AMERICAN CUISINE, REDUCED CALORIE

	1,600 Calories	1,200 Calories
Breakfast		
Cantaloupe	1 cup	½ cup
Farina, prepared with 1% low-fat milk	½ cup	½ cup
White Bread	1 slice	1 slice
Margarine	1 tsp	1 tsp
Jelly	1 tsp	1 tsp
Orange Juice	1½ cup	¾ cup
Milk, 1% low-fat	½ cup	½ cup
Lunch		
Beef Enchilada		
Tortilla, corn	2 tortillas	2 tortillas
Lean Roast Beef	2 ½ oz	2 oz
Vegetable Oil	⅔ tsp	⅔ tsp
Onion	1 T	1 T
Tomato	4 T	4 T
Lettuce	½ cup	½ cup
Chili Peppers	2 tsp	2 tsp
Refried Beans, prepared with vegetable oil	¼ cup	¼ cup
Carrots	5 sticks	5 sticks
Celery	6 sticks	6 sticks
Milk, 1% low-fat	½ cup	—
Dinner		
Chicken Taco		
Tortilla, corn	1 tortilla	1 tortilla
Chicken Breast, without skin	2 oz	1 oz
Vegetable Oil	⅔ tsp	⅔ tsp
Cheddar Cheese, low-fat, low-sodium	1 oz	½ oz
Guacamole	2 T	1 T
Salsa	1 T	1 T
Corn, seasoned with	½ cup	½ cup
margarine	½ tsp	—
Spanish Rice without meat, seasoned without margarine	½ cup	½ cup
Banana	1 large	½ large
Coffee	1 cup	1 cup
Milk 1%	1 oz	1 oz

Calories:	1,638	Calories:	1,239
Total Carb, % kcals:	56	Total Carb, % kcals:	58
Total Fat, % kcals:	27	Total Fat, % kcals:	26
*Sodium, mg:	1,616	*Sodium, mg:	1,364
SFA, % kcals:	9	SFA, % kcals:	8
Cholesterol, mg:	143	Cholesterol, mg:	91
Protein, % kcals:	20	Protein, % kcals:	19

1,600: 100% RDA met for all nutrients except: Vit E 97%, Zinc 84%
1,200: 100% RDA met for all nutrients except: Vit E 71%, Vit B₁ & B₃ 91%, Vit B₂ & Iron 90%, Calcium 92%, Magnesium 95%, Zinc 64%.
* No salt added in recipe preparation or as seasoning. Consume at least 32 oz. water.

Table 51.10.

SAMPLE MENU: LACTO-OVO VEGETARIAN CUISINE, REDUCED CALORIE

	1,600 Calories	1,200 Calories
Breakfast		
Orange	1 medium	1 medium
Pancakes, made with 1% low-fat milk, egg whites	3 4" circles	2 4" circles
Pancake Syrup	2 T	1 T
Margarine, diet	1½ tsp	1½ tsp
Milk, 1% low-fat	1 cup	½ cup
Coffee	1 cup	1 cup
Milk, 1% low-fat	1 oz	1 oz
Lunch		
Vegetable Soup, canned, low-sodium	1 cup	½ cup
Bagel	1 medium	½ medium
Processed American Cheese, low-fat and low sodium	¾ oz	—
Spinach Salad		
Spinach	1 cup	1 cup
Mushrooms	⅛ cup	⅛ cup
Salad Dressing, regular calorie	2 tsp	2 tsp
Apple	1 medium	1 medium
Iced Tea, unsweetened	1 cup	1 cup
Dinner		
Omelette		
Egg Whites	4 large eggs	4 large eggs
Green Pepper	2 T	2 T
Onion	2 T	2 T
Mozzarella Cheese, made from part-skim milk, low-sodium	1½ oz	1 oz
Vegetable Oil	1 T	½ T
Brown Rice, seasoned with	½ cup	½ cup
margarine, diet	½ tsp	½ tsp
Carrots, seasoned with	½ cup	½ cup
margarine, diet	½ tsp	½ tsp
Whole Wheat Bread	1 slice	1 slice
Margarine, diet	1 tsp	1 tsp
Fig Bar Cookie	1 bar	1 bar
Tea	1 cup	1 cup
Honey	1 tsp	1 tsp
Snack		
Milk, 1% low-fat	¾ cup	¾ cup

Calories:	1,650	Calories:	1,205
Total Carb, % kcals:	56	Total Carb, % kcals:	60
Total Fat, % kcals:	27	Total Fat, % kcals:	25
*Sodium, mg:	1,829	*Sodium, mg:	1,335
SFA, % kcals:	8	SFA, % kcals:	7
Cholesterol, mg:	82	Cholesterol, mg:	44
Protein, % kcals:	19	Protein, % kcals:	18

1,600: 100% RDA met for all nutrients except: Vit E 92%, Vit B$_3$ 97%, Vit B$_6$ 67%, Magnesium 98%, Iron 73%, Zinc 68%
1,200: 100% RDA met for all nutrients except: Vit E 75%, Vit B$_1$ 92%, Vit B$_3$ 69%, Vit B$_6$ 59%, Iron 54%, Zinc 46%
* No salt added in recipe preparation or as seasoning. Consume at least 32 oz. water.

Chapter 52

References

This chapter lists book titles, brochures, pamphlets, and articles that contain useful information on many of the topics in this sourcebook. For easy reference, the topics are organized in the same format as the chapters of the sourcebook itself. Contact information is included when available.

Part I: General Information about Obesity

"Binge Eating Disorder," NIH Publication No. 94-3589. This fact sheet describes the symptoms, causes, complications, and treatment of binge eating disorder, along with a profile of those at risk for the disorder. 1993. Available from the Weight Information Network (WIN). See the "Resources" chapter of this sourcebook for contact information.

Long, P. "The Great Weight Debate," *Health*. February/March, 1992, pp. 42-47. This article, written for the general public, discusses the controversy over which weight-for-height table is best to use. It also provides some simple guidelines for determining whether someone needs to lose weight. Available in public libraries.

Part II: Diseases Linked to Obesity

Clayman C.B., ed. *The American Medical Association Encyclopedia of Medicine*. New York: Random House, 1989. This authoritative reference guide for patients has entries on the gallbladder, gallstones, and the biliary system. It is widely available in libraries and bookstores.

"Obesity kills but you can fight back-October 26, 1999," http://www.cnn.com/HEALTH/9910/26/obesity.studies.

DeGroot, Leslie J., ed., et al. "Cushing's Syndrome," *Endocrinology. Vol. 2*. Philadelphia: W. B. Saunders Company, 1995, pp. 1741-1769.

Everhart, J.E. "Contributions of Obesity and Weight-Loss to Gallstone Disease," *Annals of Internal Medicine*. 1993, Vol. 119, pp. 1029-35. This article, written for physicians, shows how obesity as well as weight loss and low calorie diets increase the risk of gallstones.

"Gallstones," NIH Publication No. 93-2897. This fact sheet provides basic information about gallstones and treatment options. It is published by the National Institute of Diabetes and Digestive and Kidney Diseases and is available through the National Digestive Diseases Information Clearinghouse, Box NDDIC, 2 Information Way, Bethesda, MD 20892, Tel: (301) 654-3810.

Isselbacher, Kurt J., ed., et al. "Cushing's Syndrome Etiology," *Harrison's Principles of Internal Medicine*. Vol. 2, No. 13, New York: McGraw-Hill Book Company, 1994, pp. 1960-1965.

"NCI Research Report: Cancer of the Lung. Prepared by the Office of Cancer Communications, National Cancer Institute," NIH Publication No. 93-526.

Weinsier RL, et. al. "Gallstone Formation and Weight Loss," *Obesity Research*. 1993, pp. 51-56. This review article, written for physicians, examines gallstone formation rates in patients on very-low-calorie diets, including the role that fasting and diet composition may play.

Wilson, Jean D., ed, et al. "Hyperfunction: Glucocorticoids: Hypercortisolism (Cushing's syndrome)," *Williams Textbook of Endocrinology*. No. 8, Philadelphia: W.B. Saunders, 1992, pp. 536-562.

References

Part III: Managing Obesity

"Are You Eating Right?" *Consumer Reports.* October 1992, pp. 644-55. This article summarizes advice from 68 nutrition experts, including a discussion on weight control and health risks of obesity. Available from the Weight Information Network (WIN). See the "Resources" chapter of this sourcebook for contact information.

Bray, G.A. "Pathophysiology of Obesity," *American Journal of Clinical Nutrition.* 1992, Supplement to Vol. 55 (2), pp. 488S-494S. This article comes from the proceedings of an NIH Consensus Development Conference on Gastrointestinal Surgery for Severe Obesity. Written for health professionals in technical language. Available in medical libraries.

Dietary Guidelines for Americans. Fifth Edition, 2000, Home and Garden Bulletin No. 232. This pamphlet, issued by the U.S. Agriculture and Health and Human Services Departments, contains information about maintaining a healthy weight, as well as dietary and nutrition recommendations. Available through the Government Printing Office.

"Exercise and Weight Control," The President's Council on Physical Fitness and Sports, Department of Health and Human Services. This brochure discusses the difference between being "overweight" and "overfat" and the role diet and exercise can play in a weight loss program. Copies can be obtained from the President's Council on Physical Fitness and Sports, 200 Independence Ave. SW, Humphrey Bldg., Rm. 738-H, Washington, DC 20201.

Katahn, Martin. *How to Quit Smoking Without Gaining Weight.* New York: W.W., Norton & Company, 1994.

"Losing Weight: What Works, What Doesn't," and "Rating the Diets," *Consumer Reports.* June 1993, pp. 347-57. These articles report on a survey of readers' experiences with weight-loss diets, discuss research related to weight control, and outline pros and cons of different diet programs. Available in public libraries.

"Physical Activity and Weight Control," Revised 1997, NIH Publication No. 96-4031. This booklet explains how physical activity helps promote weight control and other ways it benefits one's health. It also describes the different types of physical activity and provides tips on how to become more physically active. Available from the Weight Information Network (WIN). See the "Resources" chapter of this sourcebook for contact information.

"A Report of the Surgeon General: Physical Activity and Health," 1996. Produced by the Centers for Disease Control and Prevention, this report compiles decades of research concerning physical activity and health. It addresses the nationwide health problems associated with physical inactivity and outlines the benefits of becoming more physically active. Available for $19.00 from the U.S. Government Printing Office, Superintendent of Documents, Washington, DC 20402; (202) 512-1800. Stock Number 017-023-00196-5.

"Weight Cycling," 1995, NIH Publication No. 95-3901. Based on research, this fact sheet describes the health effects of weight cycling, also known as "yo-yo" dieting, and how it affects obese individuals' future weight-loss efforts. Available from the Weight Information Network (WIN). See the "Resources" chapter of this sourcebook for contact information.

Part IV: Obesity Issues for Special Populations and the Prevention of Obesity

"Healthy Eating for a Healthy Life," AARP (American Association of Retired Persons) Fulfillment, 601 E. St., N.W., Washington, DC 20049. Ask for publication by title and stock number D15565.

Chapter 53

Resources

This chapter lists contact information for some of the government agencies, professional organizations, websites, and publications involved in weight control and obesity research and education. Information is listed alphabetically according to the name of the organization.

General Resources for Obesity and Overweight

American Dietetic Association
Consumer Education Team
216 West Jackson Boulevard
Chicago, IL 60606
(Send self addressed stamped envelope)
Phone: (800) 877-1600, ext. 5000 for publications, or
(800) 366-1655 for recorded food/nutrition messages
Website: http://www.eatright.org

American Medical Association (AMA) Website
Website: http://www.ama-assn.org

The resources listed in this section were compiled from a wide variety of sources deemed accurate. Contact information was updated and verified in April 2000. Inclusion does not constitute endorsement.

American Obesity Association
1250 24th Street, NW
Suite 300
Washington, DC 20037
Phone: (800) 98-OBESE
Fax: (202) 776-7712
Website: http://www.obesity.org

Fighting for the rights of obese persons.

The American Society of Bariatric Physicians
5600 S. Quebec Street
Suite 109A
Englewood, CO 80111
Phone: (303) 770-2526, ext. 17 (membership information only)
Phone: (303) 779-4833
Colorado residents call (303) 770-2526, ext. 10
Fax: (303) 779-4834
E-mail: bariatric@asbp.org
Website: http://www.asbp.org

Center for Food Safety and Applied Nutrition (CFSAN)
U.S. Food and Drug Administration (FDA)
200 C Street SW
Washington, DC 20204
Website: http://vm.cfsan.fda.gov

Centers for Disease Control and Prevention (CDC)
Phone: (800) 311-3435 (general inquiries)
Website: http://www.cdc.gov
For more information about nutrition and physical activity:
Phone: (888) CDC-4NRG
CDC's Nutrition and Physical Activity Website:
http://www.cdc.gov/nccdphp/dnpa

Consumer Information Center, Pueblo
Toll Free: (800) 688-9889
TTY (text telephone): (800) 326-2996
E-Mail: catalog.pueblo@gsa.gov
Website: http://www.pueblo.gsa.gov

Resources

The Council on Size and Weight Discrimination
P.O. Box 305
Mt. Marion, NY 12456
(Send self-addressed stamped envelope)
Phone: (914) 679-1209
Fax: (914) 679-1206
Website: http://www.cswd.org

Department of Nutrition Sciences
University of Alabama (Birmingham)
Birmingham, AL 35294
Phone: (205) 934-5218
Website: http://main.uab.edu

The Endocrine Society
4350 East West Highway, Suite 500
Bethesda, Maryland 20814-4410
Phone: (301) 941-0200
Fax: (301) 941-0259
E-mail: endostaff@endo-society.org
Website: http://www.endo-society.org

Federation of American Societies for Experimental Biology
Website: http://www.faseb.org/

Food and Drug Administration (FDA)
5600 Fishers Lane
Rockville, MD 20857
Phone: (888) 463-6332
Website: http://www.fda.gov

The Human Obesity Gene Map
Donald B. Brown Research Chair on Obesity
Ferdinand-Vandry Building, Room 3101J
Medicine Faculty
Université Laval
Ste-Foy, Québec G1K 7P4
Canada
Phone: (418) 656-2131
Fax: (418) 656-7898
Website: http://www.obesity.chair.ulaval.ca/Genes.html

Mayo Clinic Health Oasis
Website: http://www.mayoclinic.com

National Association to Advance Fat Acceptance (NAAFA)
P.O. Box 188620
Sacramento, CA 95818
Phone: (916) 558-6880
Fax: (916) 558-6881
Website: http://www.naafa.org

National Diabetes Information Clearinghouse
1 Information Way
Bethesda, MD 20892-3560
Phone: (301) 654-3327
Fax: (301) 907-8906
E-mail: ndic@info.niddk.nih.gov
Website: http://www.niddk.nih.gov/health/diabetes/diabetes.htm

National Digestive Diseases Information Clearinghouse
2 Information Way
Bethesda, MD 20892-3570
Phone: (301) 654-3810
Fax: (301) 907-8906
E-mail: nddic@info.niddk.nih.gov
Website: http://www.niddk.nih.gov/health/digest/digest.htm

National Heart, Lung, and Blood Institute Information Center
Bldg. 31
31 Center Drive, MSC 2486
Bethesda, MD 20892
Phone: (301) 592-8573
E-mail: nhlbiinfo@rover.nhlbi.nih.gov
Website: http://www.nhlbi.nih.gov

Resources

National Institute of Arthritis and Musculoskeletal and Skin Diseases
1 AMS Circle
Bethesda, MD 20892-3675
Toll Free: (877) 22-NIAMS
TTY (text telephone): (301) 565-2966
Phone: (301) 495-4484
Fax: (301) 718-6366
Website: http://www.nih.gov/niams

National Institute of Diabetes and Digestive and Kidney Diseases
31 Center Drive
MSC 2560
Bethesda, MD 20892
Phone: (301) 496-3583
Website: http://www.niddk.nih.gov

National Women's Health Information Center
Phone: (800) 994-9662
TDD: (888) 220-5446
E-Mail: 4woman@soza.com
Website: http://www.4woman.gov

North American Association for the Study of Obesity
8630 Fenton Street
Suite 412
Silver Spring, MD 20910
Phone: (301) 563-6526
Fax: (301) 587-2365
Website: http://www.naaso.org/obres

Partnership for Healthy Weight Management
Website: http://www.consumer.gov/weightloss/index.htm

President's Council on Physical Fitness and Sports
200 Independence Ave., SW
Humphrey Bldg., Rm. 738-H
Washington, DC 20201
Phone: (202) 690-9000

Screening for Mental Health, Inc. (Eating Disorders)
Website: http://www.nmisp.org

Shape Up America!
6707 Democracy Blvd.
Suite 306
Bethesda, Maryland 20817
E-Mail: suainfo@shapeup.org
Website: http://shapeup.org

This website is designed to provide you with the latest information about safe weight management, healthy eating, increased activity and physical fitness.

Weight-Control Information Network (WIN)
1 Win Way
Bethesda, MD 20892-3665
Phone: (202) 828-1025 or (877) 946-4627
Fax: (202) 828-1028
E-mail: win@info.niddk.nih.gov
Website: http://www.niddk.nih.gov/health/nutrit/win.htm

The Weight-Control Information Network (WIN) is a service of the National Institute of Diabetes and Digestive and Kidney Diseases (NIDDK), part of the National Institutes of Health, under the U.S. Public Health Service. Authorized by Congress (Public Law 103-43), WIN assembles and disseminates to health professionals and the public information on weight control, obesity, and nutritional disorders. WIN responds to requests for information; develops, reviews, and distributes publications; and develops communications strategies to encourage individuals to achieve and maintain a healthy weight. Publications produced by the clearinghouse are reviewed carefully for scientific accuracy, content, and readability.

You First *Health Risk Assessment website*
Phone: (800) 561-3261
Website: http://www.youfirst.com

Weight Loss Program Fraud

Federal Trade Commission
Consumer Response Center
600 Pennsylvania Avenue, NW
Washington, DC 20580
Toll Free: (877) 382-4357
Phone: (202) 326-2222
Website: http://www.ftc.gov

Food and Drug Administration
Consumer Affairs and Information
5600 Fishers Lane
Rockville, MD 2085
Phone: (888) 463-6332
Website: http://www.fda.gov

Smoking and Overweight

American Cancer Society
1599 Clifton Road, NE
Atlanta, GA 30329
Phone: (404) 320-3333 or (800) ACS-2345
Website: http://www.cancer.org

American Heart Association
National Center
7272 Greenville Avenue
Dallas, TX 75231
Phone: (800) AHA-USA1
Website: http://www.americanheart.org

American Lung Association
1740 Broadway
New York, NY 10019-4274
Phone: (212) 315-8700 or (800) LUNG-USA
E-Mail: info@lungusa.org
Website: http://www.lungusa.org

National Cancer Institute
Public Inquiries Office
Building 31, Room 10A03
31 Center Drive, MSC 2580
Bethesda, MD 20892-2530
Phone: (800) 422-6237
E-mail: cis@icicc.nci.nih.gov
Website: http://www.nci.nih.gov

Nicotine Anonymous World Service Office
P.O. Box 126338
Harrisburg, PA 17112
Phone: (415) 750-0328
E-mail: info@nicotine-anonymous.org
Website: http://www.nicotine-anonymous.org

Office on Smoking and Health
Centers for Disease Control and Prevention (CDC)
Mail Stop K-50
4770 Buford Highway, NE
Atlanta, GA 30341-3724
Phone: (770) 488-5705 or (800) CDC-1311
E-mail: ccdinfo@cdc.gov
Website: http://www.cdc.gov/tobacco

Children and Obesity

The American Academy of Pediatrics
141 Northwest Point Boulevard
Elk Grove Village, IL 60007-1098
Phone: (847) 434-4000
Fax: (847) 434-8000
E-Mail: pubrel@aap.org
Website: http://www.aap.org

Food and Nutrition Information Center
United States Department of Agriculture (USDA)
Website: http://www.nal.usda.gov/fnic

Resources

The National Center for Nutrition and Dietetics
The American Dietetic Association
216 West Jackson Boulevard
Chicago, IL 60606-6995
Phone: (312) 899-0040
Toll Free: (800) 366-1655 (consumer nutrition hotline)
Fax: (312) 899-4739
E-Mail: hotline@eatright.org
Website: http://www.eatright.org/ncnd.html

Obesity and the Elderly

Administration on Aging
Elder Care Locator
Phone: (800) 677-1116 (information about meal programs for senior citizens in your area)
Website: http://www.aoa.gov/elderpage/locator.html

National Center for Nutrition and Dietetics
(American Dietetic Association)
Phone: (800) 366-1655 (to find a registered dietitian in your area)

Cushing's Syndrome

Cushing's Support and Research Foundation, Inc.
65 East India Row, Suite 22-B
Boston, Massachusetts 02110
Phone: (617) 723-3824 or (617) 723-3674
E-Mail: csrf@world.std.com
Website: http://world.std.com/~csrf/

Pituitary Tumor Network Association
P.O. Box 1958
Thousand Oaks, CA 91358
Phone: (805) 499-2262
Fax: (805) 499-1523
Website: http://www.pituitary.com

Index

Index

Index

Page numbers followed by 'n' indicate a footnote. Page numbers in *italics* indicate a table or illustration.

A

AAFP *see* American Academy of Family Physicians
AARP *see* American Association of Retired Persons
abdominal fat, defined 277
absolute risk, defined 277
acanthosis nigricans 53
Accreditation Council for Continuing Medical Education 24
ACS *see* American Cancer Society
ACTH *see* adrenocorticotropin hormone
acupuncture 130
ADA *see* American Dietetic Association
Adipex-P (phentermine) 172
adipose tissue 277
Administration on Aging (AoA)
  contact information 341
  Older Americans Act 258
adrenal tumors 83, 87–88
adrenocortical carcinomas 83
adrenocorticotropin hormone (ACTH) 82
adults, obesity 15–21, 25

aerobic exercise
  defined 277
  see also exercise
African Americans
  heart disease 221
  hypertension 221
  obesity 219–20, 224
  television watching 253–54
age-adjusted, defined 277
age factor
  body mass index 16
  diet and nutrition 255–61
  obesity 224, 263–73
AHA *see* American Heart Association
ALA *see* American Lung Association
alcohol abuse, gout 99
alcoholism, cortisol 82
alcohol use, hypertension 65–66
algae *see* spirulina
allopurinol 102
AMA *see* American Medical Association
American Academy of Family Physicians (AAFP) 24
The American Academy of Pediatrics, contact information 340
American Association of Retired Persons (AARP)
  contact information 332
  publications 332

American Cancer Society (ACS), contact information 339
American College of Sports Medicine 247
American Dietetic Association (ADA) 24, 111, 263n
  contact information 333
  National Center for Nutrition and Dietetics, contact information 242, 341
American Druggist 195
American Family Physician 26, 91n
American Heart Association (AHA)
  contact information 339
  obesity risks 47, 56
  71st Scientific Session 55
American Home Products Corporation 183
American Indians *see* Native Americans
American Journal of Clinical Nutrition 331
American Lung Association (ALA), contact information 339
American Medical Association (AMA) 24
  contact information 333
The American Medical Association Encyclopedia of Medicine (Clayman, editor) 329
American Obesity Association (AOA) 4, 111
  Body Mass Index 53, 222
  contact information 334
  insurance denials 40
  obesity as disability 33–35
  overweight criteria 227
  publications 3n, 29n, 33n, 39n, 40, 45n, 219n, 223n
  tax deduction petition 31
American Osteopathic Association 24
American Society of Anesthesiologists (ASA) 93, 94
American Society of Bariatric Physicians (ASBP) 23
  contact information 23n, 55n, 334
  described 24
The American Surgeon 93n
Americans with Disabilities Act (ADA) 36–37, 41–42

Andersen, Ross E. 254
angina 58
animal studies
  appetite suppressant medications 176
  chromium supplements 136–37
  leptin 200
Annals of Internal Medicine 330
anorexiant, defined 277
anthropometric measurements, defined 277
antidepressants 19, 173
Anturane (sulfinpyrazone) 103
AOA *see* American Obesity Association
AoA *see* Administration on Aging
apnea *see* sleep apnea
appetite suppressant medications 171–80, 199
  bariatricians 24–25
  described 23
  questions and answers 177–80
  side effects 175–77
"appetite suppressing eyeglasses" 130
apple-shaped body 17, 20, 199, 292
"Are Health-Care Professionals Advising Obese Patients to Lose Weight?" (JAMA) 7
"Are You Eating Right?" 331
Argus Press 133n
arteriosclerosis 58
arthritis 45–46, 225
  see also osteoarthritis; rheumatoid arthritis
Arthritis Foundation 103
ASA *see* American Society of Anesthesiologists
ASBP *see* American Society of Bariatric Physicians
asthma, overweight 97–98
atherogenic, defined 278

B

back pain prevention 151
balloon, intragastric 282
bariatricians, described 23
bariatric medicine 23–28
bariatric surgery 115

Index

behavior modification 20, 24, 122
   guide 159–61
behavior therapy, defined 278
Benemid (probenecid) 103
benign intracranial hypertension *see* pseudo tumor cerebri
beta carotene 182
Better Nutrition 133n
biliopancreatic diversion
   defined 278
   depicted *214*
"Binge Eating Disorders" (NIH) 329
bioelectric impedance analysis 15
birth defects, obesity 46, 225
BMI *see* body mass index
body composition, defined 278
body fat 15–16
body mass index (BMI) *304–5*
   cancers 46–47
   defined 278
   described 4, 16
   diets 145–46
   gallstones 76
   minority populations 220
   NIH 55
   obesity medications 204
   older adults 263–64
   osteoarthritis 45
   overweight 53
   surgery recovery 93, 94
      procedures 209, 216
   twins studies 133
   weight management goals 109–10
   women 224
Bontril (phendimetrazine) 172
breast cancer 46, 225–26
The Brown University Child and Adolescent Behavior Letter 253n
Business and Health 41n

C

calcium 142, 143, 310–11
"Caloric Imbalance and Public Health Policy" (JAMA) 7
calorie intakes 17, 113, 128, 135, 166, 309
   see also diets

Camargo, Carlos 97
cancers
   adrenocortical carcinomas 83
   food labels 142
   minority populations 221
   obesity 3, 19, 46–47, 53, 226
   overweight 9, 11–12
carbohydrates 119
   defined 278
cardiovascular disease (CVD)
   defined 278
   obesity 47
   sleep apnea 69
carnitine 137
carpal tunnel syndrome (CTS), obesity 47–48
catecholamine neurotransmitters 280
causes of death, obesity 3, 225
Centers for Disease Control and Prevention (CDC)
   contact information 334
   National Center for Chronic Disease Prevention and Health Promotion 245n
   National Center for Health Statistics 94, 169, 245
   obesity research 5, 6
   Office on Smoking and Health, contact information 340
   publications 5n, 245n, 332
central abdominal obesity 134
central fat distribution, defined 278–79
cesarean delivery, obesity 91
CHD *see* coronary heart disease
"Childhood Obesity: Healthier Lifestyles Are Needed to Treat This Growing Problem" 245n
children
   obesity 26, 245–51
   overweight 235–43
      guidelines 251–53
   television watching 6, 253–54
cholecystectomy, defined 279
cholecystitis, defined 279
cholesterol 119, 135, 284–85
   defined 279
   see also high density lipoproteins; hypercholestrolemia; low density lipoproteins

347

Obesity Sourcebook, First Edition

"Exercise and Weight Control" 331
extreme obesity, defined 281

F

"The Facts about Weight Loss Products and Programs" (DHHS) 127
familial Carney's complex 88
familial Cushing's syndrome 83
families
  issues
    overweight children 237–43, 248
Fastin (phentermine) 172
fat blockers 129
fat-free, described 143
"A Fat Regulator in the Body" (Hunter) 199
"FDA Announces Withdrawal of Fenfluramine and Dexfenfluramine" 183n
"FDA Approves Orlistat for Obesity" (FDA) 181n
FDA Consumer 99n, 139n, 193n, 255n
"FDA Warns against Drug Promotion of 'Herbal Fen-Phen' for Weight Loss" (ASBP) 191n
Federal Food, Drug, and Cosmetic Act 194
Federal Register 35
Federal Trade Commission (FTC) 27
  contact information 112, 339
  false claim suits 129, 130
  jurisdiction 132
  web publications 127n
Federation of American Societies for Experimental Biology 335
femoxetine, defined 281
fenfluramine 171, 176, 177, 182, 183, 185–90
  defined 281
fen-phen 173, 183–90
  herbal 191–92
fiber 119, 131, 142
fibrinogen 135
  defined 281
financial concerns
  heart disease 55–56

financial concerns, continued
  obesity 3, 26
  older adults
    diet and nutrition 30, 258–60, 266
fixed menu diet 119
flexible diets 120–21
fluoxetine 173
  defined 282
folic acid 142
food groups *117*
Food Guide Pyramid 116–19, *117*, 166, 238
food labels 64, 139–43, 260–61
food preparation 311–13
formula diet 120, 136
Framingham Heart Study 56
fraud, weight loss programs 128–31
"Frequently Asked Questions about Bariatric Medicine and Obesity" (ASBP) 23n

G

gallbladder disease 3
  obesity 49, 226
  overweight 9, 12
"Gallstone Formation and Weight Loss" (Weinsier et al.) 330
gallstones
  causes 76, 115
  defined 282
  described 75–76
  diets 75–79, 146–47
  treatment 78–79
"Gallstones" (NIH) 330
gastric banding 205, 211
  defined 282
  depicted *212*
gastric bubble, defined 282
gastric bypass 205, 211
  defined 282
  depicted *214*
gastric exclusion, defined 282
gastric partitioning *see* gastric exclusion
gastric surgery 209–16
"Gastric Surgery for Severe Obesity" (NIH) 209

350

Index

gastroesophageal reflux 53
gastrointestinal surgery 20, 115
gastroplasty 211
   defined 283
gender factor
   Cushing's disease 82
   fen-phen usage 190
   gout 99
   obesity 220, 264–65
   sleep apnea 68
genetic factors
   Cushing's syndrome 83
   hypertension 59
   obesity 17–18, 26, 133, 134, 247–48
   overweight 71, 236
genotype, defined 283
"Getting to Know Gout" (Flieger) 99
Gila River Indian Community *see* Pima Indian studies
glucomannan 129
glucose tolerance, defined 283
Goldberg, Kohn (law firm) 42
gout
   obesity 19, 49, 99–104
   overweight 9, 12
Government Printing Office (GPO) 331, 332
"The Great Weight Debate" (Long) 329
"Growing Older, Eating Better" (Kurtzweil) 255
guar gum 129
"Guide to Behavior Change" (NHLBI) 159
"Guide to Physical Activity" (NHLBI) 149n
gynecologic complications, obesity 51, 226–27

H

hardening of the arteries *see* arteriosclerosis
Harrison's Principles of Internal Medicine 330
Harvard Medical School 97
HDL *see* high density lipoproteins

Health 329
"Health Effects of Obesity" (AOA) 45
healthy body weight 9, *10*
"Healthy Eating for a Healthy Life" (AARP) 332
heart disease 3, 5, 19, 142, 177
   hypertension 58
   lifetime risks 55–56
   obesity 135
   overweight 9, 11
   prevention 150
   valvular 188–89
Heart Disease & Stroke 28
heat disorders, obesity 49
heel spurs 53
"Helping Your Overweight Child" (NIH) 235
hemoglobin A1c, defined 283
hemorrhagic stroke, defined 283
hepatitis 50
herbal teas 193–97
herbal treatments 173, 191–92
heritability, defined 284
hernias 53
high blood cholesterol 4
   see also hypercholestrolemia
high blood pressure *see* hypertension
high-density lipoproteins (HDL) 47
   defined 284
high-protein, described 142
hirsutism 53
Hispanics
   obesity 221
   television watching 253–54
"How to Prevent High Blood Pressure" (NIH) 57
How to Quit Smoking Without Gaining Weight (Katahn) 331
Hu Hu Kam Memorial Hospital (Arizona) 232
The Human Obesity Gene Map 335
hypercapnia 53
hypercholestrolemia, defined 284
hypercortisolism 81
   see also Cushing's syndrome
"Hyperfunction: Glucocorticoids: Hypercortsolism (Cushing's syndrome)" (Wilson, editor, et al.) 330
hyperlipidemia 6

hypertension 3, 4, 19
  causes 61
  defined 284
  minority populations 221
  obesity 49
  prevention 57–66, 150
  sodium intake 142
hypertriglyceridemia, defined 284–85
hypopnea 67
  see also sleep apnea
hypothalamus 82
hypothyroidism 19
hypoxemia 68
hypoxia 53

I

IFIC *see* International Food Information Council Foundation
imaging procedures 85
immune response, obesity 50
incidence, defined 285
"Increased Incidence of Nosocomial Infections in Obese Surgical Patients" (Choban, et al.) 93n
Indian Health Service 231
Indian Health Service Hospital (Phoenix, AZ) 73
infections
  nosocomial 93
  obesity 50, 53
infertility, obesity 50
  women 226
"The Influence of Smoking Cessation on the Prevalence of Overweight in the United States" (NEJM) 170
insulin-dependent diabetes mellitus (type I diabetes), defined 285
insulin resistance 199, 200
insurance coverage, obesity 3, 39–40
interleukins 135
Internal Revenue Service (IRS) 29–30, 31
International Food Information Council Foundation (IFIC), contact information 143
Interneuron Pharmaceuticals 183
intestinal bypass surgery 210–11

Ionamin (phentermine) 172
iron 143
IRS *see* Internal Revenue Service
ischemia 283
ischemic stroke 283
  defined 285

J

JAMA see *The Journal of the American Medical Association*
jejunoileostomy *see* gastroplasty
John Wiley & Sons, Inc. 169n
Journal of Consulting and Clinical Psychology 26
Journal of Pediatrics 26
Journal of Physical Education, Recreation and Dance 26
Journal of the American Dietetic Association 28
The Journal of the American Medical Association (JAMA) 5, 6, 7, 26, 261
Journals of Gerontology 256
j-shaped relationship 285

K

kidney damage, hypertension 58

L

L-carnitine 137
LCD *see* low calorie diet
LDL *see* low density lipoproteins
legislation
  dietary supplements 194
  obesity 4, 35, 36–37, 41–42
leptin 199–201, 205, 207
leukotrienes 135
levofenfluramine 185
lifestyles
  changes
    bariatricians 23, 24
    children 245–50
    physical activity 149
    sedentary 135
    smoking cessation 163–70
    see also behavior modification

Index

"Lifetime Risks and Costs of Heart Disease Are Much Higher for Obese" (ASBP) 55n
linoleic acid 134
lipase inhibitors 181
lipoproteins, defined 285
  see also high density lipoproteins; low density lipoproteins
liver disease, obesity 50
locus, defined 285
longitudinal study, defined 286
"Losing Weight: What Works, What Doesn't" 331
low back pain, obesity 51
low-calorie diet (LCD) 24
  carnitine 137
  defined 286
low-density lipoproteins (LDL) 47
  defined 286
lower-fat diet, defined 286
L-tryptophan 192
Lyda Associates, Inc. 169n

M

macronutrients, defined 286
"magic weight loss earrings" 130
"magnet" diet pills 129
magnetic resonance imaging (MRI) 85
  defined 286
Ma Huang see ephedra
malnutrition, cortisol 82
mammegaly 53
Manisses Communications Group, Inc. 253n
Mayo Clinic
  Health Oasis
    publications 245n, 251n
    webiste 336
  heart valve disease research 176, 184, 186
Mayo Foundation for Medical Education and Research 245n, 251n
  heart valve disease research 184
Mazanor (mazindol) 172
mazindol 172
meal-replacement formulas see formula diet

Medical Economics Company 41n
medications
  bariatricians 23
  obesity 19, 26–27, 115, 171–80
    combinations 173–74
  see also *individual medications*
men
  body shapes 17
  hypertension 59
menopause, defined 286
menus 322–27
Meridia (sibutramine) 172, 203–4, 206
Mexican Americans
  diabetes 221
  obesity 219–20, 224
  television watching 253–54
MI see myocardial infarction
minerals 117
minorities, obesity 219–22
monoamine oxidase (MAO) inhibitors 179
monounsaturated fat, defined 286
MRI see magnetic resonance imaging
multiple endocrine neoplasia 83
myocardial infarction (MI), defined 287

N

NAAFA see National Association to Advance Fat Acceptance
National Association of Attorneys General (NAAG) 127n
National Association to Advance Fat Acceptance (NAAFA), contact information 336
National Cancer Institute (NCI)
  contact information 340
  Cushing's syndrome research 88
  obesity research sponsorships 21
  publications 330
National Center for Chronic Disease Prevention and Health Promotion 245n
National Center for Health Statistics (NCHS) 94
  smoking *versus* weight 169
  surveys 245

The National Center for Nutrition and Dietetics, contact information 242, 341
National Center for Research Resources (NCRR), obesity research sponsorships 21
National Cholesterol Education Program 284–85
National Diabetes Information Clearinghouse, contact information 336
National Digestive Diseases Advisory Board, National Task Force on Prevention and Treatment of Obesity 125
National Digestive Diseases Information Clearinghouse, contact information 330, 336
National Health and Nutrition Examination Survey (NHANES) 56, 245, 264
  described 287
National Heart, Lung, and Blood Institute (NHLBI)
  contact information 336
  Obesity Education Initiative 57n, 149n, 159n
  obesity research sponsorships 21
  publications 149n, 159n, 163n
National Institute of Arthritis and Musculoskeletal and Skin Diseases (NIAMS)
  contact information 337
  obesity research sponsorships 21
National Institute of Child Health and Human Development (NICHD)
  Cushing's syndrome research 88
  Developmental Endocrinology Branch 88
    contact information 89
  obesity research sponsorships 21
National Institute of Diabetes and Digestive and Kidney Diseases (NIDDK) 111
  contact information 330, 337
  mission described 21
  National Task Force on Prevention and Treatment of Obesity 21
  Obesity Resource Information Center 21

National Institute of Diabetes and Digestive and Kidney Diseases (NIDDK), continued
  publications 9n, 15n, 71n, 75n, 81n, 113n, 123n, 145n, 149n, 163n, 171n, 209n, 229n, 235n, 330
  research
    Cushing's syndrome 88
    obesity 71
    Pima Indians 229, 231
National Institute of Environmental and Health Sciences (NIEHS), obesity research sponsorships 21
National Institute of Mental Health (NIMH), obesity research sponsorships 21
National Institute of Neurological Disorders and Stroke
  Cushing's syndrome research 88
  obesity research sponsorships 21
National Institute of Nursing Research (NINR), obesity research sponsorships 21
National Institute on Aging (NIA), obesity research sponsorships 21
National Institutes of Health (NIH) 203
  Body Mass Index guidelines 55
  Center for Health Statistics 94
  Center for Research Resources 21
  clinics 232
  Digestive Diseases Information Clearinghouse contact information 336
  Heart, Lung, and Blood Institute 21, 57n, 336
  Institute of Arthritis and Musculoskeletal and Skin Diseases 21, 337
  National Institute of Diabetes and Digestive and Kidney Diseases 9n, 15n, 21, 111, 330, 337
  publications 9n, 15n, 57n, 67n, 71n, 75n, 91n, 113n, 123n, 145n, 149n, 171n, 209n, 229n, 235n, 329, 330, 331–32
  research
    Cushing's syndrome support 88
    obesity 4
    Pima Indians 231, 232, 233

Index

National Task Force on Prevention and Treatment of Obesity 21, 125
National Women's Health Information Center, contact information 337
Native Americans
 diabetes 220
 obesity 219
 see also Pima Indian studies
Natural Alternatives to Over-the-Counter and Prescription Drugs (Murray) 136
NCHS see National Center for Health Statistics
NCI see National Cancer Institute
"NCI Research Report: Cancer of the Lung" (NCI) 330
NCRR see National Center for Research Resources
NEJM see *New England Journal of Medicine*
"New Drugs, Safer Surgery May Help Overcome Overweight and Obesity" (Webb) 203
New England Journal of Medicine (NEJM) 170, 186
The New Food Label: There's Something in It for Everybody (FDA) 143
New York state, Human Rights Law 42
New York State Division of Human Rights 41
The New York Times 136
NHANES see National Health and Nutrition Examination Survey
NHLBI see National Heart, Lung, and Blood Institute
NIA see National Institute on Aging
NIAMS see National Institute of Arthritis and Musculoskeletal and Skin Diseases
NICHD see National Institute of Child Health and Human Development
Nicotine Anonymous World Services, contact information 340
nicotine replacement 167
NIDDK see National Institute of Diabetes and Digestive and Kidney Diseases
NIEHS see National Institute of Environmental and Health Sciences
NIH see National Institutes of Health
NIMH see National Institute of Mental Health
NINDS see National Institute of Neurological Disorders and Stroke
1996 Surgeon General's Report on Physical Activity and Health 6–7
NINR see National Institute of Nursing Research
non-clinical weight loss programs 114
non-insulin dependent diabetes mellitus (type 2 diabetes) 11, 150, 178
nonsteroidal anti-inflammatory drugs (NSAID), gout 102
North American Association for the Study of Obesity 111
 contact information 337
North American Primary Care Research Group 91
nosocomial infections 93
NSAID see nonsteroidal anti-inflammatory drugs
nutrition see diet and nutrition
Nutrition Facts Labels 140, 166, *303*
 see also food labels
Nutrition Research Newsletter 169n
Nutrition Today 133, 134

O

obesity
 bariatric medicine 23–28
 causes 17–19, 264–65
 children 26, 245–51, 253–54
 consequences 19–20, 45–53, 128, 265–66
 defined 5, 25, 287
 described 3–4
 extreme, defined 281
 gallstones 76
 measurement 15–17
 prevalence 25
 prevention 151
 refractory, defined 289
 research 21
 treatment 20, 23–28, 266–68
  tax deductions 29–31

"Obesity and Diabetes" (NIDDK) 71n
"Obesity and Health Insurance" (AOA) 39
"Obesity as a Medical Deduction" (AOA) 29n
"Obesity Before Pregnancy Is a Risk Factor for Cesarean Delivery" (Rose) 91n
"Obesity Epidemic Increases Dramatically in the United States" (CDC) 5
"Obesity in Minority Populations" (AOA) 219
"Obesity in Older Persons" (ADA) 263
Obesity Research 330
observational study, defined 287
obstetric complications, obesity 51, 226–27
Oby-trim (phentermine) 172
Older Americans Act 258
omega-3 fatty acids 134–35
omega-6 fatty acids 134–35
"On the Teen Scene: Food Label Makes Good Eating Easier" (Kurtzweil) 139n
orlistat 181–82, 206
  defined 287
osteoarthritis 45
  defined 287
  obesity 19
  overweight 9, 12
osteoporosis 142
  prevention 151
overweight
  causes 235–36
  defined 287
  health risks 9–13
  versus obesity 4, 53
  statistics 3

P

pain, obesity 51
Pan Am 41
pancreatitis, obesity 51–52
panic disorders, cortisol 82
panniculitis 53
Partnership for Healthy Weight Management
  contact information 337
  described 111
  publications 107n
"Pathophysiology of Obesity" (Bray) 331
pear-shaped body 17, 20, 292
Pediatric Alert 26
peripheral regions, defined 288
petrosal sinus sampling 85
pharmacotherapy, defined 288
Pharmacy Benefit Management Institute 40
phendimetrazine 172
phenotype, defined 288
phentermine 172, 173, 176, 183, 185–90
  defined 288
physical activity 261
  children 248–50
  diets 147
  hypertension prevention 63
  increase 6, 13
  program 154–55
  recommended levels 6
  smoking cessation 165–66
  weight control 149–50
  weight loss management 121–22
  weight management 108–9
  see also exercise
"Physical Activity and Weight Control" (NIH) 149n, 331
The Pima Indians, Pathfinders for Health (NIDDK) 71n, 229n
Pima Indian studies 71–74, 229–33
  see also Native Americans
pituitary adenomas 82, 86–87
Pituitary Tumor Network Association, contact information 341
Plegine (phendimetrazine) 172
Policy Analysis, Inc. 55
polynicotinate 137
polyunsaturated fat 134
  defined 288
Pondimin (fenfluramine) 171, 172, 177, 183, 185
postprandial plasma blood glucose, defined 288
PPH *see* primary pulmonary hypertension

Index

pregnancy
  appetite suppressant medications 179
  obesity 91
Prelu-2 (phendimetrazine) 172
prepackaged-meal diet 120
"Prescription Medications for the Treatment of Obesity" (NIH) 171
The President's Council on Physical Fitness and Sports contact information 331, 337
prevalence, defined 288
primary pigmented micronodular adrenal disease 83
primary pulmonary hypertension (PPH) 175–76
probenecid 103
"Promoting Lifelong Physical Activity —At a Glance!" (CDC) 245n
prospective study, defined 288
prostaglandins 135
prostate cancer 53
proteins 117–18, 142
  defined 288
pseudo Cushing's syndrome 85–86
pseudo tumor cerebri 53
psychological effects, obesity 19–20
psychological factors, obesity 18
Public Health Service 88
pulmonary disorders, obesity 19, 50

Q

"Questions and Answers about Withdrawal of Fenfluramine and Dexfenfluramine" (FDA) 185

R

randomization, defined 288–89
randomized clinical trial (RCT), defined 289
"Rating the Diets" 331
RCT *see* randomized clinical trial
RDA *see* recommended daily allowance
recessive genes, defined 289

recommended daily allowance (RDA) 123
Redux (dexfenfluramine) 171, 172, 177, 185
refractory obesity, defined 289
renal cell cancer 47
Report of the Dietary Guidelines Advisory Committee on the Dietary Guidelines for Americans 10
"A Report of the Surgeon General: Physical Activity and Health" 332
respiratory disturbance index 67
respiratory function, obesity 50
resting metabolic rate (RMR), defined 289
RGB *see* Roux-en-Y bypass
rheumatoid arthritis 46
risk, defined 289
RMR *see* resting metabolic rate
Roche Laboratories, Inc. 182
Roche Pharmaceuticals 204
Roux-en-Y bypass (RGB)
  defined 289
  depicted *213*

S

St. John's wort 192
Sanorex (mazindol) 172
saturated fat 119, 142
  defined 289–90
Screening for Mental Health, Inc. (Eating Disorders) 338
secular trends, defined 290
Seminole Electric Cooperative, Inc. 42
serotonin, defined 290
serotonin reuptake inhibitor (SSRI) 190
"Setting Goals for Weight Loss" 107n
severe arterial hypoxemia *see* hypoxemia
Shape Up America! 26
  contact information 338
shopping lists 297–302, 306–8
sibutramine 172, 175, 177, 203, 206
  defined 290
sleep apnea 9, 12, 19, 52, 67–69, 290
  defined 290
  obesity 19, 52, 67–69
  overweight 9, 12

smoking cessation
  overweight 169–70
  weight control 163–68
"Smoking Cessation and Overweight" 169
social effects, obesity 19–20
social pressure, defined 290
Social Security Administration (SSA) 33–35
socioeconomic factors, obesity 220
  women 223–24
sodium levels 63–64, 142
sphygmomanometer 59–60
spirulina 129
sporting activities 156
  see also exercise
"The Spread of Obesity in the United States" (JAMA) 7
SSRI *see* serotonin reuptake inhibitor
starch blockers 129
statistics
  obesity 3, 5
  overweight children 235
steatohepatitis 50
steroids 19
stimulant laxatives 194–96
stoma size, defined 290
stress
  cortisol 82
  smoking cessation 166–67
stress incontinence, defined 290
  see also urinary stress incontinence
stress management, defined 291
stroke 3, 19
  defined 291
  hypertension 57, 59
  obesity 52
  overweight 9, 11
  prevention 150
"stroke belt states," described 59
submaximal heart rate test
  defined 291
sugar-free, described 143
sulfinpyrazone 103
surgical procedures
  adrenal glands 88
  body mass index 93–94
  defined 291
  gallstones 78

surgical procedures, continued
  gastrointestinal 20, 115, 209–16, 282
  laparoscopy 205, 207
  obesity 52, 93–96
  sleep apnea 69
  stomach banding 205
systolic blood pressure 58, 60
  defined 291

T

target heart rate zone *153*
T-cells 200
television watching 6, 253–54
"Television-Watching Is Associated with Obesity" 253
Tenuate (diethylpropion) 172
tests, Cushing's syndrome 84–86
thrifty gene theory 71–72
tobacco use 163–64
trans fatty acids 134
triglycerides 47, 174
  defined 291
Tufts University, Program of Obesity and Metabolism 200
Tufts University Health & Nutrition Letter 97n
24-hour urinary free cortisol test 84
twins studies 133

U

"Understanding Adult Obesity" (WIN) 15n
University of Alabama (Birmingham), Department of Nutrition Sciences 111, 335
unsaturated fats 135
uric acid 100–103
urinary stress incontinence, obesity 52, 227
  see also stress incontinence
US Department of Agriculture (USDA)
  Food and Nutrition Information Center contact information 340

Index

US Department of Agriculture (USDA), continued
  Food Guide Pyramid *117*
  labeling
    food 140
    revisions 256
  publications 331
US Department of Health and Human Services (DHHS)
  Food Guide Pyramid *117*
  publications 99n, 331
  web publications 127n
US Department of Justice (DOJ)
  disabilities defined 33
  obesity and disability 33, 35
US Food and Drug Administration (FDA) 103
  Center for Drug Evaluation and Research 185n
  Center for Food Safety and Applied Nutrition 334
  contact information 335, 339
  dieter's teas 193
  food additives regulation 194
  Food Advisory Committee 194, 195, 196
  health claims 141
  herbal ingredients warnings 191
  ingredients bans 129
  jurisdiction 132
  labeling
    claims 260
    food 140, 143
    revisions 256
  MedWatch program contact information 184, 197
  obesity treatment recommendations 184, 189
  publications 127n, 139n, 181n, 255n
  Talk Papers 181n, 192
  Public Health Advisories, fen-phen and heart valve disease 186
  study reviews 187
  voluntary recalls
    appetite suppressants 172–73, 176–77
    obesity treatments 181, 183
US Government Printing Office 331, 332

V

validity, defined 291
vegetable oils 135
vertical banded gastroplasty 211
  defined 292
  depicted *212*
very low-calorie diet (VLCD) 24, 114, 128, 145–47
  defined 292
  gallstones 78
"Very Low-Calorie Diets" (NIH) 145n
very low-density lipoprotein (VLDL), defined 292
visceral fat, defined 292
vitamins 117
  orlistat 182
VLCD *see* very low-calorie diet
VLDL *see* very low-density lipoprotein
VO 2 max, defined 292

W

waist circumference 222
  defined 292
waist measurements 9, 110
waist-to-hip ratio (WHR) 17, 222
  defined 292
Wal-Mart 39–40
Warren Grant Magnuson Clinical Center (Bethesda, MD) contact information 89
weight control *see* weight management
Weight-Control Information Network (WIN) 9n, 15n, 75n, 114, 115
  contact information 338
  publications 329, 331–32
  web publications 113n, 123n, 149n, 163n, 171n, 209n, 235n
"Weight Cycling" (NIH) 332
weight-for-height chart *10*
weight-for-height tables 16
weight/health profile 109–11
"Weight-Loss Aids, with Dietary Changes, Help Us Reach Our Goal" 133n

"Weight Loss for Life" (NIH) 113n
weight loss industry 127–28
  products 127–32
  programs 24, 27–28, 123–25
    dietary changes 133–38
    gallstones 77–78
    tax deductions 29–30
    types, described 113–15
    see also diets
weight management
  exercise 149–57
  goals 107–12
  lifetime 113–22
  older adults 266–69
  tips 131–32
Weight Management and Health Insurance 40
"What Is a Bariatrician?" (ASBP) 23n
"What Is Obesity?" (AOA) 3
WHR *see* waist-to-hip ratio
Williams Textbook of Endocrinology 330
WIN *see* Weight-Control Information Network

women
  body shapes 17
  hypertension 59
  low back pain 51
  obesity 220, 223–27
"Women and Obesity" (AOA) 223
workplace discrimination, obesity 20
Wyeth-Ayerst Laboratories 40, 183

X

Xenical (orlistat) 182, 204–5, 206
X-Trozine (phendimetrazine) 172

Y

"You Can Control Your Weight As You Quit Smoking" (NIH) 163n
You First Health Risk Assessment website 338

Z

Zyloprim (allopurinol) 102

Health Reference Series
COMPLETE CATALOG

AIDS Sourcebook, 1st Edition

Basic Information about AIDS and HIV Infection, Featuring Historical and Statistical Data, Current Research, Prevention, and Other Special Topics of Interest for Persons Living with AIDS

Along with Source Listings for Further Assistance

Edited by Karen Bellenir and Peter D. Dresser. 831 pages. 1995. 0-7808-0031-1. $78.

"One strength of this book is its practical emphasis. The intended audience is the lay reader . . . useful as an educational tool for health care providers who work with AIDS patients. Recommended for public libraries as well as hospital or academic libraries that collect consumer materials."
—*Bulletin of the Medical Library Association, Jan '96*

"This is the most comprehensive volume of its kind on an important medical topic. Highly recommended for all libraries."   —*Reference Book Review, '96*

"Very useful reference for all libraries."
—*Choice, Association of College and Research Libraries, Oct '95*

"There is a wealth of information here that can provide much educational assistance. It is a must book for all libraries and should be on the desk of each and every congressional leader. Highly recommended."
—*AIDS Book Review Journal, Aug '95*

"Recommended for most collections."
—*Library Journal, Jul '95*

AIDS Sourcebook, 2nd Edition

Basic Consumer Health Information about Acquired Immune Deficiency Syndrome (AIDS) and Human Immunodeficiency Virus (HIV) Infection, Featuring Updated Statistical Data, Reports on Recent Research and Prevention Initiatives, and Other Special Topics of Interest for Persons Living with AIDS, Including New Antiretroviral Treatment Options, Strategies for Combating Opportunistic Infections, Information about Clinical Trials, and More

Along with a Glossary of Important Terms and Resource Listings for Further Help and Information

Edited by Karen Bellenir. 751 pages. 1999. 0-7808-0225-X. $78.

"Highly recommended."
—*American Reference Books Annual, 2000*

"Excellent sourcebook. This continues to be a highly recommended book. There is no other book that provides as much information as this book provides."
—*AIDS Book Review Journal, Dec-Jan 2000*

"Recommended reference source."
—*Booklist, American Library Association, Dec '99*

"A solid text for college-level health libraries."
—*The Bookwatch, Aug '99*

Cited in *Reference Sources for Small and Medium-Sized Libraries, American Library Association, 1999*

Alcoholism Sourcebook

Basic Consumer Health Information about the Physical and Mental Consequences of Alcohol Abuse, Including Liver Disease, Pancreatitis, Wernicke-Korsakoff Syndrome (Alcoholic Dementia), Fetal Alcohol Syndrome, Heart Disease, Kidney Disorders, Gastrointestinal Problems, and Immune System Compromise and Featuring Facts about Addiction, Detoxification, Alcohol Withdrawal, Recovery, and the Maintenance of Sobriety

Along with a Glossary and Directories of Resources for Further Help and Information

Edited by Karen Bellenir. 635 pages. 2000. 0-7808-0325-6. $78.

SEE ALSO *Drug Abuse Sourcebook, Substance Abuse Sourcebook*

Allergies Sourcebook

Basic Information about Major Forms and Mechanisms of Common Allergic Reactions, Sensitivities, and Intolerances, Including Anaphylaxis, Asthma, Hives and Other Dermatologic Symptoms, Rhinitis, and Sinusitis

Along with Their Usual Triggers Like Animal Fur, Chemicals, Drugs, Dust, Foods, Insects, Latex, Pollen, and Poison Ivy, Oak, and Sumac; Plus Information on Prevention, Identification, and Treatment

Edited by Allan R. Cook. 611 pages. 1997. 0-7808-0036-2. $78.

Alternative Medicine Sourcebook

Basic Consumer Health Information about Alternatives to Conventional Medicine, Including Acupressure, Acupuncture, Aromatherapy, Ayurveda, Bioelectromagnetics, Environmental Medicine, Essence Therapy, Food and Nutrition Therapy, Herbal Therapy, Homeopathy, Imaging, Massage, Naturopathy, Reflexology, Relaxation and Meditation, Sound Therapy, Vitamin and Mineral Therapy, and Yoga, and More

Edited by Allan R. Cook. 737 pages. 1999. 0-7808-0200-4. $78.

"Recommended reference source."
—*Booklist, American Library Association, Feb '00*

"A great addition to the reference collection of every type of library."
—*American Reference Books Annual, 2000*

■

Alzheimer's, Stroke & 29 Other Neurological Disorders Sourcebook, 1st Edition

Basic Information for the Layperson on 31 Diseases or Disorders Affecting the Brain and Nervous System, First Describing the Illness, Then Listing Symptoms, Diagnostic Methods, and Treatment Options, and Including Statistics on Incidences and Causes

Edited by Frank E. Bair. 579 pages. 1993. 1-55888-748-2. $78.

"Nontechnical reference book that provides reader-friendly information."
—*Family Caregiver Alliance Update, Winter '96*

"Should be included in any library's patient education section." —*American Reference Books Annual, 1994*

"Written in an approachable and accessible style. Recommended for patient education and consumer health collections in health science center and public libraries." —*Academic Library Book Review, Dec '93*

"It is very handy to have information on more than thirty neurological disorders under one cover, and there is no recent source like it." —*Reference Quarterly, American Library Association, Fall '93*

SEE ALSO Brain Disorders Sourcebook

■

Alzheimer's Disease Sourcebook, 2nd Edition

Basic Consumer Health Information about Alzheimer's Disease, Related Disorders, and Other Dementias, Including Multi-Infarct Dementia, AIDS-Related Dementia, Alcoholic Dementia, Huntington's Disease, Delirium, and Confusional States

Along with Reports Detailing Current Research Efforts in Prevention and Treatment, Long-Term Care Issues, and Listings of Sources for Additional Help and Information

Edited by Karen Bellenir. 524 pages. 1999. 0-7808-0223-3. $78.

"Provides a wealth of useful information not otherwise available in one place. This resource is recommended for all types of libraries."
—*American Reference Books Annual, 2000*

"Recommended reference source."
—*Booklist, American Library Association, Oct '99*

Arthritis Sourcebook

Basic Consumer Health Information about Specific Forms of Arthritis and Related Disorders, Including Rheumatoid Arthritis, Osteoarthritis, Gout, Polymyalgia Rheumatica, Psoriatic Arthritis, Spondyloarthropathies, Juvenile Rheumatoid Arthritis, and Juvenile Ankylosing Spondylitis

Along with Information about Medical, Surgical, and Alternative Treatment Options, and Including Strategies for Coping with Pain, Fatigue, and Stress

Edited by Allan R. Cook. 550 pages. 1998. 0-7808-0201-2. $78.

"... accessible to the layperson."
—*Reference and Research Book News, Feb '99*

■

Asthma Sourcebook

Basic Consumer Health Information about Asthma, Including Symptoms, Traditional and Nontraditional Remedies, Treatment Advances, Quality-of-Life Aids, Medical Research Updates, and the Role of Allergies, Exercise, Age, the Environment, and Genetics in the Development of Asthma

Along with Statistical Data, a Glossary, and Directories of Support Groups, and Other Resources for Further Information

Edited by Annemarie S. Muth. 628 pages. 2000. 0-7808-0381-7. $78.

■

Back & Neck Disorders Sourcebook

Basic Information about Disorders and Injuries of the Spinal Cord and Vertebrae, Including Facts on Chiropractic Treatment, Surgical Interventions, Paralysis, and Rehabilitation

Along with Advice for Preventing Back Trouble

Edited by Karen Bellenir. 548 pages. 1997. 0-7808-0202-0. $78.

"The strength of this work is its basic, easy-to-read format. Recommended."
—*Reference and User Services Quarterly, American Library Association, Winter '97*

■

Blood & Circulatory Disorders Sourcebook

Basic Information about Blood and Its Components, Anemias, Leukemias, Bleeding Disorders, and Circulatory Disorders, Including Aplastic Anemia, Thalassemia, Sickle-Cell Disease, Hemochromatosis, Hemophilia, Von Willebrand Disease, and Vascular Diseases

Along with a Special Section on Blood Transfusions and Blood Supply Safety, a Glossary, and Source Listings for Further Help and Information

Edited by Karen Bellenir and Linda M. Shin. 554 pages. 1998. 0-7808-0203-9. $78.

"Recommended reference source."
—*Booklist, American Library Association,* Feb '99

"An important reference sourcebook written in simple language for everyday, non-technical users."
—*Reviewer's Bookwatch,* Jan '99

Brain Disorders Sourcebook

Basic Consumer Health Information about Strokes, Epilepsy, Amyotrophic Lateral Sclerosis (ALS/Lou Gehrig's Disease), Parkinson's Disease, Brain Tumors, Cerebral Palsy, Headache, Tourette Syndrome, and More Along with Statistical Data, Treatment and Rehabilitation Options, Coping Strategies, Reports on Current Research Initiatives, a Glossary, and Resource Listings for Additional Help and Information

Edited by Karen Bellenir. 481 pages. 1999. 0-7808-0229-2. $78.

"Belongs on the shelves of any library with a consumer health collection." —*E-Streams,* Mar '00

"Recommended reference source."
—*Booklist, American Library Association,* Oct '99

SEE ALSO *Alzheimer's, Stroke & 29 Other Neurological Disorders Sourcebook, 1st Edition*

Breast Cancer Sourcebook

Basic Consumer Health Information about Breast Cancer, Including Diagnostic Methods, Treatment Options, Alternative Therapies, Help and Self-Help Information, Related Health Concerns, Statistical and Demographic Data, and Facts for Men with Breast Cancer Along with Reports on Current Research Initiatives, a Glossary of Related Medical Terms, and a Directory of Sources for Further Help and Information

Edited by Edward J. Prucha and Karen Bellenir. 600 pages. 2001. 0-7808-0244-6. $78.

SEE ALSO *Cancer Sourcebook for Women, 1st and 2nd Editions, Women's Health Concerns Sourcebook*

Burns Sourcebook

Basic Consumer Health Information about Various Types of Burns and Scalds, Including Flame, Heat, Cold, Electrical, Chemical, and Sun Burns Along with Information on Short-Term and Long-Term Treatments, Tissue Reconstruction, Plastic Surgery, Prevention Suggestions, and First Aid

Edited by Allan R. Cook. 604 pages. 1999. 0-7808-0204-7. $78.

"This key reference guide is an invaluable addition to all health care and public libraries in confronting this ongoing health issue."
—*American Reference Books Annual,* 2000

"This is an exceptional addition to the series and is highly recommended for all consumer health collections, hospital libraries, and academic medical centers." —*E-Streams,* Mar '00

"Recommended reference source."
—*Booklist, American Library Association,* Dec '99

SEE ALSO *Skin Disorders Sourcebook*

Cancer Sourcebook, 1st Edition

Basic Information on Cancer Types, Symptoms, Diagnostic Methods, and Treatments, Including Statistics on Cancer Occurrences Worldwide and the Risks Associated with Known Carcinogens and Activities

Edited by Frank E. Bair. 932 pages. 1990. 1-55888-888-8. $78.

Cited in *Reference Sources for Small and Medium-Sized Libraries,* American Library Association, 1999

"Written in nontechnical language. Useful for patients, their families, medical professionals, and librarians."
—*Guide to Reference Books,* 1996

"Designed with the non-medical professional in mind. Libraries and medical facilities interested in patient education should certainly consider adding the *Cancer Sourcebook* to their holdings. This compact collection of reliable information . . . is an invaluable tool for helping patients and patients' families and friends to take the first steps in coping with the many difficulties of cancer."
—*Medical Reference Services Quarterly,* Winter '91

"Specifically created for the nontechnical reader . . . an important resource for the general reader trying to understand the complexities of cancer."
—*American Reference Books Annual,* 1991

"This publication's nontechnical nature and very comprehensive format make it useful for both the general public and undergraduate students."
—*Choice, Association of College and Research Libraries,* Oct '90

New Cancer Sourcebook, 2nd Edition

Basic Information about Major Forms and Stages of Cancer, Featuring Facts about Primary and Secondary Tumors of the Respiratory, Nervous, Lymphatic, Circulatory, Skeletal, and Gastrointestinal Systems, and Specific Organs; Statistical and Demographic Data; Treatment Options; and Strategies for Coping

Edited by Allan R. Cook. 1,313 pages. 1996. 0-7808-0041-9. $78.

"An excellent resource for patients with newly diagnosed cancer and their families. The dialogue is simple, direct, and comprehensive. Highly recommended for patients and families to aid in their understanding of cancer and its treatment."
—*Booklist Health Sciences Supplement, American Library Association,* Oct '97

"The amount of factual and useful information is extensive. The writing is very clear, geared to general readers. Recommended for all levels."
—*Choice, Association of College and Research Libraries, Jan '97*

■

Cancer Sourcebook, 3rd Edition

Basic Consumer Health Information about Major Forms and Stages of Cancer, Featuring Facts about Primary and Secondary Tumors of the Respiratory, Nervous, Lymphatic, Circulatory, Skeletal, and Gastrointestinal Systems, and Specific Organs

Along with Statistical and Demographic Data, Treatment Options, Strategies for Coping, a Glossary, and a Directory of Sources for Additional Help and Information

Edited by Edward J. Prucha. 1,069 pages. 2000. 0-7808-0227-6. $78.

■

Cancer Sourcebook for Women, 1st Edition

Basic Information about Specific Forms of Cancer That Affect Women, Featuring Facts about Breast Cancer, Cervical Cancer, Ovarian Cancer, Cancer of the Uterus and Uterine Sarcoma, Cancer of the Vagina, and Cancer of the Vulva; Statistical and Demographic Data; Treatments, Self-Help Management Suggestions, and Current Research Initiatives

Edited by Allan R. Cook and Peter D. Dresser. 524 pages. 1996. 0-7808-0076-1. $78.

". . . written in easily understandable, non-technical language. Recommended for public libraries or hospital and academic libraries that collect patient education or consumer health materials."
—*Medical Reference Services Quarterly, Spring '97*

"Would be of value in a consumer health library. . . . written with the health care consumer in mind. Medical jargon is at a minimum, and medical terms are explained in clear, understandable sentences."
—*Bulletin of the Medical Library Association, Oct '96*

"The availability under one cover of all these pertinent publications, grouped under cohesive headings, makes this certainly a most useful sourcebook."
—*Choice, Association of College and Research Libraries, Jun '96*

"Presents a comprehensive knowledge base for general readers. Men and women both benefit from the gold mine of information nestled between the two covers of this book. Recommended."
—*Academic Library Book Review, Summer '96*

"This timely book is highly recommended for consumer health and patient education collections in all libraries."   —*Library Journal, Apr '96*

SEE ALSO Breast Cancer Sourcebook, Women's Health Concerns Sourcebook

Cancer Sourcebook for Women, 2nd Edition

Basic Consumer Health Information about Specific Forms of Cancer That Affect Women, Including Cervical Cancer, Ovarian Cancer, Endometrial Cancer, Uterine Sarcoma, Vaginal Cancer, Vulvar Cancer, and Gestational Trophoblastic Tumor; and Featuring Statistical Information, Facts about Tests and Treatments, a Glossary of Cancer Terms, and an Extensive List of Additional Resources

Edited by Edward J. Prucha. 600 pages. 2001. 0-7808-0226-8. $78.

SEE ALSO Breast Cancer Sourcebook, Women's Health Concerns Sourcebook

■

Cardiovascular Diseases & Disorders Sourcebook, 1st Edition

Basic Information about Cardiovascular Diseases and Disorders, Featuring Facts about the Cardiovascular System, Demographic and Statistical Data, Descriptions of Pharmacological and Surgical Interventions, Lifestyle Modifications, and a Special Section Focusing on Heart Disorders in Children

Edited by Karen Bellenir and Peter D. Dresser. 683 pages. 1995. 0-7808-0032-X. $78.

". . . comprehensive format provides an extensive overview on this subject."
—*Choice, Association of College and Research Libraries, Jun '96*

". . . an easily understood, complete, up-to-date resource. This well executed public health tool will make valuable information available to those that need it most, patients and their families. The typeface, sturdy non-reflective paper, and library binding add a feel of quality found wanting in other publications. Highly recommended for academic and general libraries. "
—*Academic Library Book Review, Summer '96*

SEE ALSO Healthy Heart Sourcebook for Women, Heart Diseases & Disorders Sourcebook, 2nd Edition

■

Caregiving Sourcebook

Basic Consumer Health Information for Caregivers, Including a Profile of Caregivers, Caregiving Responsibilities, Tips for Specific Conditions, Care Environments, and the Effects of Caregiving

Along with Legal Issues, Financial Concerns, Future Planning, a Glossary, and a Listing of Additional Resources

Edited by Joyce Brennfleck Shannon. 550 pages. 2001. 0-7808-0331-0. $78.

Colds, Flu & Other Common Ailments Sourcebook

Basic Consumer Health Information about Common Ailments and Injuries, Including Colds, Coughs, the Flu, Sinus Problems, Headaches, Fever, Nausea and Vomiting, Menstrual Cramps, Diarrhea, Constipation, Hemorrhoids, Back Pain, Dandruff, Dry and Itchy Skin, Cuts, Scrapes, Sprains, Bruises, and More

Along with Information about Prevention, Self-Care, Choosing a Doctor, Over-the-Counter Medications, Folk Remedies, and Alternative Therapies, and Including a Glossary of Important Terms and a Directory of Resources for Further Help and Information

Edited by Chad T. Kimball. 600 pages. 2001. 0-7808-0435-X. $78.

Communication Disorders Sourcebook

Basic Information about Deafness and Hearing Loss, Speech and Language Disorders, Voice Disorders, Balance and Vestibular Disorders, and Disorders of Smell, Taste, and Touch

Edited by Linda M. Ross. 533 pages. 1996. 0-7808-0077-X. $78.

"This is skillfully edited and is a welcome resource for the layperson. It should be found in every public and medical library." — *Booklist Health Sciences Supplement, American Library Association, Oct '97*

Congenital Disorders Sourcebook

Basic Information about Disorders Acquired during Gestation, Including Spina Bifida, Hydrocephalus, Cerebral Palsy, Heart Defects, Craniofacial Abnormalities, Fetal Alcohol Syndrome, and More

Along with Current Treatment Options and Statistical Data

Edited by Karen Bellenir. 607 pages. 1997. 0-7808-0205-5. $78.

"Recommended reference source."
— *Booklist, American Library Association, Oct '97*

SEE ALSO *Pregnancy & Birth Sourcebook*

Consumer Issues in Health Care Sourcebook

Basic Information about Health Care Fundamentals and Related Consumer Issues, Including Exams and Screening Tests, Physician Specialties, Choosing a Doctor, Using Prescription and Over-the-Counter Medications Safely, Avoiding Health Scams, Managing Common Health Risks in the Home, Care Options for Chronically or Terminally Ill Patients, and a List of Resources for Obtaining Help and Further Information

Edited by Karen Bellenir. 618 pages. 1998. 0-7808-0221-7. $78.

"Both public and academic libraries will want to have a copy in their collection for readers who are interested in self-education on health issues."
— *American Reference Books Annual, 2000*

"The editor has researched the literature from government agencies and others, saving readers the time and effort of having to do the research themselves. Recommended for public libraries."
— *Reference and User Services Quarterly, American Library Association, Spring '99*

"Recommended reference source."
— *Booklist, American Library Association, Dec '98*

Contagious & Non-Contagious Infectious Diseases Sourcebook

Basic Information about Contagious Diseases like Measles, Polio, Hepatitis B, and Infectious Mononucleosis, and Non-Contagious Infectious Diseases like Tetanus and Toxic Shock Syndrome, and Diseases Occurring as Secondary Infections Such as Shingles and Reye Syndrome

Along with Vaccination, Prevention, and Treatment Information, and a Section Describing Emerging Infectious Disease Threats

Edited by Karen Bellenir and Peter D. Dresser. 566 pages. 1996. 0-7808-0075-3. $78.

Death & Dying Sourcebook

Basic Consumer Health Information for the Layperson about End-of-Life Care and Related Ethical and Legal Issues, Including Chief Causes of Death, Autopsies, Pain Management for the Terminally Ill, Life Support Systems, Insurance, Euthanasia, Assisted Suicide, Hospice Programs, Living Wills, Funeral Planning, Counseling, Mourning, Organ Donation, and Physician Training

Along with Statistical Data, a Glossary, and Listings of Sources for Further Help and Information

Edited by Annemarie S. Muth. 641 pages. 1999. 0-7808-0230-6. $78.

"This book is a definite must for all those involved in end-of-life care." — *Doody's Review Service, 2000*

Diabetes Sourcebook, 1st Edition

Basic Information about Insulin-Dependent and Non-insulin-Dependent Diabetes Mellitus, Gestational Diabetes, and Diabetic Complications, Symptoms, Treatment, and Research Results, Including Statistics on Prevalence, Morbidity, and Mortality

Along with Source Listings for Further Help and Information

Edited by Karen Bellenir and Peter D. Dresser. 827 pages. 1994. 1-55888-751-2. $78.

". . . very informative and understandable for the layperson without being simplistic. It provides a comprehensive overview for laypersons who want a general understanding of the disease or who want to focus on various aspects of the disease."
—*Bulletin of the Medical Library Association, Jan '96*

Diabetes Sourcebook, 2nd Edition

Basic Consumer Health Information about Type 1 Diabetes (Insulin-Dependent or Juvenile-Onset Diabetes), Type 2 (Noninsulin-Dependent or Adult-Onset Diabetes), Gestational Diabetes, and Related Disorders, Including Diabetes Prevalence Data, Management Issues, the Role of Diet and Exercise in Controlling Diabetes, Insulin and Other Diabetes Medicines, and Complications of Diabetes Such as Eye Diseases, Periodontal Disease, Amputation, and End-Stage Renal Disease

Along with Reports on Current Research Initiatives, a Glossary, and Resource Listings for Further Help and Information

Edited by Karen Bellenir. 688 pages. 1998. 0-7808-0224-1. $78.

"This comprehensive book is an excellent addition for high school, academic, medical, and public libraries. This volume is highly recommended."
—*American Reference Books Annual, 2000*

"An invaluable reference." —*Library Journal, May '00*

Selected as one of the 250 "Best Health Sciences Books of 1999." —*Doody's Rating Service, Mar-Apr 2000*

"Recommended reference source."
—*Booklist, American Library Association, Feb '99*

". . . provides reliable mainstream medical information . . . belongs on the shelves of any library with a consumer health collection." —*E-Streams, Sep '99*

"Provides useful information for the general public."
—*Healthlines, University of Michigan Health Management Research Center, Sep/Oct '99*

Diet & Nutrition Sourcebook, 1st Edition

Basic Information about Nutrition, Including the Dietary Guidelines for Americans, the Food Guide Pyramid, and Their Applications in Daily Diet, Nutritional Advice for Specific Age Groups, Current Nutritional Issues and Controversies, the New Food Label and How to Use It to Promote Healthy Eating, and Recent Developments in Nutritional Research

Edited by Dan R. Harris. 662 pages. 1996. 0-7808-0084-2. $78.

"Useful reference as a food and nutrition sourcebook for the general consumer." —*Booklist Health Sciences Supplement, American Library Association, Oct '97*

"Recommended for public libraries and medical libraries that receive general information requests on nutrition. It is readable and will appeal to those interested in learning more about healthy dietary practices."
—*Medical Reference Services Quarterly, Fall '97*

"An abundance of medical and social statistics is translated into readable information geared toward the general reader." —*Bookwatch, Mar '97*

"With dozens of questionable diet books on the market, it is so refreshing to find a reliable and factual reference book. Recommended to aspiring professionals, librarians, and others seeking and giving reliable dietary advice. An excellent compilation." —*Choice, Association of College and Research Libraries, Feb '97*

SEE ALSO *Digestive Diseases & Disorders Sourcebook, Gastrointestinal Diseases & Disorders Sourcebook*

Diet & Nutrition Sourcebook, 2nd Edition

Basic Consumer Health Information about Dietary Guidelines, Recommended Daily Intake Values, Vitamins, Minerals, Fiber, Fat, Weight Control, Dietary Supplements, and Food Additives

Along with Special Sections on Nutrition Needs throughout Life and Nutrition for People with Such Specific Medical Concerns as Allergies, High Blood Cholesterol, Hypertension, Diabetes, Celiac Disease, Seizure Disorders, Phenylketonuria (PKU), Cancer, and Eating Disorders, and Including Reports on Current Nutrition Research and Source Listings for Additional Help and Information

Edited by Karen Bellenir. 650 pages. 1999. 0-7808-0228-4. $78.

"This reference document should be in any public library, but it would be a very good guide for beginning students in the health sciences. If the other books in this publisher's series are as good as this, they should all be in the health sciences collections."
—*American Reference Books Annual, 2000*

"Recommended reference source."
—*Booklist, American Library Association, Dec '99*

SEE ALSO *Digestive Diseases & Disorders Sourcebook, Gastrointestinal Diseases & Disorders Sourcebook*

Digestive Diseases & Disorders Sourcebook

Basic Consumer Health Information about Diseases and Disorders that Impact the Upper and Lower Digestive System, Including Celiac Disease, Constipation, Crohn's Disease, Cyclic Vomiting Syndrome, Diarrhea, Diverticulosis and Diverticulitis, Gallstones, Heartburn, Hemorrhoids, Hernias, Indigestion (Dyspepsia), Irritable Bowel Syndrome, Lactose Intolerance, Ulcers, and More

Along with Information about Medications and Other Treatments, Tips for Maintaining a Healthy Digestive

Tract, a Glossary, and Directory of Digestive Diseases Organizations

Edited by Karen Bellenir. 335 pages. 1999. 0-7808-0327-2. $48.

"Recommended reference source."
—*Booklist, American Library Association, May '00*

SEE ALSO *Diet & Nutrition Sourcebook, 1st and 2nd Editions, Gastrointestinal Diseases & Disorders Sourcebook*

■

Disabilities Sourcebook

Basic Consumer Health Information about Physical and Psychiatric Disabilities, Including Descriptions of Major Causes of Disability, Assistive and Adaptive Aids, Workplace Issues, and Accessibility Concerns

Along with Information about the Americans with Disabilities Act, a Glossary, and Resources for Additional Help and Information

Edited by Dawn D. Matthews. 616 pages. 2000. 0-7808-0389-2. $78.

"Recommended reference source."
—*Booklist, American Library Association, Jul '00*

"An involving, invaluable handbook."
—*The Bookwatch, May '00*

■

Domestic Violence & Child Abuse Sourcebook

Basic Consumer Health Information about Spousal/Partner, Child, Sibling, Parent, and Elder Abuse, Covering Physical, Emotional, and Sexual Abuse, Teen Dating Violence, and Stalking; Includes Information about Hotlines, Safe Houses, Safety Plans, and Other Resources for Support and Assistance, Community Initiatives, and Reports on Current Directions in Research and Treatment

Along with a Glossary, Sources for Further Reading, and Governmental and Non-Governmental Organizations Contact Information

Edited by Helene Henderson. 1,064 pages. 2000. 0-7808-0235-7. $78.

■

Drug Abuse Sourcebook

Basic Consumer Health Information about Illicit Substances of Abuse and the Diversion of Prescription Medications, Including Depressants, Hallucinogens, Inhalants, Marijuana, Narcotics, Stimulants, and Anabolic Steroids

Along with Facts about Related Health Risks, Treatment Issues, and Substance Abuse Prevention Programs, a Glossary of Terms, Statistical Data, and Directories of Hotline Services, Self-Help Groups, and Organizations Able to Provide Further Information

Edited by Karen Bellenir. 629 pages. 2000. 0-7808-0242-X. $78.

SEE ALSO *Alcoholism Sourcebook, Substance Abuse Sourcebook*

■

Ear, Nose & Throat Disorders Sourcebook

Basic Information about Disorders of the Ears, Nose, Sinus Cavities, Pharynx, and Larynx, Including Ear Infections, Tinnitus, Vestibular Disorders, Allergic and Non-Allergic Rhinitis, Sore Throats, Tonsillitis, and Cancers That Affect the Ears, Nose, Sinuses, and Throat

Along with Reports on Current Research Initiatives, a Glossary of Related Medical Terms, and a Directory of Sources for Further Help and Information

Edited by Karen Bellenir and Linda M. Shin. 576 pages. 1998. 0-7808-0206-3. $78.

"Overall, this sourcebook is helpful for the consumer seeking information on ENT issues. It is recommended for public libraries."
—*American Reference Books Annual, 1999*

"Recommended reference source."
—*Booklist, American Library Association, Dec '98*

■

Endocrine & Metabolic Disorders Sourcebook

Basic Information for the Layperson about Pancreatic and Insulin-Related Disorders Such as Pancreatitis, Diabetes, and Hypoglycemia; Adrenal Gland Disorders Such as Cushing's Syndrome, Addison's Disease, and Congenital Adrenal Hyperplasia; Pituitary Gland Disorders Such as Growth Hormone Deficiency, Acromegaly, and Pituitary Tumors; Thyroid Disorders Such as Hypothyroidism, Graves' Disease, Hashimoto's Disease, and Goiter; Hyperparathyroidism; and Other Diseases and Syndromes of Hormone Imbalance or Metabolic Dysfunction

Along with Reports on Current Research Initiatives

Edited by Linda M. Shin. 574 pages. 1998. 0-7808-0207-1. $78.

"Omnigraphics has produced another needed resource for health information consumers."
—*American Reference Books Annual, 2000*

"Recommended reference source."
—*Booklist, American Library Association, Dec '98*

■

Environmentally Induced Disorders Sourcebook

Basic Information about Diseases and Syndromes Linked to Exposure to Pollutants and Other Substances in Outdoor and Indoor Environments Such as Lead, Asbestos, Formaldehyde, Mercury, Emissions, Noise, and More

Edited by Allan R. Cook. 620 pages. 1997. 0-7808-0083-4. $78.

"Recommended reference source."
—*Booklist, American Library Association, Sep '98*

"This book will be a useful addition to anyone's library."
— *Choice Health Sciences Supplement, Association of College and Research Libraries, May '98*

". . . a good survey of numerous environmentally induced physical disorders . . . a useful addition to anyone's library."
— *Doody's Health Sciences Book Reviews, Jan '98*

". . . provide[s] introductory information from the best authorities around. Since this volume covers topics that potentially affect everyone, it will surely be one of the most frequently consulted volumes in the *Health Reference Series*."
— *Rettig on Reference, Nov '97*

Ethnic Diseases Sourcebook

Basic Consumer Health Information for Ethnic and Racial Minority Groups in the United States, Including General Health Indicators and Behaviors, Ethnic Diseases, Genetic Testing, the Impact of Chronic Diseases, Women's Health, Mental Health Issues, and Preventive Health Care Services

Along with a Glossary and a Listing of Additional Resources

Edited by Joyce Brennfleck Shannon. 600 pages. 2001. 0-7808-0336-1. $78.

Family Planning Sourcebook

Basic Consumer Health Information about Planning for Pregancy and Contraception, Including Traditional Methods, Barrier Methods, Hormonal Methods, Permanent Methods, Future Methods, Emergency Contraception, and Birth Control Choices for Women at Each Stage of Life

Along with Statistics, a Glossary, and Sources of Additional Information

Edited by Amy Marcaccio Keyzer. 600 pages. 2001. 0-7808-0379-5. $78.

SEE ALSO Pregnancy & Birth Sourcebook

Fitness & Exercise Sourcebook, 1st Edition

Basic Information on Fitness and Exercise, Including Fitness Activities for Specific Age Groups, Exercise for People with Specific Medical Conditions, How to Begin a Fitness Program in Running, Walking, Swimming, Cycling, and Other Athletic Activities, and Recent Research in Fitness and Exercise

Edited by Dan R. Harris. 663 pages. 1996. 0-7808-0186-5. $78.

"A good resource for general readers."
— *Choice, Association of College and Research Libraries, Nov '97*

"The perennial popularity of the topic . . . make this an appealing selection for public libraries."
— *Rettig on Reference, Jun/Jul '97*

Fitness & Exercise Sourcebook, 2nd Edition

Basic Consumer Health Information about the Fundamentals of Fitness and Exercise, Including How to Begin and Maintain a Fitness Program, Fitness as a Lifestyle, the Link between Fitness and Diet, Advice for Specific Groups of People, Exercise as It Relates to Specific Medical Conditions, and Recent Research in Fitness and Exercise

Along with a Glossary of Important Terms and Resources for Additional Help and Information

Edited by Kristen M. Gledhill. 600 pages. 2001. 0-7808-0334-5. $78.

Food & Animal Borne Diseases Sourcebook

Basic Information about Diseases That Can Be Spread to Humans through the Ingestion of Contaminated Food or Water or by Contact with Infected Animals and Insects, Such as Botulism, E. Coli, Hepatitis A, Trichinosis, Lyme Disease, and Rabies

Along with Information Regarding Prevention and Treatment Methods, and Including a Special Section for International Travelers Describing Diseases Such as Cholera, Malaria, Travelers' Diarrhea, and Yellow Fever, and Offering Recommendations for Avoiding Illness

Edited by Karen Bellenir and Peter D. Dresser. 535 pages. 1995. 0-7808-0033-8. $78.

"Targeting general readers and providing them with a single, comprehensive source of information on selected topics, this book continues, with the excellent caliber of its predecessors, to catalog topical information on health matters of general interest. Readable and thorough, this valuable resource is highly recommended for all libraries."
— *Academic Library Book Review, Summer '96*

"A comprehensive collection of authoritative information."
— *Emergency Medical Services, Oct '95*

Food Safety Sourcebook

Basic Consumer Health Information about the Safe Handling of Meat, Poultry, Seafood, Eggs, Fruit Juices, and Other Food Items, and Facts about Pesticides, Drinking Water, Food Safety Overseas, and the Onset, Duration, and Symptoms of Foodborne Illnesses, Including Types of Pathogenic Bacteria, Parasitic Protozoa, Worms, Viruses, and Natural Toxins

Along with the Role of the Consumer, the Food Handler, and the Government in Food Safety; a Glossary, and Resources for Additional Help and Information

Edited by Dawn D. Matthews. 339 pages. 1999. 0-7808-0326-4. $48.

"This book takes the complex issues of food safety and foodborne pathogens and presents them in an easily understood manner. [It does] an excellent job of covering a large and often confusing topic."
— *American Reference Books Annual, 2000*

"Recommended reference source."
—*Booklist, American Library Association, May '00*

Forensic Medicine Sourcebook

Basic Consumer Information for the Layperson about Forensic Medicine, Including Crime Scene Investigation, Evidence Collection and Analysis, Expert Testimony, Computer-Aided Criminal Identification, Digital Imaging in the Courtroom, DNA Profiling, Accident Reconstruction, Autopsies, Ballistics, Drugs and Explosives Detection, Latent Fingerprints, Product Tampering, and Questioned Document Examination

Along with Statistical Data, a Glossary of Forensics Terminology, and Listings of Sources for Further Help and Information

Edited by Annemarie S. Muth. 574 pages. 1999. 0-7808-0232-2. $78.

"There are several items that make this book attractive to consumers who are seeking certain forensic data.... This is a useful current source for those seeking general forensic medical answers."
—*American Reference Books Annual, 2000*

"Recommended for public libraries."
—*Reference & User Services Quarterly, American Library Association, Spring 2000*

"Recommended reference source."
—*Booklist, American Library Association, Feb '00*

"A wealth of information, useful statistics, references are up-to-date and extremely complete. This wonderful collection of data will help students who are interested in a career in any type of forensic field. It is a great resource for attorneys who need information about types of expert witnesses needed in a particular case. It also offers useful information for fiction and nonfiction writers whose work involves a crime. A fascinating compilation. All levels." —*Choice, Association of College and Research Libraries, Jan 2000*

Gastrointestinal Diseases & Disorders Sourcebook

Basic Information about Gastroesophageal Reflux Disease (Heartburn), Ulcers, Diverticulosis, Irritable Bowel Syndrome, Crohn's Disease, Ulcerative Colitis, Diarrhea, Constipation, Lactose Intolerance, Hemorrhoids, Hepatitis, Cirrhosis, and Other Digestive Problems, Featuring Statistics, Descriptions of Symptoms, and Current Treatment Methods of Interest for Persons Living with Upper and Lower Gastrointestinal Maladies

Edited by Linda M. Ross. 413 pages. 1996. 0-7808-0078-8. $78.

"... very readable form. The successful editorial work that brought this material together into a useful and understandable reference makes accessible to all readers information that can help them more effectively understand and obtain help for digestive tract problems."
—*Choice, Association of College and Research Libraries, Feb '97*

SEE ALSO *Diet & Nutrition Sourcebook, 1st and 2nd Editions, Digestive Diseases & Disorders Sourcebook*

Genetic Disorders Sourcebook, 1st Edition

Basic Information about Heritable Diseases and Disorders Such as Down Syndrome, PKU, Hemophilia, Von Willebrand Disease, Gaucher Disease, Tay-Sachs Disease, and Sickle-Cell Disease, Along with Information about Genetic Screening, Gene Therapy, Home Care, and Including Source Listings for Further Help and Information on More Than 300 Disorders

Edited by Karen Bellenir. 642 pages. 1996. 0-7808-0034-6. $78.

"Recommended for undergraduate libraries or libraries that serve the public."
—*Science & Technology Libraries, Vol. 18, No. 1, '99*

"Provides essential medical information to both the general public and those diagnosed with a serious or fatal genetic disease or disorder."
—*Choice, Association of College and Research Libraries, Jan '97*

"Geared toward the lay public. It would be well placed in all public libraries and in those hospital and medical libraries in which access to genetic references is limited." —*Doody's Health Sciences Book Review, Oct '96*

Genetic Disorders Sourcebook, 2nd Edition

Basic Consumer Health Information about Hereditary Diseases and Disorders, Including Cystic Fibrosis, Down Syndrome, Hemophilia, Huntington's Disease, Sickle Cell Anemia, and More; Facts about Genes, Gene Research and Therapy, Genetic Screening, Ethics of Gene Testing, Genetic Counseling, and Advice on Coping and Caring

Along with a Glossary of Genetic Terminology and a Resource List for Help, Support, and Further Information

Edited by Kathy Massimini. 650 pages. 2000. 0-7808-0241-1. $78.

Head Trauma Sourcebook

Basic Information for the Layperson about Open-Head and Closed-Head Injuries, Treatment Advances, Recovery, and Rehabilitation

Along with Reports on Current Research Initiatives

Edited by Karen Bellenir. 414 pages. 1997. 0-7808-0208-X. $78.

Health Insurance Sourcebook

Basic Information about Managed Care Organizations, Traditional Fee-for-Service Insurance, Insurance Portability and Pre-Existing Conditions Clauses, Medicare, Medicaid, Social Security, and Military Health Care

Along with Information about Insurance Fraud

Edited by Wendy Wilcox. 530 pages. 1997. 0-7808-0222-5. $78.

"Particularly useful because it brings much of this information together in one volume. This book will be a handy reference source in the health sciences library, hospital library, college and university library, and medium to large public library."
—*Medical Reference Services Quarterly, Fall '98*

Awarded "Books of the Year Award"
—*American Journal of Nursing, 1997*

"The layout of the book is particularly helpful as it provides easy access to reference material. A most useful addition to the vast amount of information about health insurance. The use of data from U.S. government agencies is most commendable. Useful in a library or learning center for healthcare professional students."
—*Doody's Health Sciences Book Reviews, Nov '97*

Healthy Aging Sourcebook

Basic Consumer Health Information about Maintaining Health through the Aging Process, Including Advice on Nutrition, Exercise, and Sleep, Help in Making Decisions about Midlife Issues and Retirement, and Guidance Concerning Practical and Informed Choices in Health Consumerism

Along with Data Concerning the Theories of Aging, Different Experiences in Aging by Minority Groups, and Facts about Aging Now and Aging in the Future; and Featuring a Glossary, a Guide to Consumer Help, Additional Suggested Reading, and Practical Resource Directory

Edited by Jenifer Swanson. 536 pages. 1999. 0-7808-0390-6. $78.

"Recommended reference source."
—*Booklist, American Library Association, Feb '00*

SEE ALSO Physical & Mental Issues in Aging Sourcebook

Healthy Heart Sourcebook for Women

Basic Consumer Health Information about Cardiac Issues Specific to Women, Including Facts about Major Risk Factors and Prevention, Treatment and Control Strategies, and Important Dietary Issues

Along with a Special Section Regarding the Pros and Cons of Hormone Replacement Therapy and Its Impact on Heart Health, and Additional Help, Including Recipes, a Glossary, and a Directory of Resources

Edited by Dawn D. Matthews. 336 pages. 2000. 0-7808-0329-9. $48.

SEE ALSO Cardiovascular Diseases & Disorders Sourcebook, 1st Edition, Heart Diseases & Disorders Sourcebook, 2nd Edition, Women's Health Concerns Sourcebook

Heart Diseases & Disorders Sourcebook, 2nd Edition

Basic Consumer Health Information about Heart Attacks, Angina, Rhythm Disorders, Heart Failure, Valve Disease, Congenital Heart Disorders, and More, Including Descriptions of Surgical Procedures and Other Interventions, Medications, Cardiac Rehabilitation, Risk Identification, and Prevention Tips

Along with Statistical Data, Reports on Current Research Initiatives, a Glossary of Cardiovascular Terms, and Resource Directory

Edited by Karen Bellenir. 612 pages. 2000. 0-7808-0238-1. $78.

SEE ALSO Cardiovascular Diseases & Disorders Sourcebook, 1st Edition, Healthy Heart Sourcebook for Women

Immune System Disorders Sourcebook

Basic Information about Lupus, Multiple Sclerosis, Guillain-Barré Syndrome, Chronic Granulomatous Disease, and More

Along with Statistical and Demographic Data and Reports on Current Research Initiatives

Edited by Allan R. Cook. 608 pages. 1997. 0-7808-0209-8. $78.

Infant & Toddler Health Sourcebook

Basic Consumer Health Information about the Physical and Mental Development of Newborns, Infants, and Toddlers, Including Neonatal Concerns, Nutrition Recommendations, Immunization Schedules, Common Pediatric Disorders, Assessments and Milestones, Safety Tips, and Advice for Parents and Other Caregivers

Along with a Glossary of Terms and Resource Listings for Additional Help

Edited by Jenifer Swanson. 585 pages. 2000. 0-7808-0246-2. $78.

Kidney & Urinary Tract Diseases & Disorders Sourcebook

Basic Information about Kidney Stones, Urinary Incontinence, Bladder Disease, End Stage Renal Disease, Dialysis, and More

Along with Statistical and Demographic Data and Reports on Current Research Initiatives

Edited by Linda M. Ross. 602 pages. 1997. 0-7808-0079-6. $78.

Learning Disabilities Sourcebook

Basic Information about Disorders Such as Dyslexia, Visual and Auditory Processing Deficits, Attention Deficit/Hyperactivity Disorder, and Autism

Along with Statistical and Demographic Data, Reports on Current Research Initiatives, an Explanation of the Assessment Process, and a Special Section for Adults with Learning Disabilities

Edited by Linda M. Shin. 579 pages. 1998. 0-7808-0210-1. $78.

Named "Oustanding Reference Book of 1999."
—*New York Public Library, Feb 2000*

"An excellent candidate for inclusion in a public library reference section. It's a great source of information. Teachers will also find the book useful. Definitely worth reading."
—*Journal of Adolescent & Adult Literacy, Feb 2000*

"Readable . . . provides a solid base of information regarding successful techniques used with individuals who have learning disabilities, as well as practical suggestions for educators and family members. Clear language, concise descriptions, and pertinent information for contacting multiple resources add to the strength of this book as a useful tool."
—*Choice, Association of College and Research Libraries, Feb '99*

"Recommended reference source."
—*Booklist, American Library Association, Sep '98*

"This is a useful resource for libraries and for those who don't have the time to identify and locate the individual publications."
—*Disability Resources Monthly, Sep '98*

Liver Disorders Sourcebook

Basic Consumer Health Information about the Liver and How It Works; Liver Diseases, Including Cancer, Cirrhosis, Hepatitis, and Toxic and Drug Related Diseases; Tips for Maintaining a Healthy Liver; Laboratory Tests, Radiology Tests, and Facts about Liver Transplantation

Along with a Section on Support Groups, a Glossary, and Resource Listings

Edited by Joyce Brennfleck Shannon. 591 pages. 2000. 0-7808-0383-3. $78.

"Recommended reference source."
—*Booklist, American Library Association, Jun '00*

Medical Tests Sourcebook

Basic Consumer Health Information about Medical Tests, Including Periodic Health Exams, General Screening Tests, Tests You Can Do at Home, Findings of the U.S. Preventive Services Task Force, X-ray and Radiology Tests, Electrical Tests, Tests of Blood and Other Body Fluids and Tissues, Scope Tests, Lung Tests, Genetic Tests, Pregnancy Tests, Newborn Screening Tests, Sexually Transmitted Disease Tests, and Computer Aided Diagnoses

Along with a Section on Paying for Medical Tests, a Glossary, and Resource Listings

Edited by Joyce Brennfleck Shannon. 691 pages. 1999. 0-7808-0243-8. $78.

"A valuable reference guide."
—*American Reference Books Annual, 2000*

"Recommended for hospital and health sciences libraries with consumer health collections."
—*E-Streams, Mar '00*

"This is an overall excellent reference with a wealth of general knowledge that may aid those who are reluctant to get vital tests performed."
—*Today's Librarian, Jan 2000*

Men's Health Concerns Sourcebook

Basic Information about Health Issues That Affect Men, Featuring Facts about the Top Causes of Death in Men, Including Heart Disease, Stroke, Cancers, Prostate Disorders, Chronic Obstructive Pulmonary Disease, Pneumonia and Influenza, Human Immunodeficiency Virus and Acquired Immune Deficiency Syndrome, Diabetes Mellitus, Stress, Suicide, Accidents and Homicides; and Facts about Common Concerns for Men, Including Impotence, Contraception, Circumcision, Sleep Disorders, Snoring, Hair Loss, Diet, Nutrition, Exercise, Kidney and Urological Disorders, and Backaches

Edited by Allan R. Cook. 738 pages. 1998. 0-7808-0212-8. $78.

"This comprehensive resource and the series are highly recommended."
—*American Reference Books Annual, 2000*

"Recommended reference source."
—*Booklist, American Library Association, Dec '98*

Mental Health Disorders Sourcebook, 1st Edition

Basic Information about Schizophrenia, Depression, Bipolar Disorder, Panic Disorder, Obsessive-Compulsive Disorder, Phobias and Other Anxiety Disorders, Paranoia and Other Personality Disorders, Eating Disorders, and Sleep Disorders

Along with Information about Treatment and Therapies

Edited by Karen Bellenir. 548 pages. 1995. 0-7808-0040-0. $78.

"This is an excellent new book . . . written in easy-to-understand language."
—*Booklist Health Sciences Supplement, American Library Association, Oct '97*

". . . useful for public and academic libraries and consumer health collections."
—*Medical Reference Services Quarterly, Spring '97*

"The great strengths of the book are its readability and its inclusion of places to find more information. Especially recommended."
—*Reference Quarterly, American Library Association, Winter '96*

"... a good resource for a consumer health library."
— *Bulletin of the Medical Library Association, Oct '96*

"The information is data-based and couched in brief, concise language that avoids jargon. ... a useful reference source." — *Readings, Sep '96*

"The text is well organized and adequately written for its target audience." — *Choice, Association of College and Research Libraries, Jun '96*

"... provides information on a wide range of mental disorders, presented in nontechnical language."
— *Exceptional Child Education Resources, Spring '96*

"Recommended for public and academic libraries."
— *Reference Book Review, 1996*

Mental Health Disorders Sourcebook, 2nd Edition

Basic Consumer Health Information about Anxiety Disorders, Depression and Other Mood Disorders, Eating Disorders, Personality Disorders, Schizophrenia, and More, Including Disease Descriptions, Treatment Options, and Reports on Current Research Initiatives

Along with Statistical Data, Tips for Maintaining Mental Health, a Glossary, and Directory of Sources for Additional Help and Information

Edited by Karen Bellenir. 605 pages. 2000. 0-7808-0240-3. $78.

Mental Retardation Sourcebook

Basic Consumer Health Information about Mental Retardation and Its Causes, Including Down Syndrome, Fetal Alcohol Syndrome, Fragile X Syndrome, Genetic Conditions, Injury, and Environmental Sources

Along with Preventive Strategies, Parenting Issues, Educational Implications, Health Care Needs, Employment and Economic Matters, Legal Issues, a Glossary, and a Resource Listing for Additional Help and Information

Edited by Joyce Brennfleck Shannon. 642 pages. 2000. 0-7808-0377-9. $78.

"From preventing retardation to parenting and family challenges, this covers health, social and legal issues and will prove an invaluable overview."
— *Reviewer's Bookwatch, Jul '00*

Obesity Sourcebook

Basic Consumer Health Information about Diseases and Other Problems Associated with Obesity, and Including Facts about Risk Factors, Prevention Issues, and Management Approaches

Along with Statistical and Demographic Data, Information about Special Populations, Research Updates, a Glossary, and Source Listings for Further Help and Information

Edited by Wilma Caldwell and Chad T. Kimball. 376 pages. 2001. 0-7808-0333-7. $48.

Ophthalmic Disorders Sourcebook

Basic Information about Glaucoma, Cataracts, Macular Degeneration, Strabismus, Refractive Disorders, and More

Along with Statistical and Demographic Data and Reports on Current Research Initiatives

Edited by Linda M. Ross. 631 pages. 1996. 0-7808-0081-8. $78.

Oral Health Sourcebook

Basic Information about Diseases and Conditions Affecting Oral Health, Including Cavities, Gum Disease, Dry Mouth, Oral Cancers, Fever Blisters, Canker Sores, Oral Thrush, Bad Breath, Temporomandibular Disorders, and other Craniofacial Syndromes

Along with Statistical Data on the Oral Health of Americans, Oral Hygiene, Emergency First Aid, Information on Treatment Procedures and Methods of Replacing Lost Teeth

Edited by Allan R. Cook. 558 pages. 1997. 0-7808-0082-6. $78.

"Unique source which will fill a gap in dental sources for patients and the lay public. A valuable reference tool even in a library with thousands of books on dentistry. Comprehensive, clear, inexpensive, and easy to read and use. It fills an enormous gap in the health care literature." — *Reference and User Services Quarterly, American Library Association, Summer '98*

"Recommended reference source."
— *Booklist, American Library Association, Dec '97*

Osteoporosis Sourcebook

Basic Consumer Health Information about Primary and Secondary Osteoporosis and Juvenile Osteoporosis and Related Conditions, Including Fibrous Dysplasia, Gaucher Disease, Hyperthyroidism, Hypophosphatasia, Myeloma, Osteopetrosis, Osteogenesis Imperfecta, and Paget's Disease

Along with Information about Risk Factors, Treatments, Traditional and Non-traditional Pain Management, a Glossary of Related Terms, and a Directory of Resources

Edited by Allan R. Cook. 600 pages. 2001. 0-7808-0239-X. $78.

SEE ALSO Women's Health Concerns Sourcebook

Pain Sourcebook

Basic Information about Specific Forms of Acute and Chronic Pain, Including Headaches, Back Pain, Muscular Pain, Neuralgia, Surgical Pain, and Cancer Pain Along with Pain Relief Options Such as Analgesics, Narcotics, Nerve Blocks, Transcutaneous Nerve Stimulation, and Alternative Forms of Pain Control, Including Biofeedback, Imaging, Behavior Modification, and Relaxation Techniques

Edited by Allan R. Cook. 667 pages. 1997. 0-7808-0213-6. $78.

"The text is readable, easily understood, and well indexed. This excellent volume belongs in all patient education libraries, consumer health sections of public libraries, and many personal collections."
—*American Reference Books Annual, 1999*

"A beneficial reference." —*Booklist Health Sciences Supplement, American Library Association, Oct '98*

"The information is basic in terms of scholarship and is appropriate for general readers. Written in journalistic style . . . intended for non-professionals. Quite thorough in its coverage of different pain conditions and summarizes the latest clinical information regarding pain treatment." —*Choice, Association of College and Research Libraries, Jun '98*

"Recommended reference source."
—*Booklist, American Library Association, Mar '98*

■

Pediatric Cancer Sourcebook

Basic Consumer Health Information about Leukemias, Brain Tumors, Sarcomas, Lymphomas, and Other Cancers in Infants, Children, and Adolescents, Including Descriptions of Cancers, Treatments, and Coping Strategies Along with Suggestions for Parents, Caregivers, and Concerned Relatives, a Glossary of Cancer Terms, and Resource Listings

Edited by Edward J. Prucha. 587 pages. 1999. 0-7808-0245-4. $78.

"A valuable addition to all libraries specializing in health services and many public libraries."
—*American Reference Books Annual, 2000*

"Recommended reference source."
—*Booklist, American Library Association, Feb '00*

"An excellent source of information. Recommended for public, hospital, and health science libraries with consumer health collections." —*E-Stream, Jun '00*

■

Physical & Mental Issues in Aging Sourcebook

Basic Consumer Health Information on Physical and Mental Disorders Associated with the Aging Process, Including Concerns about Cardiovascular Disease, Pulmonary Disease, Oral Health, Digestive Disorders, Musculoskeletal and Skin Disorders, Metabolic Changes, Sexual and Reproductive Issues, and Changes in Vision, Hearing, and Other Senses Along with Data about Longevity and Causes of Death, Information on Acute and Chronic Pain, Descriptions of Mental Concerns, a Glossary of Terms, and Resource Listings for Additional Help

Edited by Jenifer Swanson. 660 pages. 1999. 0-7808-0233-0. $78.

"Recommended for public libraries."
—*American Reference Books Annual, 2000*

"This is a treasure of health information for the layperson." — *Choice Health Sciences Supplement, Association of College & Research Libraries, May 2000*

"Recommended reference source."
—*Booklist, American Library Association, Oct '99*

SEE ALSO *Healthy Aging Sourcebook*

■

Podiatry Sourcebook

Basic Consumer Health Information about Foot Conditions, Diseases, and Injuries, Including Bunions, Corns, Calluses, Athlete's Foot, Plantar Warts, Hammertoes and Clawtoes, Club Foot, Heel Pain, Gout, and More Along with Facts about Foot Care, Disease Prevention, Foot Safety, Choosing a Foot Care Specialist, a Glossary of Terms, and Resource Listings for Additional Information

Edited by M. Lisa Weatherford. 600 pages. 2001. 0-7808-0215-2. $78.

■

Pregnancy & Birth Sourcebook

Basic Information about Planning for Pregnancy, Maternal Health, Fetal Growth and Development, Labor and Delivery, Postpartum and Perinatal Care, Pregnancy in Mothers with Special Concerns, and Disorders of Pregnancy, Including Genetic Counseling, Nutrition and Exercise, Obstetrical Tests, Pregnancy Discomfort, Multiple Births, Cesarean Sections, Medical Testing of Newborns, Breastfeeding, Gestational Diabetes, and Ectopic Pregnancy

Edited by Heather E. Aldred. 737 pages. 1997. 0-7808-0216-0. $78.

"A well-organized handbook. Recommended."
—*Choice, Association of College and Research Libraries, Apr '98*

"Reecommended reference source."
—*Booklist, American Library Association, Mar '98*

"Recommended for public libraries."
—*American Reference Books Annual, 1998*

SEE ALSO *Congenital Disorders Sourcebook, Family Planning Sourcebook*

Public Health Sourcebook

Basic Information about Government Health Agencies, Including National Health Statistics and Trends, Healthy People 2000 Program Goals and Objectives, the Centers for Disease Control and Prevention, the Food and Drug Administration, and the National Institutes of Health

Along with Full Contact Information for Each Agency

Edited by Wendy Wilcox. 698 pages. 1998. 0-7808-0220-9. $78.

"Recommended reference source."
— *Booklist, American Library Association, Sep '98*

"This consumer guide provides welcome assistance in navigating the maze of federal health agencies and their data on public health concerns."
— *SciTech Book News, Sep '98*

Reconstructive & Cosmetic Surgery Sourcebook

Basic Consumer Health Information on Cosmetic and Reconstructive Plastic Surgery, Including Statistical Information about Different Surgical Procedures, Things to Consider Prior to Surgery, Plastic Surgery Techniques and Tools, Emotional and Psychological Considerations, and Procedure-Specific Information

Along with a Glossary of Terms and a Listing of Resources for Additional Help and Information

Edited by M. Lisa Weatherford. 400 pages. 2001. 0-7808-0214-4. $48.

Rehabilitation Sourcebook

Basic Consumer Health Information about Rehabilitation for People Recovering from Heart Surgery, Spinal Cord Injury, Stroke, Orthopedic Impairments, Amputation, Pulmonary Impairments, Traumatic Injury, and More, Including Physical Therapy, Occupational Therapy, Speech/Language Therapy, Massage Therapy, Dance Therapy, Art Therapy, and Recreational Therapy

Along with Information on Assistive and Adaptive Devices, a Glossary, and Resources for Additional Help and Information

Edited by Dawn D. Matthews. 531 pages. 1999. 0-7808-0236-5. $78.

"Recommended reference source."
— *Booklist, American Library Association, May '00*

Respiratory Diseases & Disorders Sourcebook

Basic Information about Respiratory Diseases and Disorders, Including Asthma, Cystic Fibrosis, Pneumonia, the Common Cold, Influenza, and Others, Featuring Facts about the Respiratory System, Statistical and Demographic Data, Treatments, Self-Help Management Suggestions, and Current Research Initiatives

Edited by Allan R. Cook and Peter D. Dresser. 771 pages. 1995. 0-7808-0037-0. $78.

"**Designed for the layperson and for patients and their families coping with respiratory illness.... an extensive array of information on diagnosis, treatment, management, and prevention of respiratory illnesses for the general reader.**"
— *Choice, Association of College and Research Libraries, Jun '96*

"A highly recommended text for all collections. It is a comforting reminder of the power of knowledge that good books carry between their covers."
— *Academic Library Book Review, Spring '96*

"A comprehensive collection of authoritative information presented in a nontechnical, humanitarian style for patients, families, and caregivers."
— *Association of Operating Room Nurses, Sep/Oct '95*

Sexually Transmitted Diseases Sourcebook, 1st Edition

Basic Information about Herpes, Chlamydia, Gonorrhea, Hepatitis, Nongonoccocal Urethritis, Pelvic Inflammatory Disease, Syphilis, AIDS, and More

Along with Current Data on Treatments and Preventions

Edited by Linda M. Ross. 550 pages. 1997. 0-7808-0217-9. $78.

Sexually Transmitted Diseases Sourcebook, 2nd Edition

Basic Consumer Health Information about Sexually Transmitted Diseases, Including Information on the Diagnosis and Treatment of Chlamydia, Gonorrhea, Hepatitis, Herpes, HIV, Mononucleosis, Syphilis, and Others

Along with Information on Prevention, Such as Condom Use, Vaccines, and STD Education; And Featuring a Section on Issues Related to Youth and Adolescents, a Glossary, and Resources for Additional Help and Information

Edited by Dawn D. Matthews. 538 pages. 2000. 0-7808-0249-7. $78.

Skin Disorders Sourcebook

Basic Information about Common Skin and Scalp Conditions Caused by Aging, Allergies, Immune Reactions, Sun Exposure, Infectious Organisms, Parasites, Cosmetics, and Skin Traumas, Including Abrasions, Cuts, and Pressure Sores

Along with Information on Prevention and Treatment

Edited by Allan R. Cook. 647 pages. 1997. 0-7808-0080-X. $78.

"... **comprehensive, easily read reference book.**"
— *Doody's Health Sciences Book Reviews, Oct '97*

SEE ALSO Burns Sourcebook

Sleep Disorders Sourcebook

Basic Consumer Health Information about Sleep and Its Disorders, Including Insomnia, Sleepwalking, Sleep Apnea, Restless Leg Syndrome, and Narcolepsy

Along with Data about Shiftwork and Its Effects, Information on the Societal Costs of Sleep Deprivation, Descriptions of Treatment Options, a Glossary of Terms, and Resource Listings for Additional Help

Edited by Jenifer Swanson. 439 pages. 1998. 0-7808-0234-9. $78.

"This text will complement any home or medical library. It is user-friendly and ideal for the adult reader."
—*American Reference Books Annual, 2000*

"Recommended reference source."
—*Booklist, American Library Association, Feb '99*

"A useful resource that provides accurate, relevant, and accessible information on sleep to the general public. Health care providers who deal with sleep disorders patients may also find it helpful in being prepared to answer some of the questions patients ask."
—*Respiratory Care, Jul '99*

■

Sports Injuries Sourcebook

Basic Consumer Health Information about Common Sports Injuries, Prevention of Injury in Specific Sports, Tips for Training, and Rehabilitation from Injury

Along with Information about Special Concerns for Children, Young Girls in Athletic Training Programs, Senior Athletes, and Women Athletes, and a Directory of Resources for Further Help and Information

Edited by Heather E. Aldred. 624 pages. 1999. 0-7808-0218-7. $78.

"Public libraries and undergraduate academic libraries will find this book useful for its nontechnical language." —*American Reference Books Annual, 2000*

"While this easy-to-read book is recommended for all libraries, it should prove to be especially useful for public, high school, and academic libraries; certainly it should be on the bookshelf of every school gymnasium." —*E-Streams, Mar '00*

■

Substance Abuse Sourcebook

Basic Health-Related Information about the Abuse of Legal and Illegal Substances Such as Alcohol, Tobacco, Prescription Drugs, Marijuana, Cocaine, and Heroin; and Including Facts about Substance Abuse Prevention Strategies, Intervention Methods, Treatment and Recovery Programs, and a Section Addressing the Special Problems Related to Substance Abuse during Pregnancy

Edited by Karen Bellenir. 573 pages. 1996. 0-7808-0038-9. $78.

"A valuable addition to any health reference section. Highly recommended."
—*The Book Report, Mar/Apr '97*

". . . a comprehensive collection of substance abuse information that's both highly readable and compact. Families and caregivers of substance abusers will find the information enlightening and helpful, while teachers, social workers and journalists should benefit from the concise format. Recommended."
—*Drug Abuse Update, Winter '96/'97*

SEE ALSO *Alcoholism Sourcebook, Drug Abuse Sourcebook*

■

Traveler's Health Sourcebook

Basic Consumer Health Information for Travelers, Including Physical and Medical Preparations, Transportation Health and Safety, Essential Information about Food and Water, Sun Exposure, Insect and Snake Bites, Camping and Wilderness Medicine, and Travel with Physical or Medical Disabilities

Along with International Travel Tips, Vaccination Recommendations, Geographical Health Issues, Disease Risks, a Glossary, and a Listing of Additional Resources

Edited by Joyce Brennfleck Shannon. 613 pages. 2000. 0-7808-0384-1. $78.

■

Women's Health Concerns Sourcebook

Basic Information about Health Issues That Affect Women, Featuring Facts about Menstruation and Other Gynecological Concerns, Including Endometriosis, Fibroids, Menopause, and Vaginitis; Reproductive Concerns, Including Birth Control, Infertility, and Abortion; and Facts about Additional Physical, Emotional, and Mental Health Concerns Prevalent among Women Such as Osteoporosis, Urinary Tract Disorders, Eating Disorders, and Depression

Along with Tips for Maintaining a Healthy Lifestyle

Edited by Heather E. Aldred. 567 pages. 1997. 0-7808-0219-5. $78.

"Handy compilation. There is an impressive range of diseases, devices, disorders, procedures, and other physical and emotional issues covered . . . well organized, illustrated, and indexed." —*Choice, Association of College and Research Libraries, Jan '98*

SEE ALSO *Breast Cancer Sourcebook, Cancer Sourcebook for Women, 1st and 2nd Editions, Healthy Heart Sourcebook for Women, Osteoporosis Sourcebook*

Workplace Health & Safety Sourcebook

Basic Consumer Health Information about Workplace Health and Safety, Including the Effect of Workplace Hazards on the Lungs, Skin, Heart, Ears, Eyes, Brain, Reproductive Organs, Musculoskeletal System, and Other Organs and Body Parts

Along with Information about Occupational Cancer, Personal Protective Equipment, Toxic and Hazardous Chemicals, Child Labor, Stress, and Workplace Violence

Edited by Chad T. Kimball. 626 pages. 2000. 0-7808-0231-4. $78.

Worldwide Health Sourcebook

Basic Information about Global Health Issues, Including Malnutrition, Reproductive Health, Disease Dispersion and Prevention, Emerging Diseases, Risky Health Behaviors, and the Leading Causes of Death

Along with Global Health Concerns for Children, Women, and the Elderly, Mental Health Issues, Research and Technology Advancements, and Economic, Environmental, and Political Health Implications, a Glossary, and a Resource Listing for Additional Help and Information

Edited by Joyce Brennfleck Shannon. 500 pages. 2001. 0-7808-0330-2. $78.

Health Reference Series Cumulative Index 1999

A Comprehensive Index to the Individual Volumes of the Health Reference Series, Including a Subject Index, Name Index, Organization Index, and Publication Index;

Along with a Master List of Acronyms and Abbreviations

Edited by Edward J. Prucha, Anne Holmes, and Robert Rudnick. 990 pages. 2000. 0-7808-0382-5. $78.